Peripheral Neuropathies

Editors

RICHARD J. BAROHN
MAZEN M. DIMACHKIE

NEUROLOGIC CLINICS

www.neurologic.theclinics.com

Consulting Editor
RANDOLPH W. EVANS

May 2013 • Volume 31 • Number 2

ELSEVIER

1600 John F. Kennedy Boulevard ● Suite 1800 ● Philadelphia, Pennsylvania, 19103-2899

http://www.theclinics.com

NEUROLOGIC CLINICS Volume 31, Number 2
May 2013 ISSN 0733-8619, ISBN-13: 978-1-4557-7122-6

Editor: Donald Mumford

Neurologic Clinics (ISSN 0733-8619) is published quarterly by Elsevier Inc., 360 Park Avenue South, New York, NY 10010–1710. Months of issue are February, May, August, and November. Periodicals postage paid at New York, NY, and additional mailing offices. Subscription prices are $285.00 per year for US individuals, $489.00 per year for US institutions, $199.00 per year for US students, $359.00 per year for Canadian individuals, $586.00 per year for Canadian institutions, $397.00 per year for international individuals, $586.00 per year for international institutions, and $199.00 for Canadian and foreign students/residents. To receive student/resident rate, orders must be accompanied by name of affiliated institution, date of term, and the *signature* of program/residency coordinator on institution letterhead. Orders will be billed at individual rate until proof of status is received. Foreign air speed delivery is included in all *Clinics* subscription prices. All prices are subject to change without notice. **POSTMASTER:** Send address changes to *Neurologic Clinics*, Elsevier Health Sciences Division, Subscription Customer Service, 3251 Riverport Lane, Maryland Heights, MO 63043. **Customer Service: Telephone: 1-800-654-2452 (U.S. and Canada); 314-447-8871 (outside U.S. and Canada). Fax: 314-447-8029. E-mail: journalscustomerservice-usa@elsevier.com (for print support); journalsonlinesupport-usa@elsevier.com (for online support).**

Reprints. For copies of 100 or more of articles in this publication, please contact the Commercial Reprints Department, Elsevier Inc., 360 Park Avenue South, New York, New York, 10010-1710; Tel.: (+1) 212-633-3812; Fax: (+1) 212-462-1935, and E-mail: reprints@elsevier.com.

Neurologic Clinics is also published in Spanish by Nueva Editorial Interamericana S.A., Mexico City, Mexico.

Neurologic Clinics is covered in *Current Contents/Clinical Medicine, MEDLINE/PubMed (Index Medicus), EMBASE/Excerpta Medica, and PsycINFO, and ISI/BIOMED.*

Printed and bound by CPI Group (UK) Ltd, Croydon, CR0 4YY
Transferred to digital print 2013

Contributors

CONSULTING EDITOR

RANDOLPH W. EVANS, MD
Clinical Professor, Department of Neurology, Baylor College of Medicine, Houston, Texas

EDITORS

RICHARD J. BAROHN, MD
Chairman, Department of Neurology, Gertrude and Dewey Ziegler; Professor of Neurology, University Distinguished Professor, University of Kansas Medical Center, Kansas City, Kansas

MAZEN M. DIMACHKIE, MD, FAAN
Director, Neuromuscular Section; Professor of Neurology, Department of Neurology, University of Kansas Medical Center, Kansas City, Kansas

AUTHORS

ANTHONY A. AMATO, MD
Vice-chairman, Professor of Neurology, Department of Neurology, Brigham and Women's Hospital, Harvard Medical School, Boston, Massachusetts

WILLIAM DAVID ARNOLD, MD
Assistant Professor, Division of Neuromuscular Medicine, Department of Neurology, The Ohio State University, Columbus, Ohio

RICHARD J. BAROHN, MD
Chairman, Department of Neurology, Gertrude and Dewey Ziegler; Professor of Neurology, University Distinguished Professor, University of Kansas Medical Center, Kansas City, Kansas

MICHAEL P. COLLINS, MD
Associate Professor of Neurology; Director, Neuromuscular Laboratory, Medical College of Wisconsin, Milwaukee, Wisconsin

MAZEN M. DIMACHKIE, MD, FAAN
Director, Neuromuscular Section; Professor of Neurology, Department of Neurology, University of Kansas Medical Center, Kansas City, Kansas

BAKRI H. ELSHEIKH, MBBS
Associate Professor, Division of Neuromuscular Medicine, Department of Neurology, The Ohio State University, Columbus, Ohio

KENNETH C. GORSON, MD
Director, Neuromuscular Service, Professor of Neurology, Tufts University School of Medicine, St. Elizabeth's Medical Center, Boston, Massachusetts

NANCY HAMMOND, MD
University of Kansas Medical Center, Kansas City, Kansas

JONATHAN KATZ, MD
Director, Neuromuscular Service, California Pacific Medical Center, Professor of Neurology, University of California, San Francisco, California

JOHN T. KISSEL, MD
Professor of Neurology and Pediatrics, Director, Division of Neuromuscular Medicine, The Ohio State University, Columbus, Ohio

PATRICIA KLUDING, PT, PhD
Associate Professor, Department of Physical Therapy and Rehabilitation Science, University of Kansas Medical Center, Kansas City, Kansas

TODD D. LEVINE, MD
Phoenix Neurological Associates, University of Arizona College of Medicine, Phoenix, Arizona

MAMATHA PASNOOR, MD
Assistant Professor, Department of Neurology, University of Kansas Medical Center, Kansas City, Kansas

DAVID S. SAPERSTEIN, MD
Phoenix Neurological Associates, University of Arizona College of Medicine, Phoenix, Arizona

MARIO A. SAPORTA, MD, PhD
National Laboratory of Embryonic Stem Cells, Biomedical Sciences Department, Federal University of Rio de Janeiro, Rio de Janeiro, Brazil

MICHAEL E. SHY, MD
Department of Neurology, University of Iowa, Iowa City, Iowa

NICHOLAS J. SILVESTRI, MD
Assistant Professor, Department of Neurology, State University of New York at Buffalo School of Medicine and Biomedical Sciences, Buffalo, New York

JAYA R. TRIVEDI, MD, FAAN
Associate Professor, Department of Neurology and Neurotherapeutics, UT Southwestern Medical Center, Dallas, Texas

YUNXIA WANG, MD
University of Kansas Medical Center, Kansas City, Kansas

GIL I. WOLFE, MD
Professor, Department of Neurology, State University of New York at Buffalo School of Medicine and Biomedical Sciences, Buffalo, New York

Contents

Neuropathic disorders encompass those that affect the neuron's cell body or neuronopathies, those affecting the peripheral process, or peripheral neuropathies. The peripheral neuropathies can be broadly subdivided into the myelinopathies and axonopathies, conditions which can be hereditary or acquired. Each of these disorders has distinct clinical features that enable neurologists to recognize the various patterns of presentation. Once a particular pattern is established, further laboratory studies can be performed to support the clinical impression.

The question of how to evaluate peripheral neuropathies is complicated by there being hundreds of potential causes, both acquired and inherited. This article focuses on a targeted and thoughtful approach to the laboratory evaluation of patients with peripheral neuropathy, designed to allow the identification of treatable neuropathies without undue expense and risk to patients. After determining which clinical patterns are present, the patterns are used to define a discrete manageable subset of diseases underlying these neuropathies. Thinking in terms of such patterns is often more helpful than relying on electrodiagnostic studies, leading to a more accurate, cost-effective laboratory evaluation.

Neuropathic pain management is an important aspect in the management of painful peripheral neuropathy. Anticonvulsants and antidepressants have been studied extensively and are often used as first-line agents in the management of neuropathic pain. In this article, data from multiple randomized controlled studies on painful peripheral neuropathies are summarized to guide physicians in treating neuropathic pain. Treatment is a challenge given the diverse mechanisms of pain and variable responses in individuals. However, most patients derive pain relief from a well-chosen monotherapy or well-designed polypharmacy that combines agents with different mechanisms of action.

Compression neuropathy includes a heterogeneous group of focal neuropathy syndromes related to peripheral nerve compression. Although acute or chronic compression-related injury may occur in essentially any peripheral nerve, certain anatomic considerations may predispose certain nerves to intrinsic or extrinsic compression-related injury. The clinical presentations of specific compression or entrapment syndromes depend on factors such as chronicity, location, severity, and mechanism of involvement of a particular nerve. In this article the diagnosis and management strategies of the more common and well-established entrapment and compression-related neuropathy syndromes are addressed.

Diabetes is the most common cause of neuropathy in United States and neuropathies are the most common complication of diabetes mellitus, affecting up to 50% of patients with type 1 and type 2 diabetes mellitus. Symptoms usually include numbness, tingling, pain, and weakness. Dizziness with postural changes can be seen with autonomic neuropathy. Metabolic, vascular, and immune theories have been proposed for the pathogenesis of diabetic neuropathy. Axonal damage and segmental demyelination can be seen with diabetic neuropathies. Management of diabetic neuropathy should begin at the initial diagnosis of diabetes and mainly requires tight and stable glycemic control.

Diabetic neuropathies consist of a variety of syndromes resulting from different types of damage to peripheral or cranial nerves. Although distal symmetric polyneuropathy is the most common type of diabetic neuropathy, many other subtypes have been defined since the 1800s, including proximal diabetic, truncal, cranial, median, and ulnar neuropathies. Various theories have been proposed for the pathogenesis of these neuropathies. The treatment of most requires tight and stable glycemic control. Spontaneous recovery is seen in most of these conditions with diabetic control. Immunotherapies have been tried in some of these conditions however are controversial.

Chronic sensory or sensorimotor polyneuropathy is a common cause for referral to neurologists. Despite extensive diagnostic testing, up to one-third of these patients remain without a known cause, and are referred to as having cryptogenic sensory peripheral neuropathy. Symptoms progress slowly. On examination, there may be additional mild toe flexion and extension weakness. Electrophysiologic testing and histology reveals axonal neuropathy. Prognosis is usually favorable, as most patients maintain independent ambulation. Besides patient education and reassurance, management is focused on pharmacotherapy for neuropathic pain and physical therapy for balance training, and, occasionally, assistive devices.

paramount importance in diagnosing specific conditions and determining the most appropriate therapies. Knowledge regarding pathogenesis, diagnosis, and management of these disorders continues to expand, resulting in improved opportunities for identification and treatment.

NEUROLOGIC CLINICS

Preface

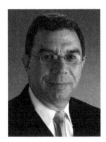 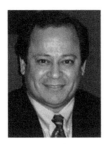

Richard J. Barohn, MD   Mazen M. Dimachkie, MD, FAAN
Editors

Patients with neuropathic disorders continue to pose challenging diagnostic and therapeutic dilemmas. We consider neuropathic disorders to include diseases that affect the lower motor neuron and sensory cell body, peripheral axon, and myelin sheath. In this current issue of *Neurologic Clinics*, we discuss a number of important issues regarding the diagnosis and treatment of these disorders. Our primary focus in these articles is on peripheral neuropathies, although we do discuss cell body diseases in the approach to patients, and we also discuss myelopathies with neuropathy (myeloneuropathies), particularly in the article on nutritional neuropathy. We have assembled a group of experts who discuss recent advances as well as practical concepts that can be used in the clinic. In this way, we hope to provide busy clinicians with up-to-date and practical information so that they can diagnose and treat their patients with neuropathic disorders better.

The contributors are in the neuromuscular services at major academic centers (such as the University of Kansas Medical Center, the Ohio State University, The University of Texas–Southwestern, SUNY Buffalo, Brigham and Women's Hospital, Tufts University, Medical College of Wisconsin, University of Iowa) and also in large tertiary care provider practice settings (California Pacific Medical Center and Phoenix Neurologic Associates). The authors are all colleagues who have worked together for many years. The group had its nucleus in Ohio and Texas and then expanded across the country. Our goal has been to push the envelope toward phenotype identification to perform selective diagnostic tests that lead us to optimal management of patients with neuromuscular disorders. We would like to express our appreciation to all of the authors who have worked so hard to make this issue a success.

Neurol Clin 31 (2013) xi–xii
http://dx.doi.org/10.1016/j.ncl.2013.02.005
0733-8619/13/$ – see front matter © 2013 Published by Elsevier Inc.

neurologic.theclinics.com

Finally, we would like to thank Abbie Whited and Amanda Grosdidier for their countless hours of outstanding support as our executive administrative assistant and research coordinator, respectively.

Richard J. Barohn, MD
Department of Neurology
University of Kansas Medical Center
3599 Rainbow Boulevard, Mail Stop 2012
Kansas City, KS 66160, USA

Mazen M. Dimachkie, MD, FAAN
Neuromuscular Section
Department of Neurology
University of Kansas Medical Center
3599 Rainbow Boulevard, Mail Stop 2012
Kansas City, KS 66160, USA

E-mail addresses:
rbarohn@kumc.edu (R.J. Barohn)
mdimachkie@kumc.edu (M.M. Dimachkie)

Pattern-Recognition Approach to Neuropathy and Neuronopathy

Richard J. Barohn, MD[a],*, Anthony A. Amato, MD[b]

KEYWORDS

- Neuropathy • Neuronopathy • Myelinopathy • Axonopathy • Plexopathy
- Radiculopathy • Mononeuritis multiplex

KEY POINTS

- The initial key to the diagnosis of neuropathy and neuronopathy is recognition of a clinical pattern.
- There are 6 key questions the clinician should consider in arriving at the pattern that fits the patient best.
- Most neuropathy and neuronopathy patients can be placed into one of 10 patterns.
- After arriving at the pattern that fits best, then the clinician can determine the most appropriate diagnostic tests and management.

INTRODUCTION

A discussion of neuropathic disorders encompasses those diseases that affect the neuron's cell body, or neuronopathies, and those affecting the peripheral process, or peripheral neuropathies (**Box 1**).[1,2] Neuronopathies can be further subdivided into those that affect only the anterior horn cells, or motor neuron disease, and those involving only the sensory neurons, also called sensory neuronopathies or gangliono-pathies. Peripheral neuropathies can be broadly subdivided into those that primarily affect myelin, or myelinopathies, and those that affect the axon, or axonopathies.

Each of these pathologic categories has distinct clinical and electrophysiologic features that allow the clinician to place a patient's disease into 1 of these groups. Therefore, the first 2 goals in the approach to a neuropathic disorder are to determine: (1) where the lesion is located; and (2) the cause of the lesion (**Box 2**).

Disclosures/Conflicts of Interest: Dr Barohn: Speaker's bureau for Genzyme and Grifols; Advisory Board for MedImmune and Novartis. Dr Amato: Medical advisory board/consultant for Amgen, Baxter, Biogen, MedImmune, Questor.
[a] Department of Neurology, University of Kansas Medical Center, 3901 Rainbow Boulevard, Mail Stop 2012, Kansas City, KS 66160, USA; [b] Department of Neurology, Brigham and Women's Hospital, Harvard Medical School, 75 Francis Street, Boston, MA 02115, USA
* Corresponding author.
E-mail address: rbarohn@kumc.edu

Box 1
Pathologic classification of neuropathic disorders

Neuronopathies (pure sensory or pure motor or autonomic):

   Sensory neuronopathies (ganglionopathies)

   Motor neuronopathies (motor neuron disease)

   Autonomic neuropathies

Peripheral neuropathies (usually sensorimotor):

   Myelinopathies

   Axonopathies

      Large- and small-fiber

      Small-fiber

For example, is the disorder hereditary or acquired? If it is acquired, is the neuropathic disorder due to a systemic dysmetabolic state? Is it drug induced or toxin induced? Is it mediated by an immune or infectious process? Or, is the cause unknown? The third goal in approaching the patient with a neuropathic disorder is to determine whether therapy is possible, and if so, what the course of therapy should be. Even if a specific therapy is not available, a management plan should be developed. These final 2 steps are often frustrating, as it is not always possible to determine the cause or alter the natural history of neuropathic disorders.

What is the chance of correctly determining the pathologic type and etiology of a neuropathic disorder? If one considers only peripheral neuropathies, some information is available. Of 205 patients referred to the Mayo Clinic with an undiagnosed peripheral neuropathy, a diagnosis was made in 76%.[3] A hereditary neuropathy was found in 42%, an inflammatory demyelinating disorder (chronic inflammatory demyelinating polyneuropathy [CIDP]) was diagnosed in 21%, and 13% were diagnosed as having a peripheral neuropathy associated with other diseases (diabetes and other metabolic disorders, nutritional deficiency, toxins, and cancer). The authors' experience of 402 consecutive patients referred to the University of Texas neuromuscular outpatient clinics in Dallas and San Antonio through 1997 for a peripheral neuropathy[4] is shown in **Table 1**. The authors recently performed a similar analysis on cohorts of neuropathy between North American (Kansas City and Dallas) and South American (Rio de Janeiro, Brazil) (NA-SA) cities.[5,6]

This NA-SA analysis underscored that a hereditary neuropathy is common, accounting for 27% in NA and 10% in SA. Acquired demyelinating polyneuropathies in tertiary care neuropathy clinics accounted for 20% in NA and 18% in SA. Diabetic neuropathies, while common (13% in NA and 23% in SA), may have been underreported in these tertiary care neuropathy center populations. (See the articles by Pasnoor and colleagues elsewhere in this issue for further exploration of this topic.) Approximately one-quarter of the patients are ultimately found to have a predominantly sensory polyneuropathy with no identifiable cause (28% in NA and 23% in SA), that is, cryptogenic sensory polyneuropathy (CSPN).[7–9] (See the article by Pasnoor and colleagues elsewhere in this issue for further exploration of this topic.) Overall, SA tertiary care centers were more likely to see patients with infections (Chagas, human T-lymphotropic virus 1, leprosy), and diabetic and hereditary disorders such as familial

Box 2
Etiology of neuropathic disorders

I. Acquired

Dysmetabolic states

    Diabetes mellitus

    Neuropathy related to renal disease

    Vitamin deficiency states (eg, vitamin B_{12} deficiency)

Immune mediated

    Guillain-Barré syndrome (GBS)

    Chronic inflammatory demyelinating polyneuropathy and variants

    Multifocal motor neuropathy

    Anti–myelin-associated glycoprotein distal acquired demyelinating symmetric neuropathy

    Radiculoplexus neuropathy: cervical, thoracic, and lumbosacral

    Vasculitis

    Sarcoidosis

Infectious

    Herpes zoster

    Leprosy, Lyme, human immunodeficiency virus (HIV), cytomegalovirus, Epstein-Barr related

Cancer-related and lymphoproliferative disorders

    Lymphoma, myeloma, carcinoma related

    Paraneoplastic subacute sensory neuronopathy

    Primary amyloidosis

Drugs or toxins

    Chemotherapy induced

    Other drugs

    Heavy metals and industrial toxins

Mechanical/compressive

    Radiculopathy

    Mononeuropathy

Unknown etiology

    Cryptogenic sensory and sensorimotor neuropathy

    Amyotrophic lateral sclerosis

II. Hereditary

Charcot-Marie-Tooth disease and related disorders

Hereditary sensory and autonomic neuropathy

Familial brachial plexopathy

Familial amyloidosis

Porphyria

Other rare peripheral neuropathies (Fabry disease, metachromatic leukodystrophy, adrenoleukodystrophy, Refsum disease, and so forth)

Motor neuron disease

  Spinal muscular atrophy

  Familial amyotrophic lateral sclerosis

  X-linked bulbospinal muscular atrophy

  Hereditary motor neuropathy

  Hereditary spastic paraplegia

amyloid neuropathies.[5,6] NA tertiary centers were more likely to see Charcot-Marie-Tooth (CMT) neuropathy. Immune and cryptogenic neuropathies were seen equally in NA and SA.

To accomplish the goal of determining the site and cause of the lesion, and, if possible, a therapy, the clinician gathers information from the history, the neurologic examination, and various laboratory studies. While gathering this information, 6 key questions are asked. From the answer to these 6 questions, the patient is placed into 9 different phenotypic patterns. Therefore, the authors call this the 3-6-10–step clinical approach to neuropathy: 3 goals, 6 key questions, 10 phenotypic patterns.

IMPORTANT INFORMATION FROM THE HISTORY AND PHYSICAL: 6 KEY QUESTIONS

The first step in this approach is to ask 6 key questions based on the patient's symptoms and signs (**Box 3**):

What Systems are Involved?

It is important to determine if the patient's symptoms and signs are pure motor, pure sensory, autonomic, or some combination of these. If the patient has only weakness without any evidence of sensory loss, a motor neuronopathy or motor neuron disease is the most likely diagnosis. The majority of patients with adult-onset motor neuron

Table 1
Breakdown by diagnosis of 402 consecutive polyneuropathy patients referred to the University of Texas at Dallas/San Antonio neuromuscular clinics

Diagnosis	No. of Patients	%
Hereditary	120	29.8
Cryptogenic sensory polyneuropathy	93	23.1
Diabetes mellitus	62	15.4
Inflammatory demyelinating polyneuropathy	53	13.1
Multifocal motor neuropathy	21	5.2
Vitamin B_{12} deficiency	9	2.2
Cryptogenic sensorimotor polyneuropathy with severe distal weakness	7	1.7
Drug-induced	6	1.5
Sensory neuronopathy (3 idiopathic, 1 anti-Hu)	4	1.0
Other[a]	27	6.7

[a] Includes: motor neuron disease plus sensorimotor polyneuropathy (SMPN) (4), SMPN associated with a solid tumor (4), mononeuritis multiplex (4), post polio with SMPN (3), vasculitis (3), infectious (3), axonal motor neuropathy (2), SMPN associated with collagen vascular disease (1), thyrotoxicosis (1), SMPN associated with leukemia (1), toxin-induced (1).

Data from Barohn RJ. Approach to peripheral neuropathy and neuronopathy. Sem Neurol 1998;18:7–18.

Box 3
Approach to neuropathic disorders: 6 key questions

1. What systems are involved?
   a. Motor, sensory, autonomic, or combinations
2. What is the distribution of weakness?
   a. Only distal versus proximal and distal
   b. Focal/asymmetric versus symmetric
3. What is the nature of the sensory involvement?
   a. Severe pain/burning or stabbing
   b. Severe proprioceptive loss
4. Is there evidence of upper motor neuron involvement?
   a. Without sensory loss
   b. With sensory loss
5. What is the temporal evolution?
   a. Acute (days to 4 weeks)
   b. Subacute (4–8 weeks)
   c. Chronic (>8 weeks)
   d. Preceding events, drugs, toxins
6. Is there evidence for a hereditary neuropathy?
   a. Family history of neuropathy
   b. Skeletal deformities
   c. Lack of sensory symptoms despite sensory signs

---

disease have evidence of both upper and lower motor neuron dysfunction on examination, that is, amyotrophic lateral sclerosis (ALS), which is the primary diagnostic hallmark of this disorder.[10] On the other hand, nearly one-third of adult patients with acquired motor neuron disease may present initially without definite upper motor neuron findings,[11,12] and these patients are often referred to as having progressive muscular atrophy (PMA). A slow pure lower motor neuron variant restricted to the arms for many years has been termed brachial amyotrophic diplegia (BAD),[13] and the version restricted to the legs has been termed leg amyotrophic diplegia (LAD).[14,15] Spinal muscular atrophy (SMA) is the autosomal recessive motor neuronopathy of childhood.[16] Patients with pure motor distal weakness with a clinical phenotype of CMT neuropathy but with no sensory involvement are now classified as hereditary motor neuropathy (HMN).[17,18] However, with advances in genetics the authors have found variable presentations, such that mutations in the same gene may cause motor and sensory CMT or a pure motor HMN; some may also be associated with upper motor neuron findings (hereditary spastic paraplegia [HSP]).

The neuropathic disorders that may present with pure motor symptoms are listed in **Box 4**. Although some peripheral neuropathies may present with only motor symptoms, the clinician can usually find evidence of sensory involvement on neurologic examination. An exception to this rule is a patient with multifocal motor neuropathy who generally has a normal sensory examination.[19] (See the article by Saporta and colleagues elsewhere in this issue for further exploration of this topic.)

Box 4
Neuropathic disorders that may have only motor symptoms at presentation

Motor neuron disease

Multifocal motor neuropathy

GBS[a]

CIDP[a]

Lead intoxication[a]

Acute porphyria[a]

Hereditary motor sensory neuropathy[a] (CMT disease)

Hereditary motor neuropathy

[a] Usually has sensory signs on examination.

Some peripheral neuropathies are associated with significant autonomic nervous system dysfunction (**Box 5**).

Inquire if the patient has had fainting spells or orthostatic lightheadedness, heat intolerance, or any bowel, bladder, or sexual dysfunction. If these symptoms are present, check for an orthostatic decrease in blood pressure without an appropriate increase in heart rate. Autonomic dysfunction in the absence of diabetes should alert the clinician to the possibility of amyloid polyneuropathy, an autoimmune small-fiber ganglionopathy, or (in a young child) hereditary sensory and autonomic neuropathy (HSAN). Rarely, idiopathic pandysautonomic syndrome can be the only manifestation of a peripheral neuropathy without other motor or sensory findings.[20,21] (see the article by Dimachkie and colleagues elsewhere in this issue for further exploration of this topic.)

What is the Distribution of Weakness?

The distribution of the patient's weakness is crucial for an accurate diagnosis, and in this regard 2 questions should be asked: (1) does the weakness only involve the distal extremity or is it both proximal and distal? and (2) is the weakness focal and asymmetric or is it symmetric? The finding of weakness in both proximal and distal muscle groups in a symmetric fashion is the hallmark for acquired immune demyelinating polyneuropathies, both the acute form (GBS) and the chronic form (CIDP).[22–25] (See the

---

Box 5
Peripheral neuropathies with autonomic nervous system involvement

Hereditary sensory autonomic neuropathy

Diabetes mellitus

Amyloidosis (familial and acquired)

GBS

Vincristine induced

Porphyria

HIV-related autonomic neuropathy

Idiopathic pandysautonomia

articles by Dimachkie and colleagues and Gorson and colleagues elsewhere in this issue for further exploration of this topic.) Patients with proximal muscle weakness will complain of difficulty raising their arms to brush their teeth or comb their hair, as well as problems climbing stairs or rising from a chair. On the neurologic examination, the clinician needs to pay particular attention for the presence of facial, neck, shoulder, and hip weakness in addition to the more distal muscle groups in the hands and feet.

Asymmetry or focality of the weakness is also a feature that can narrow the diagnostic possibilities (**Box 6**).

ALS can present with either prominent neck extensor weakness (head drop) or prominent tongue and pharyngeal weakness (dysarthria and dysphagia). The latter is the so-called bulbar presentation. These focal symmetric weakness patterns can also be seen in neuromuscular junction disorders (myasthenia gravis, Lambert-Eaton myasthenic syndrome) and some myopathies, particularly isolated neck extensor myopathy.[26] Therefore, these patterns are considered an overlap with myopathic disorder.

Other overlap patterns with muscle disease are seen with pure motor symmetric proximal to distal limb weakness. When this occurs on a neuropathic basis, the primary consideration is SMA. But of course, this is also the limb-girdle pattern seen in many myopathies. Pure motor distal symmetric weakness is the presentation for hereditary motor neuropathy, as already noted, but this pattern can also be seen in distal myopathies and, rarely, myasthenia gravis.[27,28]

Some neuropathic disorders may present with unilateral leg weakness. If sensory symptoms and signs are absent, and an elderly patient presents with painless foot drop evolving over weeks or months, motor neuron disease is the leading and most worrisome diagnostic possibility. On the other hand, if a patient presents with subacute or acute sensory and motor symptoms of one leg, lumbosacral radiculopathies, plexopathies, vasculitis, and compressive mononeuropathy need to be considered. Similarly, if the clinical manifestations are pure motor weakness in one arm or hand, motor neuron disease is probably the leading consideration. If sensory symptoms are also present, cervical radiculopathy, brachial plexopathy, or a mononeuropathy are likely possibilities. Hereditary neuropathy with predisposition to pressure palsies (HNPP) or familial brachial plexus neuropathies are also conditions that can present with focal, asymmetric leg or arm weakness.[29] Leprosy often presents with asymmetric sensory or sensorimotor features, and one needs to have a high index of suspicion for this disorder, particularly in immigrant populations from developing countries.[30] Unilateral combined motor and sensory presentations in a single extremity are usually due to a simple entrapment or compressive neuropathy or radiculopathy (See the article by Arnold and colleagues in this issue for further exploration of this topic).

The importance of finding symmetric proximal and distal weakness in a patient who presents with both motor and sensory symptoms cannot be overemphasized, because this identifies the important subset of patients who may have a treatable acquired demyelinating neuropathic disorder, that is, acute or CIDP. On the other hand, if a patient with both symmetric sensory and motor findings has weakness involving only the distal lower and upper extremities, the disorder generally reflects a primarily axonal peripheral neuropathy and is much less likely to represent a treatable entity.

Exceptions

There are important exceptions to this generalization that symmetric distal sensory and motor weakness reflects an axonal process that is likely to be unresponsive to

---

Box 6
Neuropathic disorders that produce asymmetric/focal weakness

Motor neuron disease

    ALS

Radiculopathy: cervical or lumbosacral

    Root compression from osteoarthritis

    Root compression from herniated disc

    Herpes zoster focal paresis (with rash)

    Meningeal carcinomatosis and lymphomatosis

    Sarcoid

    Amyloid

    Chronic immune sensory polyradiculopathy

Plexopathy: cervical, thoracic, or lumbosacral

    Immune-mediated/Idiopathic

    Neoplastic infiltration

    Diabetic radiculoplexopathy (primarily lumbosacral)

    Familial brachial plexopathy

    Hereditary neuropathy with liability to pressure palsy

Mononeuropathy multiplex due to:

    Vasculitis

    Multifocal motor neuropathy

    Multifocal acquired demyelinating sensory and motor neuropathy (MADSAM)

    Multifocal acquired motor axonopathy (MAMA)

    Lyme disease

    Sarcoid

    Leprosy

    HIV infection

    Hepatitis B and C

    Cryoglobulinemia

    Amyloidosis

    Hereditary neuropathy with liability to pressure palsy

Compressive/entrapment mononeuropathies

    Median neuropathy

    Ulnar neuropathy

    Peroneal neuropathy

---

therapy, and that acquired demyelinating neuropathies present with proximal and distal symmetric weakness. Patients with multifocal motor neuropathy and multifocal acquired demyelinating sensory and motor (MADSAM) neuropathy have distal, asymmetric extremity involvement, but these disorders respond to immunosuppressive therapy.[19,24,31] (See the articles by Saporta and colleagues and Arnold and colleagues elsewhere in this issue for further exploration of this topic.) In addition, the acquired demyelinating neuropathies associated with immunoglobulin M–κ monoclonal antibodies, which are typically targeted to myelin-associated glycoprotein, have the curious pattern of predominantly distal symmetric sensory loss and weakness, with little or no proximal weakness. This condition is now known as DADS-M (distal acquired demyelinating symmetric with monoclonal gammopathy) neuropathy.[24,32]

Another important exception to the rule that distal, symmetric sensory and motor sensory and motor loss is unresponsive to immunosuppressive therapy is the occasional patients with vasculitis of the peripheral nervous system. Approximately 20% to 30% of patients with vasculitis of the peripheral nervous system may present with a distal, symmetric motor, and sensory dysfunction[33] rather than with asymmetric, multiple mononeuropathies. The clue to diagnosing these patients is the subacute evolution over weeks with severe pain and prominent motor involvement, features that help to make the distinction from metabolic, toxic, or hereditary disorders (See the article by Collins and colleagues in this issue for further exploration of this topic).

What is the Nature of the Sensory Involvement?

When taking the history from a patient with a peripheral neuropathy, it is important to determine whether the patient has loss of sensation (numbness), altered sensation (tingling), or pain. Sometimes patients may find it difficult to distinguish between uncomfortable tingling sensations (dysesthesias) and pain. Neuropathic pain can be burning, dull, and poorly localized (protopathic pain), presumably transmitted by polymodal C nociceptor fibers, or sharp and lancinating (epicritic pain), relayed by Aδ fibers.

Complaints of numbness or tingling, and the type of neuropathic pain while implicating sensory involvement, are in general not very helpful in suggesting a specific diagnosis, as these symptoms can accompany many peripheral neuropathies. However, 2 sensory features may be helpful to the clinician in arriving at a diagnosis. If severe pain is one of the patient's symptoms, certain peripheral neuropathies should be considered (**Box 7**).

The CSPN and neuropathy due to diabetes mellitus are the most common neuropathies associated with severe pain.[7–9] In addition, painful peripheral neuropathies attributable to peripheral nerve vasculitis or GBS are important to recognize because these disorders are treatable. The pain in vasculitic neuropathy is generally distal and asymmetric in the most severely involved extremity. Some patients with GBS have severe back pain associated with symmetric numbness and paresthesias in the extremities. The pain associated with CSPN and diabetic distal sensory neuropathy

---

Box 7
Peripheral neuropathies often associated with pain

Cryptogenic sensory or sensorimotor neuropathy

Diabetes mellitus

Vasculitis

GBS

Amyloidosis

Toxic (arsenic, thallium)

HIV-related distal symmetric polyneuropathy

Fabry disease

is symmetric and is usually worse in the feet. Another painful form of diabetic neuropathy is lumbosacral radiculoplexopathy (also known as diabetic amyotrophy), whereby patients may present with the abrupt onset of back, hip, or thigh pain that may precede weakness by days or weeks.[34] (See the article by Pasnoor and colleagues elsewhere in this issue for further exploration of this topic.)

The other important sensory abnormality that significantly narrows the differential diagnosis is severe proprioceptive loss. This disorder is sometimes difficult to discern from the history, but complaints of loss of balance (especially in the dark), incoordination of the limbs, or symptoms suggesting disequilibrium may be helpful. Although the symptoms of gait unsteadiness are common to many neuropathies with sensory involvement, if the neurologic examination reveals a dramatic asymmetric loss of proprioception with significant vibration loss and normal strength, the clinician should immediately consider a sensory neuronopathy (ie, ganglionopathy). In addition to the severe proprioceptive and vibration deficits, sensory neuronopathies usually have a panmodality sensory loss in the affected extremities. Light touch and pain sensation are also affected, owing to injury of all sensory cell bodies. The various causes of sensory neuronopathy are listed in **Box 8**.

A variant of CIDP termed chronic immune sensory polyradiculopathy (CISP) manifests as a sensory ataxia and clinically resembles a sensory neuronopathy/ganglionopathy.[35] Normal sensory nerve action potentials (because the lesion is proximal to the ganglion cells) differentiate this disorder from sensory neuronopathy. Clinicians probably have encountered such patients in the past, being perplexed by the preserved sensory nerve action potentials (SNAPs).[36,37] The discordance between the sensory ataxia and loss of reflexes but normal SNAPs should make one consider CISP. Although the SNAPs may be normal, often the H-reflexes are prolonged or absent, as perhaps are more proximal potentials on somatosensory evoked potentials, owing to proximal demyelination of the sensory roots. Cerebrospinal fluid protein may be elevated. In addition, enlarged and enhancing nerve roots may be appreciated on magnetic resonance imaging. Root biopsies have demonstrated demyelination and inflammation. Most of these patients respond to immunomodulating therapy, similar to CIDP patients. Therefore, CISP should be in the differential of severe ataxia, proprioceptive loss, and areflexia.

Of course, profound proprioception and vibration loss can also be due to posterior column damage from disorders such as combined system degeneration. However, myelopathy of the posterior column is generally symmetric, in general is less profound than in most patients with true dorsal root ganglion loss, and is often associated with evidence of upper motor neuron abnormality (see later discussion). One notable exception is vitamin E deficiency, which can affect both sensory nerves and posterior columns and can produce a profound symmetric proprioceptive deficit.[38]

Box 8
Causes of sensory neuronopathy (ganglionopathy)

Cancer (paraneoplastic)

Sjögren syndrome

Idiopathic sensory neuronopathy

Cisplatinum and other analogues

Vitamin B_6 toxicity

HIV-related sensory neuronopathy

The modalities of light touch, pain sensation (with an unused safety pin), vibration, and proprioception should be assessed in all 4 limbs in a patient with a peripheral neuropathy. The authors have found the use of nylon monofilaments of different tensile strengths very useful in assessing and grading the loss of touch sensation.[30,39] Another useful quantitative bedside test that is easy to perform is maximal timed vibratory testing with a 128-Hz tuning fork. The examination technique consists of striking the tuning fork to obtain a maximal vibratory stimulus and immediately applying the top of the handle to the interphalangeal joint of the great toe. Using a clock, one determines how long the patient can perceive the vibratory stimulus. In children and young adults, this maximal vibratory stimulus is appreciated for at least 15 seconds over the great toe. As patients age, this time decreases even in the absence of overt peripheral neuropathy. As a basic rule of thumb, a 1-second loss of vibration perception per decade is allowed. Thus, it is not uncommon for a 70-year-old patient to have only 9 or 10 seconds of maximal vibration perception over the great toe. Both graded monofilament and timed vibration testing can be easily rechecked at each follow-up visit to monitor the course.

On the other hand, the authors believe that it is extremely difficult to determine with any degree of certainty whether temperature sensation deficits are present with bedside testing, and therefore do not routinely check this modality. It is suspected that temperature sensation can only be assessed reliably with computerized quantitative sensory testing (QST). QST has now become commercially available through several manufacturers.[40] However, the authors' experience in measuring QST for temperature and vibration thresholds in more than 800 neuropathy patients was disappointing in ultimately assisting in diagnosis and management.[41] At present, the authors do not believe that QST is useful in routine clinical practice.

In general, the authors have found the concept of trying to place patients into categories of "large-fiber" and "small-fiber" sensory involvement rarely to be clinically useful in establishing a diagnosis or in management. If a careful bedside examination is performed, most patients with sensory loss associated with the more common categories of peripheral neuropathy (eg, CSPN and diabetes) will clinically have diminished light touch, pin, and vibration sensation, with proprioception affected in more severe cases.[7–9] (See the article by Pasnoor and colleagues elsewhere in this issue for further exploration of this topic.) In addition, QST for vibration and temperature thresholds in these common disorders usually shows abnormalities in both modalities. In truth, selective involvement of small sensory fibers for pain and temperature sensation is uncommon and is seen in rare disorders such as hereditary sensory neuropathy, Fabry disease, and some cases of amyloidosis, but also is seen in some patients with CSPN who have normal nerve conduction studies, reflexes, and vibration. Epidermal nerve quantification by skin biopsy is used by some to confirm a small-fiber neuropathy, but often simply confirms the clinical suspicion obtained from the history and clinical examination.[42–44] The value of skin biopsies lies more in their potential as an objective marker for research studies.[42,45]

Is There Evidence of Upper Motor Neuron Involvement?

In patients with symptoms of signs suggestive of lower motor neuron abnormality without sensory loss, the presence of concomitant upper motor neuron signs is the hallmark of ALS.[10,11] As noted earlier, these patients typically present with asymmetric, distal weakness without sensory loss. Pure upper motor neuron involvement (limb or bulbar) is the presentation for primary lateral sclerosis (PLS),[46,47] as well as hereditary spastic paraparesis.

Box 9
Ten patterns of neuropathic disorders

Pattern 1: Symmetric proximal and distal weakness with sensory loss

Consider:

   Inflammatory demyelinating polyneuropathy (GBS and CIDP)

Pattern 2: Symmetric distal sensory loss with or without distal weakness

Consider:

   Cryptogenic sensory polyneuropathy (CSPN)

   Metabolic disorders

   Drugs, toxins

   Hereditary (CMT, amyloidosis, and others)

Pattern 3: Asymmetric distal weakness with sensory loss

Multiple nerves, consider:

   Vasculitis

   HNPP

   MADSAM neuropathy

   Infectious (leprosy, Lyme, sarcoid, HIV)

Single nerves/regions, consider:

   Compressive mononeuropathy and radiculopathy

Pattern 4: Asymmetric proximal and distal weakness with sensory loss

Consider:

   Polyradiculopathy or plexopathy due to diabetes mellitus, meningeal carcinomatosis or lymphomatosis, sarcoidosis, amyloidosis, Lyme, idiopathic, hereditary (HNPP, familial)

Pattern 5: Asymmetric distal weakness without sensory loss

Consider:

1. With upper motor neuron findings

   a. Motor neuron disease/ALS/PLS

2. Without upper motor neuron findings

   a. PMA

      i. BAD

      ii. LAD

   b. Multifocal motor neuropathy

   c. MAMA

   d. Juvenile monomelic amyotrophy

Pattern 6: Symmetric sensory loss and distal areflexia with upper motor neuron findings

Consider:

   B_{12} deficiency and other causes of combined system degeneration with peripheral neuropathy

   Copper deficiency (including zinc toxicity)

   Inherited disorders (adrenomyeloneuropathy, metachromatic leukodystrophy, Friedreich ataxia)

Pattern 7: Symmetric weakness without sensory loss[a]

Consider:

1. Proximal and distal weakness

  a. SMA

2. Distal weakness

  a. Hereditary motor neuropathy

Pattern 8: Focal midline proximal symmetric weakness[a]

Consider:

  Neck extensor weakness: ALS

  Bulbar weakness: ALS, PLS

Pattern 9: Asymmetric proprioceptive sensory loss without weakness

Consider:

  Sensory neuronopathy (ganglionopathy) (see **Box 9**)

  CISP

Pattern 10: Autonomic symptoms and signs

Consider:

  Neuropathies associated with autonomic dysfunction (see **Box 6**)

[a] Overlaps with myopathies and neuromuscular junction disorders.

On the other hand, if the patient presents with symmetric distal sensory symptoms and signs suggestive of a distal sensory neuropathy, but there is additional evidence of symmetric upper motor involvement, the physician should consider a disorder such as combined system degeneration with neuropathy. The most common cause for this pattern is vitamin B_{12} deficiency, but other causes of combined system degeneration with neuropathy should be considered (eg, copper deficiency, HIV infection, severe hepatic disease, or adrenomyeloneuropathy).[48–52] In the authors' experience, these patients may be distinguished from typical CSPN patients by the presence of crossed adductor reflexes or mild spread of reflexes in the arms, in the setting of absent ankle reflexes. This scenario in a patient who presents with distal sensory loss and unsteadiness should lead to an intensive search for vitamin B_{12} deficiency (ie, assessing for elevated serum methylmalonic acid and homocysteine levels), if the B_{12} level is in the lower limit of normal range. In addition, some of these patients develop sensory symptoms in the hands before they begin in the feet, otherwise known as the numb hand syndrome.[48–50,52]

A similar myeloneuropathy or myelopathy may occur secondary to copper deficiency.[53–56] (See the article by Hammond and colleagues elsewhere in this issue for further exploration of this topic.) Patients present with lower limb paresthesias, weakness, spasticity, and gait difficulties. Sensory loss is impaired distally, reflexes are brisk (but may be absent at the ankles), and plantar responses may be extensor. Electrophysiologic studies often show an axonal sensorimotor neuropathy. Patients may have neutropenia, microcytic anemia, and a pancytopenia. The copper deficiency may be due to prior gastric surgery. The use of denture adhesives containing zinc has also been associated with copper deficiency.[57] In such cases, zinc levels are elevated and the metal may compete with copper, leading to the syndrome. Treatment consists

Table 2
Clinical patterns of neuropathic disorders

	Weakness				Sensory Symptoms	Severe Proprioceptive Loss	UMN Signs	Autonomic Symptoms/ Signs	Diagnosis
	Proximal	Distal	Asymmetric	Symmetric					
Pattern 1: symmetric proximal and distal weakness with sensory loss	+	+		+	+				GBS/CIDP
Pattern 2: distal sensory loss with/without weakness		+		+	+				CSPN, metabolic, drugs, hereditary
Pattern 3: distal weakness with sensory loss		+	+		+				Multiple: vasculitis, HNPP, MADSAM, infection Single: mononeuropathy, radiculopathy
Pattern 4: asymmetric proximal and distal weakness with sensory loss	+	+	+		+				Polyradiculopathy, plexopathy
Pattern 5: asymmetric distal weakness without sensory loss	+	+	+				±		LMN and UMN – ALS Pure UMN – PLS Pure LMN – MMN, PMA, BAD, LAD, MAMA

Pattern						Examples
Pattern 6: symmetric sensory loss and upper motor neuron signs	+	+	+	+		B12 deficiency, copper deficiency, Friedreich ataxia, adrenomyeloneuropathy
Pattern 7a: symmetric weakness without sensory loss	±	+	+	+		Proximal and distal SMA, Distal Hereditary motor neuropathy
Pattern 8a: focal midline proximal symmetric weakness	Neck/extensor +, Bulbar +	+	+	+	+	ALS
Pattern 9: asymmetric proprioceptive loss without weakness	+	+	+			Sensory neuronopathy (ganglionopathy)
Pattern 10: autonomic dysfunction					+	HSAN, diabetes, GBS, amyloid, porphyria, Fabry

Abbreviations: ALS, amyotrophic lateral sclerosis; BAD, brachial amyotrophic diplegia; CIDP, chronic inflammatory demyelinating polyneuropathy; CSPN, cryptogenic sensory polyneuropathy; GBS, Guillain-Barré syndrome; HNPP, hereditary neuropathy with liability to pressure palsy; HSAN, hereditary sensory and autonomic neuropathy; LAD, leg amyotrophic diplegia; MADSAM, multifocal acquired demyelinating sensory and motor; MAMA, multifocal acquired motor axonopathy; MMN, multifocal motor neuropathy; PMA, progressive muscular atrophy; SMA, spinal muscular atrophy; UMN, upper motor neuron.

a Overlap patterns with myopathy/neuromuscular junction disorders.

of either daily oral copper supplements or, in severe cases, intravenous copper therapy.

What is the Temporal Evolution?

Of obvious importance is the onset, duration, and evolution of symptoms and signs. Does the disease have an acute (days to 4 weeks), subacute (4–8 weeks), or chronic (>8 weeks) course? Is the course monophasic, progressive, or relapsing? Neuropathies with acute and subacute presentations include GBS, vasculitis, and diabetic lumbosacral radiculoplexopathy. A relapsing course can be present in CIDP and porphyria. It is also important to inquire about preceding or concurrent infections, associated medical conditions, drug use including over-the-counter vitamin preparations (B_6), alcohol, and dietary habits.

Is There Evidence for a Hereditary Neuropathy?

Finally, a hereditary cause for a peripheral neuropathy should not be overlooked.[18,58,59] In both the Mayo Clinic and University of Texas series, hereditary neuropathy accounted for the largest group of neuropathy patients referred to a tertiary referral center.[2–5] Although this may not be true in general neurology practice, it is still important for the clinician to look for the clues that suggest a hereditary neuropathy. In patients with a chronic, very slowly progressive distal weakness over many years, with very little in the way of sensory symptoms, the clinician should pay particular attention to the family history and inquire about foot deformities in immediate relatives. Patients with hereditary neuropathy often will present with significant foot drop, with no sensory symptoms, but significant vibration loss in the toes. In addition, episodes of recurrent compressive mononeuropathies may indicate an underlying hereditary predisposition to pressure palsies. On examining the patient, the clinician must look carefully at the feet for arch and toe abnormalities (high or flat arches, hammer toes), and look at the spine for scoliosis. In suspicious cases, it may be necessary to perform both neurologic and electrophysiologic studies on family members (See the article by Saporta and colleagues elsewhere in this issue for further discussion of this topic).

PHENOTYPE PATTERNS OF NEUROPATHIC DISORDERS

After answering the 6 key questions obtained from the history and neurologic examination outlined here, one can classify neuropathic disorders into several patterns based on sensory and motor involvement and the distribution of signs (**Box 9, Table 2**). Each syndrome has a limited differential diagnosis. A final diagnosis is arrived at by using other clues such as the temporal course, presence of other disease states, family history, and information from laboratory studies. The authors use this pattern-recognition approach to neuropathic disorders routinely in patients, and suspect that many clinicians use a similar approach without being aware of it. Although this may seem like an oversimplification, the recognition of these patterns will usually push the clinician very close to the final diagnosis. After placing a patient in 1 of the 10 phenotype patterns, one can more appropriately begin the laboratory evaluation and potential treatments.[59] (See the articles by Levine and colleagues and Trivedi and colleagues elsewhere in this issue for further exploration of this topic.)

REFERENCES

1. Amato AA, Russell J. Neuromuscular disease. New York: McGraw-Hill; 2008. p. 3–69.

2. Amato AA, Barohn RJ. Peripheral neuropathy. In: Longo DL, Fauci AS, Kasper DL, et al, editors. Harrison's principles of internal medicine. 18th edition. New York (NY): The McGraw-Hill Companies, Inc; 2012. p. 3448–72.

3. Dyck PJ, Oviatt KF, Lambert EH. Intensive evaluation of referred unclassified neuropathies yields improved diagnosis. Ann Neurol 1981;10:222–6.

4. Barohn RJ. Approach to peripheral neuropathy and neuronopathy. Semin Neurol 1998;18:7–18.

5. Khan S, Pasnoor M, Mummaneni RB, et al. North America and South America (NA-SA) Neuropathy Project [Abstract]. J Child Neurol 2006;21(3).

6. Pasnoor M, Nascimento O, Trivedi J, et al. North America and South America (NA-SA) Neuropathy Project. Int J Neurosci, in press.

7. Grahmann F, Winterholler M, Neundorfer B. Cryptogenetic polyneuropathies: an out-patient follow-up study. Acta Neurol Scand 1991;84:221–5.

8. Wolfe GI, Barohn RJ. Cryptogenic sensory and sensorimotor polyneuropathies. Semin Neurol 1998;18:105–12.

9. Wolfe GI, Baker NS, Amato AA, et al. Chronic cryptogenic sensory polyneuropathies: clinical and laboratory characteristics. Arch Neurol 1999;56:540–7.

10. Jackson CE, Bryan WW. Amyotrophic lateral sclerosis. Semin Neurol 1998;18: 27–40.

11. Barohn RJ. Clinical spectrum of motor neuron disorders. In: Miller AE, editor. Continuum: lifelong learning in neurology. Minneapolis: Lippincott Williams & Wilkins; 2009. p. 111–31.

12. Tan E, Lynn DJ, Amato AA, et al. Immunosuppressive treatment of motor neuron syndromes: attempts to distinguish a treatable disorder. Arch Neurol 1994;51: 194–200.

13. Katz JS, Wolfe GI, Anderson PB, et al. Brachial amyotrophic diplegia: a slowly progressive motor neuron disorder. Neurology 1999;53:1071–6.

14. Rosenfeld J, Chang SW, Jackson CE, et al. Lower extremity amyotrophic diplegia (LAD): a new clinical entity in the spectrum of motor neuron disease. Neurology 2002;58:A411–2.

15. Muzyka IM, Dimachkie MM, Barohn RJ, et al. Lower extremity amyotrophic diplegia (LAD): prevalance and pattern of weakness. J Clin Neuromuscul Dis 2010;11(3):14–5.

16. Iannaccone ST. Spinal muscular atrophy. Semin Neurol 1998;18:19–26.

17. Workshop report, 2nd Workshop of the European CMT Consortium: 53rd ENMC International Workshop on Classification and Diagnostic Guidelines for Charcot-Marie-Tooth Type 2 (CMT2-HMSN II) and Distal Hereditary Motor Neuropathy (Distal HMN-Spina CMT), 26-28 September 1997, Naarden, The Netherlands. Neuromuscul Disord 1998;8:426–31.

18. Nanjiani Z, Nations SP, Elliott JL, et al. Distal hereditary motor neuropathy: a distinct form of Charcot-Marie-Tooth disease [abstract]. J Child Neurol 2000; 15:200–2001.

19. Katz JS, Wolfe GI, Bryan WW, et al. Electrophysiologic findings in multifocal motor neuropathy. Neurology 1997;48:700–7.

20. Hart RG, Kanter MC. Acute autonomic neuropathy: two cases and a clinical review. Arch Intern Med 1990;150:2373–6.

21. Suarez GA, Fealey RD, Camilleri M, et al. Idiopathic autonomic neuropathy: clinical, neurophysiologic, and follow-up studies on 27 patients. Neurology 1994;44:1675–82.

22. Barohn RJ, Kissel JT, Warmolts JR, et al. Chronic inflammatory demyelinating polyneuropathy. Clinical characteristics, course, and recommendations for diagnostic criteria. Arch Neurol 1989;46:878–84.

23. Barohn RJ, Saperstein DS. Guillain-Barré syndrome and chronic inflammatory demyelinating polyneuropathy. Semin Neurol 1998;18:49–62.
24. Saperstein DS, Katz JS, Amato AA, et al. Clinical spectrum of chronic acquired demyelinating polyneuropathies. Muscle Nerve 2001;24(3):311–24.
25. Dimachkie MM, Barohn RJ. Acute inflammatory demyelinating neuropathies and variants. In: Tawil RN, Venance S, editors. Neurology in practice: neuromuscular disorders. Oxford (UK): Wiley-Blackwell; 2011. p. 183–9.
26. Katz JS, Wolfe GI, Burns DK, et al. Isolated neck extensor myopathy: a common cause of dropped head syndrome. Neurology 1996;46:917–21.
27. Saperstein DS, Amato A, Barohn RJ. Clinical and genetics aspects of the distal myopathies. Muscle Nerve 2001;24:1440–50.
28. Nations SP, Wolfe GI, Amato AA, et al. Distal myasthenia gravis. Neurology 1999; 52:632–4.
29. Amato AA, Gronseth GS, Callerame KJ, et al. Tomaculous neuropathy: a clinical and electrophysiological study in patients with and without 1.5-Mb deletions in chromosome 17p11.2. Muscle Nerve 1996;19:16–22.
30. Nations SP, Katz JS, Lyde CB, et al. Leprous neuropathy: an American perspective. Semin Neurol 1998;18:113–24.
31. Saperstein DS, Amato A, Wolfe GI, et al. Multifocal acquired demyelinating sensory and motor neuropathy: the Lewis-Sumner syndrome. Muscle Nerve 1999;22:560–6.
32. Katz JS, Saperstein DS, Gronseth G, et al. Distal acquired demyelinating symmetric (DADS) neuropathy. Neurology 2000;54:615–20.
33. Kissel JT, Slivka AP, Warmolts JR, et al. The clinical spectrum of necrotizing angiopathy of the peripheral nervous system. Ann Neurol 1985;18:251–7.
34. Barohn RJ, Zahenk Z, Warmolts JR, et al. The Bruns-Garland syndrome (diabetic amyotrophy): revisited 100 years later. Arch Neurol 1991;48:1130–5.
35. Sinnreich M, Klein CJ, Daube JR, et al. Chronic immune sensory polyradiculopathy: a possibly treatable sensory ataxia. Neurology 2004;63:1662–9.
36. Greenfield F, Bryan WW, Katz JS, et al. Chronic sensory ataxia: an unusual case [abstract]. J Child Neurol 1995;10:161.
37. Manek S, Nations SP, Wolfe GI, et al. Idiopathic chronic sensory ataxia: where is the lesion? [abstract]. J Child Neurol 2000;15:193.
38. Jackson CE, Amato AA, Barohn RJ. Case of the month: isolated vitamin E deficiency. Muscle Nerve 1996;19:1161–5.
39. Caputo GM, Cavanaugh PR, Ulbrecht JS, et al. Assessment and management of foot disease in patients with diabetes. N Engl J Med 1994;331:854–60.
40. Yarnitsky D. Quantitative sensory testing. Muscle Nerve 1997;20:198–204.
41. Saperstein DS, Wolfe GI, Longeria O, et al. Quantitative sensory testing in a large cohort of neuropathy patients [abstract]. Muscle Nerve 2001;24:1417–8.
42. Barohn RJ. Intra-epidermal nerve fiber assessment: a new window on peripheral neuropathy. Arch Neurol 1998;88:1505–20.
43. England JD, Gronseth GS, Franklin G, et al. Practice parameter: the evaluation of distal symmetric polyneuropathy: the role of autonomic testing, nerve biopsy, and skin biopsy (an evidence-based review). Report of the American Academy of Neurology, the American Association of Neuromuscular and Electrodiagnostic Medicine, and the American Academy of Physical Medicine and Rehabilitation. Muscle Nerve 2009;39:106–15.
44. England JD, Gronseth GS, Franklin G, et al. Evaluation of distal symmetric polyneuropathy: the role of laboratory and genetic testing (an evidence-based review). Muscle Nerve 2009;39:116–25.

45. Kluding PM, Pasnoor M, Singh R, et al. The effect of exercise on neuropathic symptoms, nerve function, and cutaneous innervation in people with diabetic peripheral neuropathy. J Neurol Neurosurg Psychiatr 2012;26:424–9.
46. Singer MA, Kojan S, Barohn RJ, et al. Primary lateral sclerosis: clinical and laboratory findings in 25 patients. J Clin Neuromuscul Dis 2005;7:1–9.
47. Singer MA, Statland JM, Wolfe GI, et al. Primary lateral sclerosis. Muscle Nerve 2007;35(3):291–302.
48. Saperstein DS, Barohn RJ. Polyneuropathy due to nutritional and vitamin deficiency. In: Dyck PJ, Thomas PK, editors. Peripheral neuropathy. Philadelphia: Elsevier Saunders; 2005. p. 2051–62.
49. Saperstein DS, Barohn RJ. Peripheral neuropathy due to cobalamin deficiency. Curr Treat Options Neurol 2002;4:197–201.
50. Saperstein DS, Wolfe GI, Gronseth GS, et al. Challenges in the identification of cobalamin deficiency polyneuropathy. Arch Neurol 2003;60:1296–301.
51. Kojan S, Cheema Z, Nations SP, et al. Neurophysiologic abnormalities in adrenomyeloneuropathy: selective central and peripheral nervous system involvement. J Child Neurol 2000;15:197.
52. Jackson CE, Barohn RJ. Lesion localization of the number hand syndrome in B12 deficiency [abstract]. Muscle Nerve 1993;16:1111–2.
53. Greenberg SA, Briemberg HR. A neurological and hematological syndrome associated with zinc excess and copper deficiency. J Neurol 2004;251:111–4.
54. Hedera P, Fink JK, Bockenstedt PL, et al. Myelopolyneuropathy and pancytopenia due to copper deficiency and high zinc levels of unknown origin: further support for existence of a new zinc overload syndrome. Arch Neurol 2003;60: 1303–6.
55. Kumar N, Gross JB, Ahlskog JE. Copper deficiency myelopathy produces a clinical picture like acute combined degeneration. Neurology 2004;63:33–9.
56. Kumar N. Copper deficiency myelopathy (human swayback). Mayo Clin Proc 2006;81(10):1371–84.
57. Nations SP, Boyer PJ, Love LA, et al. Denture cream: an unusual source of excess zinc, leading to hypocupremia and neurologic disease. Neurology 2008;71(9): 639–43.
58. Mendell JR. Charcot-Marie-Tooth neuropathies and related disorders. Semin Neurol 1998;18:41–8.
59. Saporta AS, Sottile SL, Miller LJ, et al. Charcot-Marie-Tooth disease subtypes and genetic testing strategies. Ann Neurol 2011;69:22–33.

Laboratory Evaluation of Peripheral Neuropathy

Todd D. Levine, MD, David S. Saperstein, MD*

KEYWORDS

- Peripheral neuropathy • Nerve conduction studies • Electromyography
- Autonomic testing

KEY POINTS

- Laboratory workup for peripheral neuropathy should be guided by the clinical pattern.
- The components of nerves involved and the time course of symptoms are important factors used to categorize patients.
- Nerve conduction studies are important but play a secondary role to clinical patterns when generating a differential diagnosis.

Peripheral neuropathies are very common, with an estimated prevalence of 2% to 3% of the general population, 8% in patients older than 55 years, and 24% in patients older than 65.[1,2] The question of how to evaluate these patients is complicated by there being hundreds of potential causes, both acquired and inherited. The evaluation of these patients can be very time consuming and expensive. Furthermore, patients and neurologists may question the benefit of identifying a cause of a neuropathy when the majority of acquired, and all inherited, forms have no specific therapy. One must also consider that between one-third and one-half of all neuropathies, even after thorough evaluation, will remain idiopathic.[3] Neurologists often adopt an approach either of ordering all of the possible tests ("shotgun" approach) or of ordering very few tests ("targeted" approach).

This review focuses on a targeted and thoughtful approach to the laboratory evaluation of patients with peripheral neuropathy, designed to allow the identification of treatable neuropathies without undue expense and risk to patients. However, it is important to keep one issue in mind: if one completes the evaluation of a patient with peripheral neuropathy and believes the neuropathy to be idiopathic, it is imperative to continue to follow the patient intermittently. Most idiopathic neuropathies are very

Disclosure: Drs Levine and Saperstein have financial interest in a laboratory that processes skin biopsies for small fiber neuropathy testing.
Phoenix Neurological Associates, University of Arizona College of Medicine, 5090 North 40th Street, Suite 250, Phoenix, AZ 85018, USA
* Corresponding author.
E-mail address: david.saperstein@gmail.com

Neurol Clin 31 (2013) 363–376
http://dx.doi.org/10.1016/j.ncl.2013.01.004
0733-8619/13/$ – see front matter © 2013 Elsevier Inc. All rights reserved.

slowly progressive and typically do not involve much weakness.[3] If a patient is thought to have an idiopathic neuropathy that is progressive and disabling, particularly in terms of weakness, he or she deserves further evaluation that may include lumbar puncture, nerve biopsy, or other invasive testing. One should be loath to leave a patient with a diagnosis of idiopathic neuropathy in the face of a progressive, disabling course.

A common approach to the differential diagnosis of peripheral neuropathies relies on the results of nerve conduction studies and electromyography (NCS/EMG). The proper use and interpretation of NCS/EMG is vital to the evaluation of such patients. However, these tests can be technically challenging and often patients will exhibit both axonal and demyelinating changes, making interpretation difficult. In the authors' experience, clinicians are often inappropriately diverted toward incorrect and unnecessary diagnostic approaches when using a diagnostic algorithm that starts with NCS/EMG. The authors favor an approach that begins with determining which clinical pattern is present. This method relies predominantly on information obtained from the history and, to a lesser extent, the physical examination. Once the clinical pattern of the neuropathy is identified, further testing, to include NCS/EMG and laboratory testing, can be obtained in a strategic manner.

Potential tests to evaluate patients with peripheral neuropathy include routine laboratory tests, autoantibody testing, genetic testing, lumbar puncture, nerve biopsy, skin biopsy, autonomic testing, and quantitative sensory testing. The approach to choosing among testing options begins by asking the following questions:

- Is the disease process acute, subacute, or chronic?
- Is the disease process affecting motor nerves, sensory nerves, autonomic nerves, or a combination?
- If the disease process is purely sensory, does it affect small fibers, large fibers, or both?
- Is the disease process predominantly distal or proximal?
- Is the disease process symmetric or asymmetric?
- Is the disease process purely lower motor neuron or are there upper motor neuron findings as well?

For example, an "acute, symmetric, motor neuropathy" comprises a completely different set of diagnostic considerations to a "chronic, symmetric, sensory neuropathy." Applying these few adjectives in the assessment of a patient's neuropathy will thus allow for a focused approach to selecting diagnostic tests.

CHRONIC DISTAL SYMMETRIC SENSORY NEUROPATHY

The most commonly encountered neuropathy pattern is a chronic, distal, symmetric, sensory neuropathy. Electrodiagnostic testing may show mild signs of motor involvement in these patients, such as low compound motor action potentials or mildly slowed motor conduction velocities. However, clinically these patients do not complain of or show significant weakness. The evaluation of these patients should include the laboratory tests listed in **Table 1**.

Even with as simple a list as this, there is controversy. There is an argument that an abnormal 2-hour glucose tolerance test showing impaired glucose tolerance (IGT) does not necessarily mean that this is the cause of the neuropathy.[4] This question is difficult to unravel statistically, because as much as 15% of the United States population is estimated to have IGT while 8% of the population has neuropathy.[5] Thus it would be expected that 15% of neuropathy patients would have IGT simply by coincidence, making a statistical association between IGT and neuropathy very difficult.

Table 1
Chronic distal symmetric sensory neuropathy

Potential Etiology	Tests to Order
Diabetes mellitus	Fasting glucose, 2-h oral glucose tolerance test, HgbA1c[a]
Impaired glucose tolerance	2-h glucose tolerance test[a]
Vitamin B_{12} deficiency	B_{12} level and methylmalonic acid[a]
Paraproteinemia	Serum immunofixation[a] Serum free light chain analysis MAG antibodies (if IgM paraprotein and prolonged distal motor latencies)

Abbreviations: HgbA1c, hemoglobin A_{1c}; IgM, immunoglobulin M; MAG, myelin-associated glycoprotein.
[a] Recommended by the American Academy of Neurology practice parameter.[9]

However, if one is faced with a patient with an elevated body mass index or other comorbid conditions associated with the IGT, it makes sense to treat the IGT in the hope of delaying progression of the neuropathy. The IGT patient is already known to be at risk of developing diabetes and that this risk will be associated with potential progression of the neuropathy. So why not intervene now, before more damage has occurred? There are studies showing that treating IGT patients with glucose-lowering medications prevents progression to diabetes,[6,7] but the issue remains unresolved at present.

In terms of testing for vitamin B_{12} deficiency, it important to recognize that a normal serum B_{12} level may not exclude a clinically relevant vitamin B_{12} deficiency.[8] Therefore, a more sensitive test for vitamin B_{12} deficiency, elevated serum methylmalonic acid, is recommended.[9,10] In most situations, an elevated level of serum methylmalonic acid indicates insufficient vitamin B_{12}, and such patients should be treated for B_{12} deficiency. However, volume depletion, renal insufficiency and, rarely, genetic disorders, can cause elevated levels of methylmalonic acid independent of vitamin B_{12} deficiency.[11] Elevated homocysteine levels may also help identify vitamin B_{12} deficiency, although other factors, such as folate or pyridoxine deficiency and genetic polymorphisms, may also cause such elevations. Treatment of vitamin B_{12} deficiency can usually be accomplished with oral therapy, giving 1000 µg of vitamin B_{12} per day.[10] Levels of methylmalonic acid and homocysteine can be rechecked after several weeks and, if the levels normalize, oral therapy can be continued.[12] However, if levels of methylmalonic acid and homocysteine do not correct after 3 months of oral therapy, the patient should be switched to parenteral replacement of vitamin B_{12}. A Schilling test is rarely performed or needed.[13] It is important that patients remain on vitamin B_{12} replacement therapy even if they do not notice immediate improvement. Improvement can take many months or may not occur at all; however, vitamin B_{12} treatment may prevent or slow progression of the neuropathy.[14]

The authors do not advocate the routine testing of other B vitamins. In the absence of dietary risk factors, such testing is usually not helpful or leads to false-positive results. The authors have seen several patients with neuropathy whose referring physicians found elevated vitamin B_6 levels in patients not taking any supplements, which in their experience has not been clinically relevant.

In detecting paraproteins, the authors prefer serum immunofixation over serum protein electrophoresis. It is not clear whether these are equivalent techniques,[15] but there is at least one report suggesting that serum immunofixation has a higher yield in assessing patients with peripheral neuropathy.[16] There certainly is no need to order both tests. The addition of a quantitative immunoglobulin panel, however, can be useful in helping the clinician determine whether a paraprotein is associated with elevated levels of that class of immunoglobulin or depressed levels of another immunoglobulin class. If abnormal levels of other immunoglobulins are present, or if patients have markedly elevated total immunoglobulins, this raises the possibility of an underlying malignancy such as multiple myeloma, Waldenstrom macroglobulinemia, or lymphoma. In these cases patients should evaluated by a hematologist to determine whether they should undergo a bone marrow biopsy, and this should be performed before starting any immunomodulatory therapy for treatment of the neuropathy. The addition of a serum free light chain analysis has also recently been shown to increase the sensitivity for plasma cell dyscrasias such as amyloid, and negates the need for 24-hour urine studies.[17]

Finally, patients with an immunoglobulin M (IgM) paraprotein and a neuropathy characterized by predominant large-fiber loss presenting as ataxia, numbness, and tremor likely have a distinct neuropathy syndrome, which is often associated with antibodies against myelin-associated glycoprotein (MAG). This subject is discussed in detail in the section on other ataxic neuropathies.

SMALL-FIBER NEUROPATHY

If patients present with sensory symptoms but have intact deep tendon reflexes and normal vibration and joint position sense, one should entertain the possibility of a small-fiber neuropathy (SFN). Patients with SFN can present in a typical distal symmetric sensory pattern. However, their symptoms can also be multifocal and proximal, such that isolated SFN can present as chest or trunk pain, face and scalp pain, or very asymmetrically, involving only a single limb.[18–20] In these cases it can often be mistaken for complex regional pain syndrome, reflex sympathetic dystrophy, fibromyalgia, radiculopathy, or other chronic pain disorders. Such patients may even be suspected of having nonorganic disease. The diagnosis of SFN can be confirmed on a skin biopsy assessed for intraepidermal nerve-fiber density (IENFD).[21] The biopsy procedure can be quickly and easily performed in the office or clinic, and there are several commercial laboratories that perform this widely available test. When performing skin biopsy for measurement of IENFD it is best to biopsy a distal site and a proximal site, especially in cases of widespread bilateral symptoms, thus allowing one to determine whether the patient has a typical length-dependent or non–length-dependent SFN. Patients with a non–length-dependent SFN are more likely to have an autoimmune process.[22,23] Although skin biopsy is a very sensitive test for SFN, not all patients will have a decreased IENFD. There are also concerns for false-positive results. The overall sensitivity and specificity of IENFD testing are 80% and 90%.[21]

SFN can also be diagnosed in some cases by means of autonomic testing, specifically quantitative sudomotor axon reflex testing (QSART).[24,25] However, QSART is not abnormal in all cases of SFN.[19] Furthermore, this test is usually only available in specialized centers, making skin biopsy testing more accessible to most clinicians.

Once a diagnosis of SFN is made, the patient should be further evaluated as outlined in **Table 2**. In some cases of SFN where testing is unrevealing, especially if the neuropathy is non–length dependent or has come on abruptly, one could consider performing a lumbar puncture to look for increased protein or immune activity, such as an elevated rate of immunoglobulin G (IgG) synthesis. These findings would help support an autoimmune etiology, and may suggest the possibility of using immunomodulating therapies.[26,27]

Patients with SFN may also have significant autonomic complaints and findings. In this scenario amyloidosis is a consideration. In these patients the search for amyloid is

Table 2
Evaluation of small-fiber neuropathy

Potential Etiology	Tests to Order
Diabetes mellitus	Fasting glucose, 2-h oral glucose tolerance test, HgbA1c
Impaired glucose tolerance	2-h glucose tolerance test, HgbA1c
Sjögren syndrome	SS-A, SS-B, salivary gland biopsy
Sarcoidosis	Serum angiotensin-converting enzyme
Primary systemic amyloidosis	Serum immunofixation Quantitative immunoglobulins Serum free light chain Consider tissue biopsy (fat pad, rectal, skin, or other affected tissue)
Familial amyloidosis	Transthyretin (TTR) gene sequencing
Fabry disease	Serum α-galactosidase level

quite complex, as the yield of testing is very poor if serum immunofixation and quantitative immunoglobulins are normal. However, one should consider genetic testing for transthyretin gene mutations as well as pursuing a pathologic diagnosis with tissue: fat-pad biopsies or aspirates, rectal biopsy, and biopsies of affected organs such as heart or kidney can be performed if the suspicion is high.

The genetic disorder known as Fabry disease can present as episodic attacks of severe neuropathic pain that is often precipitated by exercise, heat, stress, or alcohol. The pain is mostly located on the palms and soles of the feet, and presents as early as age 10 years, with a mean age of 20 years.[28] Large-fiber damage is very uncommon, but skin biopsy will show a marked decreased in IENFD.[29] Patients can have other neurologic issues such as strokes or hearing loss, and frequently have angiokeratomas on their skin. This diagnosis is confirmed by measuring α-galactosidase levels in the peripheral blood.

Despite a thorough workup, no clear cause will be identified in approximately half of patients with SFN.[20,24] A recent study found a gain of function mutation in the SCN9A gene (which codes for the voltage-gated sodium channel Nav(V)1.7) in 8 out of 28 (28.5%) patients who otherwise appeared to have an idiopathic SFN.[30] Different SCN9A mutations cause inherited erythromelalgia and a rare pain syndrome called paroxysmal extreme pain disorder. Larger studies evaluating the frequency of SCN9A mutations in patients with SFN are needed. However, genetic testing for this gene is available from several commercial laboratories, making this a reasonable test to obtain in patients with SFN in whom no other cause can be identified.

ATAXIC SENSORY NEUROPATHY

The third type of predominantly sensory neuropathy predominantly affects the large fibers and can present as significant balance difficulties and ataxia out of proportion to the small-fiber complaints. When the clinical picture is non–length dependent or is acute or subacute in onset, the site of abnormality is usually the cell body in the dorsal root ganglion rather than nerve axons. This entity is referred to as sensory neuronopathy. Electrodiagnostically, sensory neuronopathies are associated with a diffuse absence of sensory responses with relative sparing of motor responses. This condition can be idiopathic, a manifestation of a paraneoplastic syndrome, or caused by vitamin E deficiency, excessive levels of vitamin B_6, or Sjögren syndrome (**Table 3**). Therefore, evaluation should include levels of vitamin E and B_6 as well as anti-Hu and

Table 3 Evaluation of sensory ataxia	
Potential Etiology	Tests to Order
Vitamin B_{12} deficiency	Vitamin B_{12}, methylmalonic acid, homocysteine
Sjögren syndrome	SS-A, SS-B, salivary gland biopsy
HIV	HIV serology
Paraneoplastic	Hu serology
Vitamin E deficiency	Vitamin E levels
Tabes dorsalis	FTA-Abs or MHA-TP
Vitamin B_6 toxicity	Vitamin B_6 levels
CISP	Somatosensory evoked potentials, gadolinium MRI of nerve roots, CSF

Abbreviations: CISP, chronic immune sensory polyradiculopathy; CSF, cerebrospinal fluid; FTA-Abs, fluorescent treponemal antibody absorption; HIV, human immunodeficiency virus; MHA-TP, micro-hemagglutination assay for Treponema pallidum; MRI, magnetic resonance imaging.

SS-A/SS-B antibodies. Malignancy remains a consideration even if anti-Hu antibodies are absent, and whole-body computed tomography or positron emission tomography scanning should be considered. Further evaluation for Sjögren syndrome with lip biopsy can be pursued in certain cases.[31,32]

Some patients with an ataxic neuropathy will have peripheral neuropathy and not neuronopathy. Vitamin B_{12} deficiency can cause this clinical picture; testing for this should be pursued as discussed earlier. A common cause of an ataxic sensory neuropathy in older individuals is demyelinating neuropathy associated with an IgM paraprotein. This condition is known in the literature by several names, including IgM neuropathy, anti-MAG neuropathy, distal acquired demyelinating symmetric (DADS) neuropathy, and chronic inflammatory sensory polyradiculoneuropathy (CIDP) with a monoclonal protein.[33,34]

Patients with a demyelinating neuropathy with an IgM monoclonal protein exhibit a rather homogeneous clinical picture: older age, male predominance, ataxia, tremor, prolonged distal latencies out of proportion to slow conduction velocities, infrequent motor conduction block and, mainly, a κ light chain.[34] Approximately half of patients will have antibodies against MAG.[34] There is no definitive evidence that patients with anti-MAG antibodies differ from those without, with respect to clinical course or response to therapies. This entity should be considered distinct from CIDP because the clinical course and response to immune-modulating therapies are markedly different.[33,34]

There are some conditions that may mimic a sensory neuronopathy or ataxic sensory neuropathy. A rare example is tabes dorsalis, a manifestation of tertiary syphilis that affects the dorsal column of the spinal cord. Testing only rapid plasma reagin (RPR) is not sufficient, as RPR titers often normalize over time.[35] Appropriate testing for late mani-festations of syphilis requires a treponemal-based immune test such as the fluorescent treponemal antibody absorption test or microhemagglutination assay for Treponema pallidum.[35] If a patient clearly has a neuropathy based on clinical examination and NCS/EMG testing, then testing for syphilis is of extremely low yield and is not needed.[36]

If sensory responses are preserved on NCS but patients have profound large-fiber involvement. one should consider a relatively recently described entity: chronic immune sensory polyradiculopathy (CISP).[37] CISP produces gait ataxia and large-fiber sensory loss, and frequently causes falls. Patients will often have abnormal somatosensory evoked potentials, enlarged nerve roots on magnetic resonance imaging, and elevated cerebrospinal fluid (CSF) protein.[37] Partial biopsy of a nerve root can also be performed to assist diagnosis, but this procedure is available only at specialized centers. CISP is an important disease to recognize, as patients typically respond well to immunomodulatory therapy.

PURE MOTOR NEUROPATHY

Pure motor neuropathies can present acutely, subacutely, or chronically (**Table 4**). To consider a patient as having a pure motor neuropathy, one obviously must exclude motor neuronopathy (amyotrophic lateral sclerosis [ALS] and other motor neuron diseases) and myelopathy. The distinguishing clinical feature of a pure motor neuropathy is the absence of sensory signs or symptoms and decreased reflexes. Pure motor weakness with preserved reflexes or hyperreflexia would prompt one to order imaging and NCS/EMG to define the pathophysiology.

Acute motor axonal neuropathy (AMAN) is typically postinfectious and is related to a gastrointestinal infection with *Campylobacter jejuni* or upper respiratory infection with *Haemophilus influenzae*. Patients often develop IgG antibodies to the GM1 ganglioside, which resembles an antigen on the bacteria. AMAN is more common among Asians and Mexicans.[38–40] Recovery is typically slower and not as complete compared with the more typical, demyelinating form of Guillain-Barré syndrome (GBS). As with typical GBS, patients with AMAN have elevated CSF protein with few or no white blood cells. If the CSF white blood cell count is significantly elevated, one should consider the polymerase chain reaction for West Nile virus, as this can also present as an acute, pure motor neuropathy.[41]

Multifocal motor neuropathy (MMN) presents subacutely or chronically, and typically presents as weakness in the arms, particularly wrist and finger extensors. Anti-GM1 IgM antibodies can serve as a diagnostic marker, but these are not present in all patients.[34] The initial descriptions of MMN emphasized conduction block, which is an important diagnostic indicator but is not present in all cases of MMN, although other features of demyelination are frequently present.[42] Other motor neuropathies to consider include ALS, which should be easy to distinguish because of the hyperreflexia in the distribution of the weakness. Kennedy disease is a slowly progressive inherited motor neuropathy whereby patients will typically have gynecomastia and very prominent fasciculations.

MIXED MOTOR AND SENSORY NEUROPATHIES

This classification refers to mixed motor and sensory symptoms. One cause is polyradiculopathies, whereby patients have either positive or negative sensory symptoms

Table 4 Evaluation of pure motor neuropathies	
Potential Etiology	**Tests to Order**
Acute motor axonal neuropathy (AMAN)	CSF, GM1 antibodies
Multifocal motor neuropathy (MMN)	GM1 antibodies Serum immunofixation Quantitative immunoglobulins
Amyotrophic lateral sclerosis (ALS)	Imaging, NCS/EMG
Kennedy Disease	Androgen receptor gene
West Nile virus	CSF for West Nile PCR

Abbreviations: EMG, electromyography; NCS, nerve conduction studies; PCR, polymerase chain reaction.

but may have normal sensory NCS. Again this highlights the importance of the history, which can be more sensitive than electrodiagnostic tests. As is the case with other categories, these disorders can present acutely, subacutely, or chronically.

The acute mixed motor and sensory neuropathies are most often autoimmune in origin (**Table 5**). GBS and acute motor sensory axonal neuropathy (AMSAN) are distinguished from each other by the changes seen on NCS/EMG. AMSAN typically follows infection with *C jejuni*, and GBS is more typical after an upper respiratory infection. In either case the most important test to order is lumbar puncture. This test is performed not so much to confirm a diagnosis, as early in the course of the disease patients may have relatively little change in their CSF. Rather, CSF should be analyzed to help exclude neoplastic or infectious causes. GBS and AMSAN both present with relatively symmetric, progressive weakness with sensory signs and symptoms. Pain may also be a prominent complaint, particularly along the spine and back.

If the acute presentation is multifocal then one should consider the possibility of mononeuritis multiplex. Mononeuritis multiplex is typically caused by a vasculitis, so one needs to test for systemic vasculitides, viral hepatitis, cryoglobulins, and human immunodeficiency virus. In a scenario of mononeuritis multiplex where the serologies are negative, a nerve biopsy should be performed to definitively diagnose vasculitis before beginning treatment with corticosteroids or another immunomodulatory treatment.

Subacute mixed neuropathies comprise a group of diseases in which the motor and sensory symptoms are progressive for more than 6 weeks (**Table 6**). Polyradiculoneuropathies caused by infectious, inflammatory, or malignant processes can cause this clinical pattern. Therefore, analysis of CSF for infectious and malignant causes may be necessary. Even if NCS are not definitely demyelinating, if the disease process is progressive over weeks to months then one should consider a thorough evaluation for a potentially immune-mediated neuropathy by analyzing CSF and possibly performing a nerve biopsy. If there are clear demyelinating changes seen on NCS, the differential can be limited to CIDP, multifocal acquired demyelinating sensory and motor (MADSAM) neuropathy, DADS neuropathy, or hereditary neuropathy with liability to pressure palsies (HNPP).[34] These distinctions are made based on the distribution findings: symmetric and generalized (CIDP), symmetric and distal (DADS), or multifocal (MADSAM or HNPP). Evaluation of these patients should include serum immunofixation, serum free light chains, quantitative immunoglobulins, and possibly CSF. If the demyelinating changes are notable for prolonged distal motor latencies, testing for MAG antibodies may be useful (although this disorder is typically slowly progressive and chronic). Prolonged distal latencies in combination with multifocal clinical findings and evidence for entrapment neuropathies suggest HNPP, and should be further explored with genetic testing.

The chronic mixed motor and sensory neuropathies are diseases that are typically slowly progressive, and also suggest the possibility of an inherited disorder. Obtaining family history, examining the patient's feet for evidence of pes cavus or hammertoes

Table 5	
Evaluation of acute mixed motor sensory neuropathies	
Potential Etiology	**Tests to Order**
Guillain-Barré syndrome	CSF
AMSAN	CSF
Mononeuritis multiplex	ESR, ANA, ANCA, hepatitis B and C serologies, cryoglobulins, HIV, nerve biopsy

Abbreviations: AMSAN, acute motor sensory axonal neuropathy; ANA, antinuclear antibodies; ANCA, antineutrophil cytoplasmic antibodies; ESR, erythrocyte sedimentation rate.

Table 6
Evaluation of subacute mixed motor and sensory neuropathies

Potential Etiology	Tests to Order
CIDP	CSF, nerve biopsy in some cases
MADSAM	CSF nerve biopsy in some cases
DADS	CSF, serum immunofixation, quantitative immunoglobulins, serum free light chains
MAG neuropathy	MAG titers
HNPP	PMP22 deletion
Lyme disease	Lyme serology, CSF
Sarcoid	Serum ACE, CSF
West Nile virus	West Nile serologies, CSF
Lymphomatous/carcinomatous meningitis	CSF with cytology (may need to be repeated)
Negative results, but progressive disease	Sural nerve biopsy

Abbreviations: ACE, angiotensin-converting enzyme; CIDP, chronic inflammatory sensory polyradiculoneuropathy; DADS, distal acquired demyelinating symmetric neuropathy; HNPP, hereditary neuropathy with liability to pressure palsies; MADSAM, multifocal acquired demyelinating sensory and motor neuropathy.

can all be helpful in suggesting an inherited disorder. The evaluation for these chronic diseases is the most varied. **Table 7** outlines the most important tests but, as mentioned previously, if the evaluation is negative and the disease continues to progress then the evaluation for subacute neuropathies should be undertaken, including CSF analysis to look for evidence of increased immune activity. If the CSF is normal, a sural nerve biopsy should be performed. However, the yield of a nerve biopsy in this situation is low, probably less than 15%.[43]

MYELONEUROPATHY

A myeloneuropathy should be considered when there are lower extremity findings of peripheral neuropathy coupled with features suggesting a spinal cord lesion: sensory

Table 7
Evaluation of chronic mixed motor and sensory neuropathies

Potential Etiology	Tests to Order
Diabetes	Fasting glucose, HgbA1c
Impaired glucose tolerance	2-h glucose tolerance test
B_{12} deficiency	Vitamin B_{12}, methylmalonic acid, homocysteine
Paraproteinemia	Serum immunofixation Quantitative immunoglobulins Serum free light chains MAG titers
Charcot-Marie-Tooth 1	PMP duplication, PMP deletion, Cx32, MPZ, MFN2
Charcot-Marie-Tooth 2	EGR2, FIG4, GARS, GDAP1, HSPB1, LMNA, MFNA2, MPZ, Periaxin, RAB7
Sjögren syndrome	SS-A, SS-B
If tests are normal but if disease is progressive	CSF, sural nerve biopsy

Table 8
Evaluation of myeloneuropathy

Potential Etiology	Tests to Order
Concomitant myelopathy and neuropathy	Spinal MRI
Vitamin B_{12} deficiency	B_{12} level, methylmalonic acid, homocysteine
Copper deficiency	Serum copper and zinc
Hereditary spastic paraplegia	Genetic testing

level, increased muscle tone, brisk lower extremity reflexes, or Babinski signs (**Table 8**). The differential for a purely motor myeloneuropathy is motor neuron disease and hereditary spastic paraplegia. Myeloneuropathy with sensory and motor features can also be caused by hereditary spastic paraplegia, but more commonly is due to a structural or metabolic cause.[44] Because peripheral neuropathy and spondylotic cervical myelopathy are both common in older individuals, both may occur in the same patient. Vitamin B_{12} deficiency is a well-appreciated cause of myeloneuropathy.

Much less common and less well appreciated is myelopathy caused by copper deficiency.[44,45] Most patients who develop copper deficiency have had previous gastric surgery or have some other risk factor for malabsorption. In some cases copper deficiency is produced by increased zinc intake, which can result from use of nutritional supplements or excessive use of denture cream.[46] Treatment with intravenous or oral copper may reverse these patient's deficits. Autoimmune disorders, such as sarcoidosis, can produce both myelopathy and peripheral neuropathy in the same patient.

AUTONOMIC NEUROPATHY

The final group of diseases is those with prominent autonomic, or solely autonomic dysfunction (**Table 9**). These peripheral neuropathies typically present as sensory rather than motor neuropathies, accompanied by systemic symptoms such as cardiac symptoms (orthostasis, tachyarrhythmia or bradyarrhythmia, and postural instability), gastrointestinal symptoms (early satiety, bloating, constipation and/or diarrhea, malnutrition, and weight loss), or genitourinary symptoms (abnormalities or urinary or sexual function). Thermoregulation issues can occur, with impaired sweating or loss of the ability to perspire.

Autonomic neuropathies can present acutely, either in isolation, as in acute autoimmune autonomic neuropathy, or in combination with GBS. Autonomic neuropathies can often be paraneoplastic, associated with breast, lung, prostate, or bladder cancer.

Table 9
Evaluation of acute or chronic autonomic neuropathies

Potential Etiology	Tests to Order
Acute autonomic ganglionopathy	Acetylcholine receptor ganglionic antibodies, voltage-gated potassium autoantibodies, GAD-65 antibodies, Hu
Guillain-Barré syndrome	CSF
Diabetes	Fasting glucose, HgbA1c
Primary systemic amyloidosis	Serum immunofixation, quantitative immunoglobulins, serum free light chains Tissue biopsy: skin, fat, rectal, or other affected organ
Sjögren syndrome	SS-A, SS-B
Familial amyloidosis	TTR gene sequencing

Subacute and chronic autoimmune neuropathies also occur. Autonomic reflex testing can very helpful in assessing such patients although, as stated earlier, this test is frequently not readily available to most clinicians. Because many patients will have associated small-fiber sensory involvement, skin biopsy to evaluate IENFD density can be helpful. Autoimmune disorders can produce autonomic neuropathies. Serum tests for ganglionic acetylcholine receptor and voltage-gated potassium-channel antibodies are commercially available. If autoantibodies are detected, immunomodulating therapy can be called upon.[47]

SUMMARY

This article outlines a useful approach to the laboratory evaluation of patients with peripheral neuropathy. The authors have intentionally avoided a detailed discussion of how to use the results of NCS/EMG. The goal has been to demonstrate that the vast majority of decision making can be performed based on the patient's history and physical examination. There certainly are situations, such as distinguishing axonal from demyelinating Charcot-Marie-Tooth disease, or segregating AMAN, GBS, and AMSAN, whereby NCS are crucial. However, the basis of deciding which test to order revolves around the understanding of the time course and listening to the patients describe their symptoms. These evaluations can be done stepwise, ordering simple tests in each section first and then progressing forward if the results are negative. With most neuropathies, if the neuropathy is undiagnosed after serologic evaluation and the patient's symptoms and signs are progressive, more aggressive tests should be considered, including CSF analysis and, perhaps, muscle and nerve biopsy.

Case study

A 74 year old man presents for evaluation of numbness and tingling in his extremities. The symptoms began 8 months ago. He recalls a rather abrupt onset of numbness of tingling in his hands and feet concurrently. Symptoms are symmetrical and have been slowly progressing. His past medical history is unremarkable and he is on no medications. There is no family history of neurological problems. Examination is notable for decreased pinprick and light touch sensation in a symmetrical stocking/glove distribution to the mid-thighs/wrists. Vibratory and joint position sense are decreased at the great toes. Romberg sign is present. Deep tendon reflexes are absent in the ankles and grade 2+ elsewhere. Plantar responses are flexor bilaterally. Casual gait is fine but the patient cannot tandem walk. Nerve conduction studies show a mild to moderately severe axonal sensorimotor polyneuropathy affecting the upper and lower extremities. EMG is normal. Laboratory testing reveals normal CBC and chemistry panels, thyroid function tests and vitamin B12 is 300 pg/mL (normal 243-894 pg/mL).

Further testing reveals elevated serum methylmalonic acid and homocysteine levels. Anti-intrinsic factor antibodies were positive. The patient is treated with oral vitamin B12 at a dose of 2000 mcg per day. Repeat testing in 2 months shows normal methylmalonic acid and homocysteine levels and a serum B12 level of 788 pg/mL. There is no immediate response, but at after a year, there is mildly improved sensation.

Comment

This patient has features that suggest he does not have a typical distal symmetrical sensory neuropathy: the onset of symptoms are abrupt and the sensory loss is not length-dependent. Both of these features are suggestive of vitamin B12 deficiency. Clinically relevant deficiency can occur in the absence of hematological abnormalities and features of myelopathy. Serum vitamin B12 levels are not adequately sensitive for identifying deficiency. Methylmalonic acid and homocysteine are more sensitive and specific for identifying vitamin B12 deficiency. Another important point is that, even in pernicious anemia, high-dose daily oral vitamin B12 can be adequate therapy.

REFERENCES

1. England JD, Asbury AK. Peripheral neuropathy. Lancet 2004;363:2151–61.
2. Mold JW, Vesely SK, Keyl BA, et al. The prevalence, predictors, and consequences of peripheral sensory neuropathy in older patients. J Am Board Fam Pract 2004;17:309–18.
3. Wolfe GI, Baker NS, Amato AA, et al. Chronic cryptogenic sensory polyneuropathy: clinical and laboratory characteristics. Arch Neurol 1999;56:540–7.
4. Dyck PJ, Dyck PJ, Klein CJ, et al. Does impaired glucose metabolism cause polyneuropathy? Review of previous studies and design of a prospective controlled population-based study. Muscle Nerve 2007;36:536–41.
5. Rao S, Disraeil P, McGregor T. Impaired glucose tolerance and impaired fasting glucose. Am Fam Physician 2004;69:1961–8.
6. Knowler WC, Barrett-Connor E, Fowler SE, et al. Reduction in the incidence of type 2 diabetes with lifestyle intervention or metformin. N Engl J Med 2002;346: 393–403.
7. Zeymer U, Schwarzmaier-D'assie A, Petzinna D, et al. Effect of acarbose treatment on the risk of silent myocardial infarctions in patients with impaired glucose tolerance: results of the randomised STOP-NIDDM trial electrocardiography substudy. Eur J Cardiovasc Prev Rehabil 2004;11:412–5.
8. Lindenbaum J, Savage DG, Stabler SP, et al. Diagnosis of cobalamin deficiency: II. Relative sensitivities of serum cobalamin, methylmalonic acid, and total homocysteine concentrations. Am J Hematol 1990;34:99–107.
9. England JD, Gronseth GS, Franklin G, et al. Practice parameter: evaluation of distal symmetric sensory polyneuropathy: role of laboratory and genetic testing (an evidence based review). Neurology 2009;72:185–92.
10. Savage DG, Lindenbaum J, Stabler SP, et al. Sensitivity of serum methylmalonic acid and total homocysteine determinations for diagnosing cobalamin and folate deficiencies. Am J Med 1994;96:239–46.
11. Carmel R. Current concepts in cobalamin deficiency. Annu Rev Med 2000;51: 357–75.
12. Stabler SP. Screening the older population for cobalamin (vitamin B12) deficiency. J Am Geriatr Soc 1995;43:1290–7.
13. Swain R. An update of vitamin B12 metabolism and deficiency states. J Fam Pract 1995;41:595–600.
14. Saperstein DS, Wolfe GI, Gronseth GS, et al. Challenges in the identification of cobalamin-deficiency polyneuropathy. Arch Neurol 2003;60:1296–301.
15. Bossuyt X, Bogaerts A, Schiettekatte G, et al. Serum protein electrophoresis and immunofixation by a semiautomated electrophoresis system. Clin Chem 1998; 44(5):944–9.
16. Vrethem M, Larsson B, von Schenck H, et al. Immunofixation superior to agarose electrophoresis in detecting small M-components in patients with polyneuropathy. J Neurol Sci 1993;120:93–8.
17. Dispensieri A, Kyle R, Merlini G, et al. International Myeloma Working Group Guidelines for serum free light chain analysis in multiple myeloma and related disorders. Leukemia 2009;23:215–24.
18. Wojcicka A, Kinsella LJ. Are fleeting paresthesias due to anxiety or small fiber neuropathy? A reappraisal using skin biopsy. Neurology 2008;70(Suppl): P01.137.
19. Devigili G, Tugnoli V, Penza P, et al. The diagnostic criteria for small fibre neuropathy: from symptoms to neuropathology. Brain 2008;131:1912–25.

20. Saperstein DS, Levine TD, Levine M, et al. Usefulness of skin biopsies in the evaluation and management of patients with suspected small fiber neuropathy. Int J Neurosci 2013;123(1):38–41.
21. Lauria G, Hsieh ST, Johansson O, et al. European Federation of Neurological Societies/Peripheral Nerve Society Guideline on the use of skin biopsy in the diagnosis of small fiber neuropathy. Report of a joint task force of the European Federation of Neurological Societies and the Peripheral Nerve Society. J Peripher Nerv Syst 2010;15:79–92.
22. Gorson KC, Herrmann DN, Thiagarajan R, et al. Non-length dependent small fibre neuropathy/ganglionopathy. J Neurol Neurosurg Psychiatry 2008;79:163–9.
23. Khan S, Zhou L. Characterization of non length dependent small fiber neuropathies. Muscle Nerve 2012;45:86–91.
24. Periquet I, Novak V, Collins M, et al. Painful sensory neuropathy: prospective evaluation using skin biopsy. Neurology 1999;53:1641–7.
25. Low VA, Sandroni P, Fealey RD, et al. Detection of small-fiber neuropathy by sudomotor testing. Muscle Nerve 2006;34:57–61.
26. Dabby R, Gilad R, Sadeh M, et al. Acute steroid responsive small-fiber sensory neuropathy: a new entity? J Peripher Nerv Syst 2006;11:47–52.
27. Levine T, Saperstein D. Improvement in small fiber neuropathies following immunomodulatory therapy. Neurology 2011;76(Suppl 4):A109.
28. Biegstraaten M, Hollak CE, Bakkers M, et al. Small fiber neuropathy in Fabry disease. Mol Genet Metab 2012;106:135–41.
29. Scott LJ, Griffin JW, Luciano C, et al. Quantitative analysis of epidermal innervation in Fabry disease. Neurology 1999;52:1249–54.
30. Faber CG, Hoeijmakers JG, Ahn HS, et al. Gain of function Nav1.7 mutations in idiopathic small fiber neuropathy. Ann Neurol 2012;71:26–39.
31. Gorson KC, Ropper AH. Positive salivary gland biopsy, Sjögren syndrome, and neuropathy: clinical implications. Muscle Nerve 2003;28:553–60.
32. Leger JM, Bouche P, Cervera P, et al. Primary Sjögren's syndrome in chronic polyneuropathy presenting in middle or old age. J Neurol Neurosurg Psychiatry 1994;57:1276–7.
33. Katz JS, Saperstein DS, Gronseth GS, et al. Distal acquired demyelinating symmetrical neuropathy. Neurology 2000;54:615–20.
34. Saperstein DS, Katz JS, Amato AA, et al. Clinical spectrum of chronic acquired demyelinating polyneuropathies. Muscle Nerve 2001;24:311–24.
35. Larsen SA, Steiner BM, Rudolph AH. Laboratory diagnosis and interpretation of tests for syphilis. Clin Microbiol Rev 1995;8:1–21.
36. Saperstein DS, Grogan PM, Gronseth GS, et al. The yield of routine laboratory tests in the evaluation of peripheral neuropathy patients in a general neurology setting. Neurology 2006;66(Suppl 2):A84.
37. Sinnreich M, Klein CJ, Daube JR, et al. Chronic immune sensory polyradiculopathy: a possibly treatable sensory ataxia. Neurology 2004;63:1662–9.
38. Sekiguchi Y, Uncini A, Yuki N, et al. Antiganglioside antibodies are associated with axonal Guillain-Barré Syndrome: a Japanese Italian collaborative study. J Neurol 2012;259:1181–90.
39. Nachamkin I, Azarte Barbosa P, Ung H, et al. Pattern of Guillain Barré syndrome in children: results from a Mexican population. Neurology 2007;69:1665–71.
40. Jackson CE, Barohn RJ, Mendell JR. Acute paralytic syndrome in three American men. Comparison with Chinese cases. Arch Neurol 1993;50:732–5.
41. Burton JM, Kern RZ, Halliday W, et al. Neurological manifestations of West Nile virus infection. Can J Neurol Sci 2004;31:185–93.

42. Katz JS, Wolfe GI, Bryan WW, et al. Electrophysiologic findings in multifocal motor neuropathy. Neurology 1997;48:700–7.
43. Gabriel CM, Howard R, Kinsella N, et al. Prospective study of the usefulness of sural nerve biopsy. J Neurol Neurosurg Psychiatry 2000;69:442–6.
44. Kumar N. Metabolic and toxic myelopathies. Semin Neurol 2012;32:123–36.
45. Saperstein DS, Barohn RB. Polyneuropathy due to nutritional and vitamin deficiency. In: Dyck PJ, Thomas PK, editors. Peripheral neuropathy. 4th edition. Philadelphia: Elsevier Saunders; 2005. p. 2051–62.
46. Nations SP, Boyer PJ, Love LA, et al. Denture cream: an unusual source of excess zinc, leading to hypocupremia and neurologic disease. Neurology 2008;71: 639–43.
47. Sharp L, Vernino S. Paraneoplastic neuromuscular disorders. Muscle Nerve 2012;46:839–40.

Treatment of Painful Peripheral Neuropathy

Jaya R. Trivedi, MD[a],*, Nicholas J. Silvestri, MD[b], Gil I. Wolfe, MD[b]

KEYWORDS

- Peripheral neuropathy • Neuropathic pain • Antidepressants • Anticonvulsants
- Opiates

KEY POINTS

- Neuropathic pain is a common problem, and it affects patients physically, emotionally, and socially.
- First-line and second-line neuropathic pain medications include antidepressants, anticonvulsants, and opiate analgesics.
- Duloxetine (Cymbalta) and pregabalin (Lyrica) are the only drugs approved for use in painful diabetic neuropathy. Other drugs are used off-label in treating painful polyneuropathy.
- Neurologists should tailor therapy for each individual based on coexisting medical conditions, cost, and drug-drug interactions.

INTRODUCTION

Neuropathic pain was recently redefined as pain resulting directly from a lesion or disease affecting the somatosensory system.[1] The injury or dysfunction may involve peripheral or central nervous system structures. Neuropathic pain is common, estimated to affect 1.5% of the US population.[2] When disorders that are not categorized as conventional neuropathic pain states are included, the prevalence is even higher.[3] Poorly controlled neuropathic pain is associated with mood and sleep disturbance and an impaired ability to work and participate in social and recreational activities.[4]

Peripheral nerve disorders are the major cause of neuropathic pain encountered by neurologists and other clinicians.[5] Even after extensive evaluation, a cause for the polyneuropathy may remain unknown in most patients, especially when small fibers

Funding sources: None.
Conflict of interest: None (J.R.T, N.J.S); G.I.W. has served as an advisor and speaker on behalf of Eli Lilly & Co.
[a] Department of Neurology & Neurotherapeutics, UT Southwestern Medical Center, 5323 Harry Hines Boulevard, Dallas, TX 75390, USA; [b] Department of Neurology, State University of New York at Buffalo School of Medicine and Biomedical Sciences, 100 High Street, Buffalo, NY 14203–1126, USA
* Corresponding author.
E-mail address: jaya.trivedi@utsouthwestern.edu

are exclusively or predominantly involved.[6,7] In such settings, a diagnosis of idiopathic or cryptogenic sensory polyneuropathy is made.[8–10] Of the identifiable causes, diabetes is the most common cause of painful polyneuropathy, but there are many other causes of painful polyneuropathies and mononeuropathies. For simplicity, in this review, the terms neuropathy and peripheral neuropathy are used in place of polyneuropathy, which implies a generalized, symmetric disorder of peripheral nerves.

The frequency, intensity, and quality of neuropathic pain, although subject to individual variability, differ with the cause. Postherpetic neuralgia is defined by a neuropathic pain experience, and 90% of patients with Fabry disease have pain[11] that classically is lancinating and lightninglike, aggravated by cold or exertion. Neuropathic pain is present in 65% to 80% of idiopathic polyneuropathies,[12] and up to one-third of diabetic patients[5] and patients with AIDS,[13] but is uncommon in paraprotein-associated neuropathies.

SYMPTOMS AND SIGNS OF NEUROPATHIC PAIN

The symptoms of neuropathic pain are often referred to as positive sensory symptoms of neuropathy. Negative symptoms and signs refer to reports of numbness and the finding of reduced or absent sensation on examination. Spontaneous (stimulus-independent) and stimulus-evoked pain can be distinguished by history and sensory examination, often coexist in individuals, and are likely to represent different pathophysiologic mechanisms.[14] Spontaneous pain may be constant or intermittent. It is not unusual for patients to experience both persistent burning pain and superimposed episodes of shooting or lancinating discomfort.

Paresthesias are abnormal spontaneous stimulus-independent sensations, often described as tingling; they are often compared with a limb that has fallen asleep. Descriptors of spontaneous painful sensation vary widely in patients with neuropathy and include burning, stabbing, stinging, squeezing, aching, cramping, shooting, and freezing. Pins and needles, broken glass, and vicelike sensations may be elicited by history. Stimulus-evoked pain is also common and is experienced in a variety of forms. Dysesthesia refers to an unpleasant abnormal sensation that can be spontaneous or evoked, allodynia refers to pain after contact with a stimulus that is not normally noxious, and hyperalgesia refers to exaggerated pain from a noxious stimulus.[1] Hyperpathia is a complex sensory experience characterized by an abnormally painful reaction to a stimulus, especially a repetitive stimulus, in a patient who initially perceives the stimulus as less intense. A variety of positive symptoms often coexist in an individual. Given the length-dependent pattern of many peripheral neuropathies, neuropathic pain symptoms tend to predominate in the distal limbs, typically involving the feet to a greater degree than the hands.[8] Sensory neuropathy seems to be the most common cause for the painful or burning-foot presentation. In a cohort of 117 patients presenting with painful, burning feet, 89% had objective evidence of peripheral neuropathy based on a variety of studies including electrophysiologic testing and intraepidermal nerve fiber density on punch skin biopsy.[6]

NEUROPATHIC PAIN MECHANISMS

The pathophysiologic basis of neuropathic pain is complex and not fully understood. Some background, however, is helpful in strategizing treatment approaches. Peripheral mechanisms include altered sensitivity and activation of C nociceptor terminals resulting in ectopic discharges in damaged or regenerating fibers, recruitment of silent nociceptors, and spontaneous discharges in more proximal segments of the sensory nerve, including the dorsal root ganglion.[14,15] Change in expression and permeability of voltage-gated sodium channels seems to be a common event in these peripheral alterations,[16] and several agents (tricyclic antidepressants, carbamazepine, topiramate, lamotrigine, mexiletine) have activity at these sodium channels. Damaged peripheral nerve fibers express α-adrenoreceptors and exhibit heightened sensitivity to sympathetic stimulation, raising the possibility of a sympathetically mediated component to neuropathic pain states.[17]

Waves of increased peripheral nerve activity move centrally, producing central sensitization in second-order and third-order neurons in the spinal cord and relay stations in the brain, respectively. The process of central sensitization alters the way neurons respond to subsequent sensory input.[18,19] These alterations include the enlargement of peripheral receptive fields to stimuli, enhanced responses to suprathreshold inputs, and generation of action potentials by previously subthreshold inputs. Central sensitization seems to result from increased and prolonged release of excitatory amino acids such as glutamate and neuropeptides.[14] For instance, enhanced release of substance P as a result of prolonged activity along nociceptive pathways can potentiate activation of postsynaptic N-methyl-D-aspartate (NMDA) receptors. Subsequently, additional ion channels open, intracellular calcium concentrations build, and action potential generation is potentiated in central sensory pathways.[20] Neuropeptides may diffuse through the dorsal horn, sensitizing neurons that would otherwise be bystanders, producing the phenomenon of enlarged peripheral receptive fields, thus causing a perception of pain over a wider distribution and of greater intensity. Some of the newer agents used for neuropathic pain (gabapentin, pregabalin, lamotrigine, topiramate, tramadol, venlafaxine) are believed to inhibit central sensitization by blocking the activity of glutamate, excitatory neuropeptides, and presynaptic calcium channels, and enhancing inhibitory pathways mediated by serotonin, norepinephrine, and γ-aminobutyric acid (GABA).

A variety of pathophysiologic processes may be active in an individual patient, and the same mechanisms may not be present in all patients who share a specific neuropathic pain state. This variability likely accounts for some of the heterogeneity of patient responses to therapeutic interventions.[21]

CLINICAL TRIALS AND DRUG INDICATIONS

Most randomized, controlled, pharmacologic studies on neuropathic pain have evaluated antidepressants and anticonvulsants. Clinical trials on neuropathic pain share many challenges and shortcomings:

- Response to placebo is considerable, typically observed in one-third[22–24] to more than one-half of subjects.[25]
- Although statistically significant differences may be demonstrated between active treatment and placebo arms, the actual clinical benefit of a 1-point or 2-point drop on an 11-point Likert scale for pain intensity may be debated.
- Although they provide objective data, neurophysiologic outcome measurements have not been helpful.[26]
- There is conflicting efficacy data for some agents.[27,28]
- Controlled studies are short, usually ranging from 6[23,24,29,30] to 8 weeks,[22,25] providing little insight into the longer-term persistence of a response.
- The effect of medications on different aspects of neuropathic pain (eg, steady vs episodic, spontaneous vs stimulus evoked) is rarely analyzed.[31]
- There are few studies using combinations of agents, and there are no US Food and Drug Administration (FDA) approved polypharmacy strategies for neuropathic pain management.

Another consideration for US clinicians is that labeled indications in the United States are limited to duloxetine and pregabalin for painful diabetic neuropathy, carbamazepine (Tegretol) for trigeminal neuralgia, and gabapentin (Neurontin), pregabalin, and lidocaine and high-dose capsaicin patches for postherpetic neuralgia. Some countries permit more liberal indications that cover neuropathic pain in general, whereas others require labeling for only specific forms.[32]

Various outcome measures have been used in neuropathic pain studies. Visual analog scales (VAS) or 10-point and 11-point scales such as the Likert scale (0 = no pain, 10 = worst possible pain) are conventional primary outcome measures. Patients record their pain levels in daily diaries, and mean values over a specified interval are compared with baseline values. The short-form McGill pain questionnaire (SF-MPQ),[33] which consists of 15 pain descriptors (11 sensory [eg, throbbing, shooting, stabbing, sharp]; 4 affective [eg, tiring-exhausting, sickening, fearful, punishing-cruel]) graded from 0 to 3, has served as either a primary or secondary outcome. Although these instruments provide reliable and valid measurements of pain intensity and unpleasantness, they do not address other aspects of the neuropathic pain experience.[33] As a result, a variety of quality-of-life and daily activity measures have been introduced, especially in more recent trials. The Wisconsin Brief Pain Questionnaire, a survey that includes 11-point rating scales for worst pain, pain right now, and average pain and assesses the effect of pain on mood, sleep, and daily activities, has been used on occasion.[34] Other secondary outcome measures provide global impressions of change from the standpoint of both study subject and clinician. Quality-of-life instruments used in neuropathic pain studies include the General Health Self-Assessment form and the Short Form-36 Quality of Life Questionnaire. Galer and Jensen[35] have developed and validated the Neuropathic Pain Scale, the first survey designed primarily for neuropathic pain. This scale includes items that address pain intensity, temporal patterns, and ratings for various descriptors of the neuropathic pain experience. The Neuropathic Pain Scale can generate distinct patterns for different neuropathic pain syndromes, a finding that has potential implications for underlying pain mechanisms and treatment.

TRICYCLIC ANTIDEPRESSANTS

Tricyclic antidepressants presumably exert their analgesic effect by modulating voltage-gated sodium channels and inhibiting the reuptake of the biogenic amines norepinephrine and serotonin. They are the most extensively studied agents for neuropathic pain, especially in diabetic neuropathy.[21,36] Efficacy for the individual agents is roughly similar,[24,37] although tricyclics with mixed serotonergic and noradrenergic reuptake inhibition (eg, amitriptyline, imipramine, and clomipramine) have been marginally more effective than those with relatively selective noradrenergic effects (desipramine, nortriptyline, and maprotiline).[38] Patients may preferentially respond to one tricyclic antidepressant over another, so that sequential therapeutic trials may be needed.[39]

Tricyclics have been effective in relieving pain in patients with and without depression, with an analgesic action that is independent of mood alteration and that becomes clinically evident as early as 1 to 2 weeks.[40,41] Tricyclics have been effective in both diabetic and nondiabetic forms of painful neuropathy.[38] The degree of analgesic response has correlated directly with serum tricyclic levels in some,[40,42] but not all studies.[24,38,39,43] Tricyclics have demonstrated greater therapeutic effects than selective serotonin reuptake inhibitors (SSRIs) such as paroxetine

(Paxil, Pexeva), but suboptimal plasma concentrations may be partly to blame for this observation.[26]

Neither amitriptyline (Elavil) at dosages up to 100 mg/d nor a standardized acupuncture regimen. either alone or in combination, was more effective than placebo in randomized trials of human immunodeficiency virus (HIV)-related painful neuropathy.[27,44] Possible explanations for these negative trials include mechanistic factors in HIV-related neuropathy that are more resistant to tricyclic actions, the modest doses used, and failure of amitriptyline to have a persistent benefit in studies of longer duration.

The clinical impression that antidepressants are more effective for burning pain, whereas anticonvulsants are preferred for shooting lancinating pain has not been verified in clinical trials; the benefit of tricyclics is not dependent on the quality of pain.[24,41]

Shortcomings of studies include dropout rates of 30% or more, often due to adverse events,[26,40] a small number of participants, and treatment duration as short as 2 weeks. In addition, many of the earlier crossover trials did not use washout periods between the various interventions.[26,39,42,45] As is true for most agents, the use of tricyclic antidepressants in neuropathic pain is off-label. Low doses (10–25 mg) can be given at bedtime, and slowly increased by 10 to 25 mg every 1 to 2 weeks up to 100 to 150 mg as tolerated. Slower titration rates may be better tolerated by the elderly. Daily tricyclic doses between 75 and 150 mg are likely to be within the effective range for most patients.[24] The main side effects of tricyclics include dry mouth, sedation, urinary retention, cardiac arrhythmia, orthostatic hypotension, dizziness, constipation, and weight gain.[5,46] The secondary amines (nortriptyline, desipramine) tend to be less sedating and have less anticholinergic activity. Tricyclic antidepressants are contraindicated in patients with cardiac arrhythmia, congestive heart failure, recent myocardial infarction, drug sensitivity, narrow-angle glaucoma, and urinary retention. Drug interactions may occur from concurrent use of central nervous system depressants or anticholinergic agents. Tricyclics should be used with caution in elderly patients who are often especially sensitive to adverse effects.

SSRIS

SSRIs have been less effective than tricyclic antidepressants in controlled studies of neuropathic pain (**Table 1**). Although both imipramine and paroxetine demonstrated benefit compared with placebo in painful diabetic neuropathy, the tricyclic was significantly more efficacious than paroxetine on both an observer and self-rating scale.[26] Scores for dysesthesia, hypesthesia, and sleep disturbance did not improve on paroxetine. However, paroxetine was better tolerated. Citalopram (Celexa) was of mild benefit in painful diabetic neuropathy.[47] No relation between drug level and analgesic effect was observed. The rs6318 (Cys23Ser) single nucleotide polymorphism in the serotonin receptor2C gene was associated with 75% moderate or better pain relief with escitalopram.[48] In another trial, fluoxetine (Prozac, Rapiflux, Sarafem, Selfemra) was no more effective than placebo in providing pain relief except in a subgroup of patients with depression.[24] Because fluoxetine has an active metabolite with a long half-life, the study's crossover design may have clouded a distinction between the active drug and placebo.[37]

Adverse events for the SSRIs tend to be mild and include somnolence or insomnia, asthenia, nausea, diarrhea, sweating, dry mouth, decreased libido, and impotence. Because neuropathic pain trials suggest that the rate of major side effects for SSRIs is half that observed for tricyclics,[41] the SSRIs may be preferred in some patients despite lower efficacy,[47] particularly if there is coexisting depression.

Table 1
Randomized placebo-controlled trials of other antidepressants[a]

Reference No.	Cause of Neuropathy	Drug	Daily Dose (mg)	n	Design	Primary Outcome	Result of Primary Outcome (P Value)	Improved on Active Drug (%)	Improved on Placebo (%)
26	DM	Paroxetine	40	20	Crossover 2 wk	VAS score	.0121	50	15
24	DM	Fluoxetine[b]	40	46	Crossover 6 wk	Pain intensity score	.34	48	41
47	DM	Citalopram	40	15	Crossover 3 wk	Six-item observer scale	.02	N/A	N/A
30	Various	Bupropion SR (Wellbutrin SR)	300	41	Crossover 6 wk	Wisconsin Brief Pain Questionnaire	<.001	73	10
56	Various	Venlafaxine (Effexor)	225	32	Crossover 4 wk	10-point rating scales	.004	27	7
49	DM	Duloxetine	20, 60, 120	457	Parallel 12 wk	11-point Likert scale	<.005 for 60, 120 mg	49–52	26
50	DM	Duloxetine	60, 120	348	Parallel 12 wk	11-point Likert scale	<.001	39–50	30

Abbreviations: DM, diabetes mellitus; N/A, not available.
[a] Main adverse events were mouth dryness (up to 37%), nausea (up to 24%), somnolence/fatigue (up to 28%), and insomnia (up to 20%).
[b] Placebo contained benztropine to mimic side effects.

ATYPICAL ANTIDEPRESSANTS
Duloxetine

Duloxetine was released in the fall of 2004, and was the first FDA-approved agent for the treatment of diabetic peripheral neuropathic pain. Like venlafaxine, its analgesic effects are believed to be related to potentiation of descending inhibition via blocking of serotonin and norepinephrine reuptake. Duloxetine has a higher, more balanced affinity at these transporter sites than previous generations of antidepressants. In several diabetic neuropathy trials, delayed-release duloxetine at dosages of 60 and 120 mg/d was more effective than placebo in reducing pain severity scores, with significant separation seen as early as 1 week[49,50] (data on file, Lilly Research Laboratories). A lower 20 mg/d dosage was not efficacious. Patients with major depression were excluded. The daily dosage of 120 mg was no more effective than 60 mg/d and caused more side effects. Significant improvement in several secondary outcomes was also observed, including night pain severity, the SF-MPQ, and a brief inventory on the effects of pain on daily activities and mood.

The main adverse events were nausea, which tended to occur in the first week and last for about 6 days, somnolence, and dizziness. Approximately 15% of patients in the duloxetine arms dropped out because of adverse events. Duloxetine is metabolized by the liver and has potential interactions with drugs that inhibit 1A2 and 2D6 isoenzymes, including tricyclics, phenothiazines, fluoroquinolones, and type 1C antiarrhythmics. Contraindications include concomitant use of monoamine oxidase inhibitors and uncontrolled narrow-angle glaucoma. No specific laboratory monitoring is recommended, and duloxetine did not seem to significantly affect diabetes management. It is not recommended in the setting of severe renal or chronic hepatic insufficiency. Although it is labeled at a dosage of 60 mg/d, 20 and 30 mg capsules are available, and titrating up from lower doses may be better tolerated from the standpoint of nausea.

Bupropion

Prominent adverse events and poor tolerability of tricyclic antidepressants have prompted investigation of atypical antidepressants with unique pharmacologic profiles (see **Table 1**). Bupropion is a second-generation nontricyclic antidepressant that specifically inhibits neuronal norepinephrine uptake. It is a weak inhibitor of dopamine reuptake. Unlike tricyclic agents, it does not have significant affinity for muscarinic, histaminergic, or α-adrenergic receptors, and is often better tolerated.[51] The sustained-release form of bupropion has been subjected to a double-blind, randomized, crossover trial in 41 patients with various forms of painful neuropathy.[30] Among the patients, 70% had either idiopathic, diabetic, paraprotein-related neuropathies, or lumbar radiculopathy. Pain relief was significant at week 2 and persisted until week 6 (see **Table 1**). A 30% reduction in pain scores relative to placebo was observed, similar to tricyclic studies. Quality-of-life measures also improved, and the drug was relatively well tolerated. Only 2 patients (5%) dropped out of the study because of medication-related side effects.[30] Only 1 of 11 patients who had discontinued tricyclics because of side effects was unable to tolerate bupropion.

The main side effects of bupropion are dry mouth, headache, nausea, insomnia, and tremor. Bupropion is contraindicated in patients with a known seizure disorder and those taking a monoamine oxidase inhibitor. Bupropion should not be used in individuals with a current or previous diagnosis of bulimia or anorexia nervosa because of a higher incidence of seizures in this population.[52]

Venlafaxine

Venlafaxine is an antidepressant that strongly inhibits the reuptake of both serotonin and norepinephrine, but has minimal muscarinic and histaminergic activity compared with tricyclics.[53] In a preliminary report of a large study of 244 patients, venlafaxine extended-release was superior to placebo in nondepressed patients with painful diabetic neuropathy.[54] Effective dosages were 150 to 225 mg/d. A double-blind placebo-controlled study showed significantly improved pain reduction, mood, and quality of life when venlafaxine was added to gabapentin for painful diabetic neuropathy.[55] Dosages of up to 150 mg/d were used.

Venlafaxine was compared with imipramine in a randomized, double-blind, placebo-controlled, 3-way crossover study (see **Table 1**). At the end of the 4-week treatment periods, both venlafaxine and imipramine were superior to placebo in reducing pain scores.[56] There was no difference in efficacy between venlafaxine and imipramine. This study is one of the few to compare responses in diabetic and nondiabetic subgroups. There was a trend for diabetic patients to experience greater pain relief than patients with other forms of painful neuropathy, although this has not been the experience from other trials.[37]

Side effects of venlafaxine include nausea, dizziness, somnolence, insomnia, sexual dysfunction, and dry mouth. Tolerability of venlafaxine may not be superior to tricyclics as the severity of side effects was similar in the comparative trial with imipramine.[56] More patients withdrew from the study as a consequence of venlafaxine. Concomitant use of a monoamine oxidase inhibitor is a contraindication.

ANTICONVULSANTS
Gabapentin

Gabapentin (Neurontin, Fanatrex, Gabarone, Gralise, Horizant) is a popular first-line anticonvulsant used in the treatment of neuropathic pain.[37] Gabapentin was developed as a structural GABA analogue, and in vivo studies demonstrated increased cerebral GABA concentrations within hours after a single dose[57] and with longer-term administration in healthy subjects and patients with epilepsy.[57,58] Several other cellular mechanisms of action have been proposed, including competition with L-type amino acids for active transport, high-affinity binding to the $\alpha_2\delta$ subunit of voltage-activated calcium channels, inhibition of voltage-activated sodium channels, increased serotonin concentrations, reduction in monoamine neurotransmitters, and prevention of neuronal death.[59] The primary mechanism responsible for gabapentin's analgesic effect remains uncertain, but high-affinity calcium channel binding is the leading candidate.

Several randomized, double-blind, placebo-controlled studies of gabapentin have been conducted in painful peripheral neuropathy. Backonja and colleagues[22] studied 165 patients with diabetic neuropathy. Gabapentin was titrated from 900 to 3600 mg/d over a period of 4 weeks or to the maximally tolerated dosage. The primary outcome measure was daily pain severity as measured on an 11-point Likert scale. Mean daily pain scores were significantly lower in the gabapentin-treated group ($P<.001$).[22] All secondary outcome measures assessing sleep, mood, and quality of life also improved significantly in the gabapentin arm.

Other randomized, double-blind, placebo-controlled studies of gabapentin have produced conflicting results.[60,61] Serpell and colleagues[61] enrolled patients with a variety of neuropathic pain syndromes, mostly complex regional pain syndrome (28%); only 2% had diabetic neuropathy. Pain scores did not improve after 6 weeks. In a study of 18 patients with Guillain-Barré syndrome (GBS) admitted to an intensive care unit, there was a significant decrease in fentanyl requirements over a 7-day period in those receiving gabapentin as opposed to placebo.[60] A later study on GBS by this group demonstrated greater efficacy for gabapentin 300 mg 3 times a day than carbamazepine 100 mg 3 times a day in reducing pain and use of fentanyl in a brief placebo-controlled study.[62] Two studies, one open-label and the other a randomized, double-blind, crossover trial, have compared gabapentin with tricyclics.[63,64] In the open-label study,[64] gabapentin was superior to amitriptyline in pain reduction (P<.026), whereas the blinded trial found the 2 drugs to be equivalent.[63]

An analysis of 5 randomized placebo-controlled trials provides direction on gabapentin dosing for neuropathic pain. The conclusion was that gabapentin should be dosed at 300 mg on day 1, 600 mg on day 2, and 900 mg on day 3. Subsequent titration to 1800 mg/d was recommended to achieve greater efficacy, with dosages up to 3600 mg/d needed in some patients.[65] However, dosages as low as 900 mg/d were effective in a placebo-controlled crossover study of painful diabetic neuropathy and slow titration is recommended in elderly or frail individuals.[66]

Gabapentin is usually well tolerated. Side effects include sedation, fatigue, dizziness, confusion, tremor, weight gain, peripheral edema, and headache. Contraindications and drug interactions are few. Gabapentin is eliminated by renal excretion, and its clearance is reduced in patients with renal insufficiency, especially those with a creatinine clearance level less than 60 mL/min.[22] Cimetidine alters the renal excretion of gabapentin. Bioavailability is reduced by concomitant administration of magnesium-based or aluminum-based antacids.[46]

Lamotrigine

Lamotrigine (Lamictal) is a novel anticonvulsant that acts on voltage-sensitive sodium channels to stabilize neuronal membranes and inhibit neurotransmitter release, principally glutamate.[67] Several randomized, placebo-controlled, double-blind studies of lamotrigine have been performed on various painful neuropathies. Although there are conflicting results, most trials support its use for neuropathic pain management. An early placebo-controlled double-blind study of 100 patients with undefined causes of neuropathic pain failed to demonstrate an analgesic benefit at a dosage of 200 mg/d.[68] However, individual disease subgroups were not analyzed. Later studies have evaluated the efficacy of lamotrigine in HIV-related[13,69] and diabetic neuropathy.[29] The first trial on painful HIV neuropathy enrolled 42 subjects, of whom 13 did not complete the study. Among the remaining 29 subjects, 20 received placebo and 9 received lamotrigine.[69] Patients receiving up to 300 mg/d of lamotrigine had a greater reduction in average pain compared with the placebo group (P = .03). However, an overestimation of the treatment effect was possible because 11 of 20 patients randomized to the active arm dropped out. Nearly half of the dropouts were a result of skin rash. This investigator group performed a larger HIV neuropathy trial in which patients were stratified according to whether they were using neurotoxic antiretroviral therapy (ART; didanosine, zalcitabine, or stavudine).[13] Lamotrigine was titrated to a dosage of 400 mg/d, but a slower titration was used. The change in the Gracely Pain Scale slope for average pain indicated that lamotrigine was more effective in reducing pain in patients receiving ART (P = .004), but was no more effective than placebo in patients not on these agents. The drug was well tolerated; adverse events, including rash, were similar to placebo. No serious rash was reported in contrast to the previous study, likely as a result of the slower titration. In a study on diabetic neuropathy, lamotrigine was beneficial at a dosage of 200–400 mg/d and adverse events were not problematic using a slow titration.[29] Lamotrigine 300 mg daily administrated for 10 weeks was more effective than placebo for neuropathy pain due to chemotherapy.[70]

Recommended lamotrigine dosing is 25 mg at night for 2 weeks, increasing weekly by 25 to 50 mg to a maximum dosage of 400 mg/d. Side effects include mild to serious rash, including Stevens-Johnson syndrome, dizziness, unsteadiness, drowsiness, and diplopia.[46] Rashes are more common in children and with rapid titration. Lamotrigine should be discontinued at the first sign of a drug-related rash. If concomitantly used with valproic acid, titration should be even slower, beginning at 25 mg every other day, with maintenance dosing generally not exceeding 200 mg/d.

Topiramate

Topiramate (Top Amax, Topiragen) is a broad-spectrum anticonvulsant that seems to inhibit voltage-gated sodium and calcium channels and glutamate-mediated neurotransmission. Although a small double-blind pilot trial of topiramate suggested efficacy,[71] 3 simultaneous placebo-controlled trials of topiramate that enrolled 1259 patients with painful diabetic neuropathy failed to demonstrate a significant analgesic effect.[72] Using a different study design, an independent multicenter trial that included 323 patients with diabetic neuropathy did demonstrate improved pain control with topiramate.[73] Sleep disruption and mental components of the SF-36 Health Survey also improved significantly compared with placebo ($P = .020$ and .023, respectively).

The most common adverse events were diarrhea, loss of appetite, and somnolence.[73] Nearly 25% of topiramate-treated patients dropped out of the study early because of adverse events, a potential drawback of this particular agent. Nausea, somnolence, and dizziness were the most frequent treatment-limiting side effects, each leading to discontinuation in 2% to 3% of participants. Patients receiving topiramate had an average weight loss of 2.6 kg compared with a gain of 0.2 kg on placebo. Weight loss occurred in 76% of subjects receiving topiramate, in contrast to the weight gain that is common to other anticonvulsant agents, and is of potential benefit in overall diabetes management. HbA_{1C} levels improved slightly in the topiramate arm.

Possible explanations for the disparate results from topiramate trials include lower baseline pain scores, more dramatic placebo responses, and the availability of rescue medication in the negative studies. Pain surveys used in the positive study were also more specific regarding the timing and location of pain, perhaps enhancing the ability to discriminate between placebo and active drug.

Carbamazepine/Oxcarbazepine

Carbamazepine (Carbatrol, Epitol, Equetro, Tegretol) is an iminostilbene derivative chemically related to tricyclic antidepressants.[74] It stabilizes membranes by inhibiting voltage-gated sodium channels.[75] Although it has been studied extensively in trigeminal neuralgia and is labeled for this indication, data regarding its effect on peripheral neuropathy is limited. Two early double-blind crossover studies found carbamazepine to be effective in painful diabetic neuropathy at dosages of 600 mg/d.[76,77] However, these were small studies, and each treatment phase lasted only 1 to 2 weeks, casting doubt on the results. Moreover, validated primary outcome measures were not used. Adverse events were frequent, although minor and transient, and included somnolence, dizziness, nausea, vomiting, gait changes, and urticaria. Other side effects of carbamazepine include hyponatremia, leukopenia, thrombocytopenia, and hepatic dysfunction.[48]

Oxcarbazepine (Trileptal) is structurally similar to carbamazepine, but has distinct pharmacokinetic and pharmacodynamic properties.[78] Like carbamazepine, oxcarbazepine slows the recovery rate of voltage-activated sodium channels, but it also inhibits high-threshold N-type and P-type calcium channels and reduces glutamatergic transmission. Whereas carbamazepine is metabolized via oxidation to 10,11-epoxide, the metabolite responsible for most side effects, oxcarbazepine undergoes reductive metabolism to a 10-monohydroxy derivative.[78] This reductive metabolism results in minimal involvement of hepatic cytochrome P450–dependent enzymes, less autoinduction, and fewer drug interactions. As a result, oxcarbazepine boasts a safety advantage over carbamazepine. Unlike carbamazepine, oxcarbazepine does not have a black box warning for aplastic anemia or agranulocytosis and is generally better tolerated.[79] Data from an open-label prospective study indicate that oxcarbazepine significantly improves pain scores in patients with diabetic neuropathy.[80] In a placebo-controlled study, 347 patients with painful diabetic neuropathy were randomized to oxcarbazepine 600 mg/d, 1200 mg/d, 1800 mg/d, or placebo for 16 weeks.[81] The primary outcome was change in VAS from baseline to the last week of the study. Although this outcome did not reach statistical significance, oxcarbazepine 1200 and 1800 mg/d did offer better pain control compared with placebo. Dropout rates were high at 23.5% and 41.4% in the 1200 and 1800 mg/d groups, respectively. The higher dropout rate in the 1800 mg/d group was related to rapid titration. In another placebo-controlled study, oxcarbazepine 1200 mg/d was not found to be effective in treating neuropathic pain.[82] Adverse effects of oxcarbazepine include dizziness, nausea, vomiting, constipation, fatigue, ataxia, headache, somnolence, tremor, diarrhea, and confusional state.[81]

Valproic Acid

Valproic acid (Depakene, Depakote, Epilim, Stavzor) has been shown to increase GABA content in the brain and prolong the repolarization phase of voltage-sensitive sodium channels.[83] There is only 1 randomized controlled trial on painful peripheral neuropathy. This study of 52 patients with diabetic neuropathy demonstrated significant improvement in pain in the valproate-treated group compared with placebo at 1 month.[84] Valproate was well tolerated at 1200 mg/d in divided doses; only 1 patient developed increased liver enzymes.

Pregabalin

An analogue of GABA, pregabalin, has been shown to have analgesic, anticonvulsant, and anxiolytic activity, although via GABA-independent mechanisms. Similar to gabapentin, it binds potently to the $\alpha_2\delta$ subunit of voltage-activated calcium channels, reducing the release of several excitatory neurotransmitters. Unlike gabapentin, pregabalin exhibits linear pharmacokinetics across the conventional dose range, and can be initiated at a therapeutic dose without a titration. Pregabalin significantly reduced mean pain scores at a dosage of 100 mg 3 times a day versus placebo in painful diabetic neuropathy.[85] No titration was used, and significant pain relief was observed by the end of the first week. Secondary efficacy variables also improved significantly, including the SF-MPQ, sleep outcomes, pain domains in the SF-36, tension-anxiety and total mood scores, and both patient-rated and clinician-rated global impressions. Other studies on diabetic neuropathy have demonstrated efficacy versus placebo using fixed or flexible dosing regimens ranging from 150 to 600 mg/d,[86–88] whereas 75 mg daily did not differ from placebo in 1 study[86] and 150 mg in another study.[87] As a result, increasing the dosage to 300 mg/d or higher in partial or nonresponders who tolerate the medication seems warranted. The onset of pain relief is usually by the end of day 2.[89]

   The main adverse events of pregabalin were dizziness (up to 39%), somnolence (up to 22%), infection (15%), and peripheral edema (up to 17%), a profile similar to gabapentin. The frequency of side effects increases with higher doses. Adverse events were mostly mild to moderate in severity, and overall the agent seems to be well tolerated.[85,86] Infections were mainly in the upper respiratory tract. Eleven to 15% of pregabalin-treated patients discontinued the studies because of adverse events.

Pregabalin was released in the fall of 2005 with indications for both painful diabetic neuropathy and postherpetic neuralgia. It is a Schedule V medication in the United States because of a low frequency of euphoria, insomnia, and headache with sudden discontinuation, and surveys of nondependent sedative or hypnotic users.

Lacosamide

Lacosamide (Vimpat) is an anticonvulsant that has a unique inhibitory action in promoting slow inactivation of voltage-gated sodium channels, in contrast to other anticonvulsants that act on sodium channels by modifying fast inactivation.[90] Lacosamide also has antinociceptive effects and has been studied in diabetic neuropathy.[91,92] Diabetic patients with at least moderate neuropathic pain were randomized to placebo or lacosamide 400 mg or 600 mg per day over a 6-week titration and 12-week maintenance periods.[91] Of 357 patients randomized, 246 completed the study. The primary outcome measure was change in the average daily Numeric Pain Rating Score from baseline to the last 4 weeks. There was no significant reduction in pain on lacosamide 400 mg or 600 mg daily in the last 4 weeks compared with baseline ($P = .12, P = .18$), possibly because of increased placebo response in the last 4 weeks. However, lacosamide 400 mg and 600 mg daily doses were significantly more effective in the titration ($P = .03, P = .006$), maintenance ($P = .01, P = .005$), and entire treatment ($P = .03, P = .02$) periods compared with placebo. In other placebo-controlled studies, lacosamide 400 mg per day was reported to be safe and effective in patients with diabetic neuropathy.[92,93]

Across studies, more side effects are observed on the 600 mg/d dosage compared with 200 mg and 400 mg daily, with withdrawal rates more than 40% on the higher dose.[92,93] Adverse events include dizziness, nausea, tremor, headache, and fatigue.

TRAMADOL

Tramadol (Ultram, Rybix, Ryzolt), a centrally acting non-narcotic analgesic medication with monoaminergic and opiate effects, has been used in Europe since the late 1970s and was first marketed in the United States in 1995. It has low-affinity binding to μ-opioid receptors coupled with mild inhibition of norepinephrine and serotonin reuptake.[94] However, 1 of its metabolites (o-desmethyltramadol) is a more potent μ-opioid agonist. Development of tolerance and dependence seem to be unusual events.[95] Tramadol has been effective in blinded placebo-controlled studies of painful diabetic neuropathy and other forms of painful neuropathy (**Table 2**).[23,96] Pain relief was manifest as early as 2 weeks, showing even greater effect by 4 weeks before a plateau was observed.[23] Overall health and social functioning improved significantly, although sleep indices did not. In a 6-month open-label extension that enrolled 120 patients from the randomized trial, tramadol provided sustained relief of neuropathic pain.[97] Eighty-five patients completed the 6-month extension. By 30 days, average pain intensity scores for the former placebo patients were similar to those who had always received active drug. The frequency and severity of adverse events did not seem to increase with time. In a smaller, placebo-controlled, crossover study (see **Table 2**), tramadol produced significant reductions in ratings for spontaneous and touch-evoked pain as well as dynamic allodynia by electronic toothbrush stimulation.[96] Although side effects from tramadol were frequent in this trial, they tended to be mild and did not correlate with the analgesic response.

Table 2
Randomized placebo-controlled trials of analgesics[a]

Reference No.	Cause of Neuropathy	Drug	Daily Dose (mg)	n	Design	Primary Outcome	Result of Primary Outcome (P Value)	Improved on Active Drug (%)	Improved on Placebo (%)
23	DM	Tramadol	210 average	131	Parallel 6 wk	5-point Likert scale	<.001	68	36
96	Various	Tramadol	200–400	34	Crossover 4 wk	10-point rating scale	.001	32	9
98	DM	Oxycodone (Dazidox, ETH-Oxydose, Endocodone, Oxecta, Oxy IR, Oxycontin, Percolone, Roxicodone)	37 average	159	Parallel 6 wk	11-point rating scale	.002	N/A	N/A
99	DM	Morphine SR + gabapentin	60 morphine; 2400 GBP	35	Crossover 5 wk	11-point rating scale	<.05[b]	78	31
102	HIV	Cannabis	3.56% tetrahydroc-annabinoid tid × 5 d	50	Parallel 5 d	VAS	.03	52	24

Abbreviations: DM, diabetes mellitus; GBP, gabapentin; N/A, not available.
[a] Main adverse events were tiredness (up to 56%), mouth dryness (up to 50%), constipation (up to 44%), dizziness (up to 44%), and nausea (up to 36%).
[b] P value versus placebo and both morphine SR and gabapentin monotherapies at higher doses.

Tramadol dosing usually begins at 50 mg twice a day. The dose can be titrated upwards at increments of 50 mg every 3 to 7 days, using a 3 times a day or 4 times a day schedule. The maximum recommended dosage is 100 mg 4 times a day. Frequently reported side effects include constipation, headache, and nausea. Sedation and dizziness have been less common, reported by less than 15% of patients,[23,97] suggesting that tramadol may be better tolerated than tricyclics in some individuals. Tramadol is contraindicated in patients with previous hypersensitivity to opioid analgesics. It should be avoided in the setting of ongoing alcohol abuse, hypnotics, centrally acting analgesics, opioids, or psychotropic drugs. Increased risk of central nervous system depression or seizures has been described with concurrent use of other centrally acting drugs including neuroleptics and all major families of antidepressants. Other potential drug interactions include carbamazepine, digoxin, and warfarin. The abuse potential of tramadol seems to be low, but this agent is best avoided in patients with a previous history of addiction.[97] Because tramadol is metabolized in the liver and is partially excreted unchanged in the urine, the dosage should be reduced in patients with either hepatic (maximum dosage of 50 mg twice daily) or renal insufficiency (maximum dosage of 100 mg twice daily).

OPIATE ANALGESICS

Although the efficacy of opiates in neuropathic pain was disputed into the 1990s,[31] later studies support these agents as a reasonable therapeutic alternative (see **Table 2**). Before 2003, controlled data for opiates in neuropathic pain states was limited to postherpetic neuralgia.[100] Controlled-release oxycodone at dosages ranging from 10 to 99 mg/d demonstrated efficacy in painful diabetic neuropathy in a double-blind placebo-controlled study.[98] Significant improvement in all pain outcomes and sleep quality was seen within 1 week of therapy, excluding the worst pain category. The reduction in pain intensity occurred in the setting of relatively low average daily doses (37 mg), one-third of the maximum allowed per study protocol. The median time to achieve mild pain relief (an average pain intensity rating of ≤ 4 on the 11-point scale) was 6 days for oxycodone and 17 days for placebo. Measures for physical function and both general and mental health did not differ significantly between the 2 treatment arms, however.

In a randomized double-blind trial of levorphanol in 81 patients with either refractory chronic peripheral or central neuropathic pain, reduction of pain intensity was significantly greater with high-strength (0.75 mg) than low-strength (0.15 mg) doses.[101] The degree of pain reduction was 36% in the high-strength group versus 21% on low-dose capsules. The level of pain reduction was not associated with previous opioid use. A drawback of high-strength dosing was the greater degree of adverse events. Only patients receiving the high-dose tablets reported anger, irritability, mood or personality change, generalized weakness, confusion, and dizziness. The study withdrawal rate of 35% was also greater in the high-strength group.[101] Withdrawal rates between 20 and 25% are typical in opioid studies.[98,100]

A placebo-controlled combination study of sustained-release morphine and gabapentin versus monotherapy with either agent in painful diabetic neuropathy and postherpetic neuralgia is of particular importance (see **Table 2**).[99] The study found that combination therapy at lower doses for each agent achieved significantly better analgesia than either agent alone or placebo. Except for higher frequencies of constipation than gabapentin and dry mouth than morphine used alone, the combination was well tolerated. This trial supports the rational polypharmacy approach to treating neuropathic pain, demonstrating that combination therapies can have superior thera-peutic profiles to agents used individually.

The frequency of adverse events is high in patients treated with opiate analgesics, ranging from 76%[100] to 96%[98] in studies. Constipation, sedation, and nausea are most commonly reported. Neither opioid tolerance nor physical dependence was observed,[98] although longer-term studies have yet to be performed. Similar to trama-dol, opioids should be used with extreme caution in patients with a history of addictive behavior. Patients should be counseled on the potential for drug tolerance and addic-tion, although such behavior has been uncommon in the experience of specialists using chronic opioids in this population.[5] Longer-acting agents are preferred for chronic therapy, including extended-release oxycodone, morphine, and methadone. Dosing varies depending on the agent. In general, the dose should be slowly titrated upwards until there is pain relief and improvement in function. Effective daily doses may be rela-tively low: 30 to 60 mg for extended-release oxycodone and 1 to 15 mg for methadone. Prophylactic laxative therapy should be considered when starting these agents. Opioids are contraindicated in patients with significant respiratory depression, obstructive pulmonary disease, and paralytic ileus. Opioids interact with central nervous system depressants, therefore concomitant use should be avoided.

CANNABINOIDS

Cannabis sativa has been used to treat pain for many years. In a randomized, double-blind, placebo-controlled study of HIV-associated sensory neuropathy, 25 subjects smoked cannabis (3.56% tetrahydrocannabinoid) 3 times daily for 5 days in the active treatment arm and 25 subjects smoked placebo cigarettes (see **Table 2**).[102] Smoking cannabis significantly reduced daily pain by 34% ($P = .03$). Greater than 30% pain reduction was noted in 52% in the cannabis group compared with 24% in the placebo group ($P = .04$). Side effects noted were anxiety, sedation, confusion, and dizziness.

MEXILETINE

Trials of mexiletine (Mexitil), a class IB antiarrhythmic agent and oral analogue of lido-caine, have generated conflicting data in studies involving patients with dia-betic,[103–105] alcoholic,[106] and HIV-related neuropathy.[27,107] In a crossover study of diabetic painful neuropathy, in which mexiletine was titrated up to a daily dose of 10 mg/kg, the VAS score and clinical symptom scale showed significant improvement ($P<.02$ and $P<.01$, respectively) compared with placebo.[104] A larger study involving 126 diabetics also suggested improvement in sleep disturbance and nocturnal pain at 675 mg/d.[103] In contrast, Stracke and colleagues[105] failed to differentiate between mexiletine and placebo in either the VAS or McGill Pain Scale, although a subanalysis did suggest that stabbing or burning pain, heat sensations, and formication improved. Clinical trials that enrolled patients with HIV-related neuropathy have failed to demon-strate any benefit for mexiletine at dosages up to 600 mg/d.[27,107]

The starting dosage is 150 mg/d, with titration up to 10 mg/kg/d divided into 3 daily doses. The main side effects include nausea, vomiting, dizziness, tremor, nervousness, headache, and liver function abnormalities. Mexiletine is contraindicated in patients with second-degree or third-degree atrioventricular blockade or cardiogenic shock.[52]

CAPSAICIN

Capsaicin, an alkaloid extracted from chili peppers that depletes substance P from sensory nerves, has had a favorable effect in most diabetic neuropathy trials but not in other painful neuropathies, but favorable response rates have been high for vehicle placebos in capsaicin studies ranging from 50% to 60%. In diabetic neuropathy studies, the proportion of patients with improved pain control has ranged from 60% to 90%.[25,108,109] Ability to sleep, work, and perform other daily activities also improved significantly on capsaicin.[109,110] A major concern raised with regard to capsaicin trials is inadequate blinding from the burning sensation induced during early capsaicin application. The 1 study that used an active placebo as a control failed to demonstrate a significant effect for capsaicin.[28] Another study found capsaicin to be no more effective than placebo in painful, HIV-associated, distal, symmetric, peripheral neuropathy.[111] Significantly higher pain scores were reported in the capsaicin group at the end of the first week of this 4-week trial. Favorable response rates have been high for vehicle placebos in capsaicin studies.

Substance P is considered to be the primary neurotransmitter for polymodal nociceptive afferent fibers. In addition to substance P depletion, capsaicin may cause epidermal nerve fiber degeneration, contributing to its analgesic effects.[112]

Capsaicin 0.075% cream is available over the counter and should be applied to the painful region 3 to 4 times daily. It should be used in well-ventilated areas, and patients should avoid rubbing their eyes after use. Nonsteroidal antiinflammatory agents may be used if the initial burning from capsaicin is intense. This side effect is reported by most patients, but usually improves over several weeks as nociceptor membranes become desensitized and substance P levels are depleted.[108,109,113] Other side effects include sneezing, coughing, rash, and skin irritation. There are no significant interactions with other medications.

NGX-4010 (Qutenza), a high-concentration capsaicin proprietary matrix-formulated dermal patch (8% capsaicin), rapidly delivers therapeutic dose of capsaicin in a single treatment. A randomized, controlled, double-blind study of NGX-4010 revealed significant reduction in pain over 12 weeks in patients with HIV neuropathy ($P = .0026$).[114] Site reactions included pain and local erythema. To avoid unblinding with use of topical high-concentration capsaicin, low-concentration capsaicin was used as control. Although there was an increased incidence of site reactions and increase in pain 2 days after application compared with controls, similar changes in pain during week 1 and the substantial difference in analgesia starting at week 2 provide evidence for successful blinding. Various patch application durations were used (30, 60, and 90 minutes). A dose response was not observed as there were significant improvements with the 30-minute and 90-minute applications, but not the 60-minute application. In another study of NGX-4010 in painful HIV neuropathy, the active treatment group had 29.5% pain reduction versus 24.5% with the placebo group ($P = .097$).[115] A high-concentration capsaicin patch, Qutenza, is labeled and marketed for postherpetic neuralgia.

LEVODOPA

There has been only 1 double-blind placebo-controlled study of levodopa in painful neuropathy.[116] This study enrolled 25 patients with diabetic peripheral neuropathy. Compared with placebo, VAS scores decreased significantly in the active arm by week 2, persisting until week 4 ($P = .004$). The levodopa dosage used in the study was 100 mg 3 times a day. No adverse events were reported.

DEXTROMETHORPHAN

Dextromethorphan is a low-affinity NMDA glutamate receptor antagonist. A small crossover study that enrolled 14 patients with diabetic neuropathy revealed significant improvement in pain at a mean dosage of 381 mg/d compared with placebo ($P =$ .014).[117] Adverse events were frequent in the active arm, including sedation, dizziness, lightheadedness, and ataxia. Sixteen percent of patients dropped out due to sedation or ataxia. There were virtually no adverse events reported on placebo, suggesting that patients may have been unblinded by the treatment.[117] A subsequent parallel study of 19 patients who used lorazepam as a sedating placebo demonstrated a trend for dextromethorphan in reducing pain intensity, but this was not statistically significant.[118] In the responder subgroup, however, a dose-response effect on pain intensity was seen at higher doses. Sedation occurred in 71% of patients receiving dextromethorphan.

BOTULINUM TOXIN

Experimental evidence suggests that botulinum toxin A (Botox, Dysport, Myobloc) not only inhibits release of acetylcholine at the neuromuscular junction but also modulates the firing of sensory afferent fibers. In a double-blind crossover study involving 18 participants with diabetic neuropathy, there was a significant reduction in VAS score at weeks 1, 4, 8, and 12 after injection of botulinum toxin A compared with placebo ($P<.05$).[119] Improvement in sleep quality was also noted at 4 weeks after injection. No major complications were reported.

OTHERS
QR-333

This topical compound, which contains quercetin, a flavonoid with aldose reductase inhibitor effects, in addition to vitamin D_3 and ascorbyl palmitate, was compared with a placebo cream in diabetic neuropathy in a preliminary safety study. The topical agent was well tolerated with reduced numbness, jolting pain, and allodynia related to socks or bedsheets.[120] However, only the allodynia measure was significantly better than placebo, and larger studies are needed.

α-Lipoic Acid

α-Lipoic acid, an antioxidant compound commonly purchased over the counter by patients with diabetic neuropathy, has been studied in class I and class II studies, generally showing modest benefit. A dosage of 600 mg/d was found to be statistically superior to placebo in reducing the pain components of the Total Symptom Score (TSS) in patients with diabetic neuropathy in a 5-week study.[121] Paresthesias and numbness did not improve. Higher doses of 1200 and 1800 mg were no more effective and had greater propensity for side effects including nausea, vomiting, and vertigo.

Nonpharmacologic Approaches

The evidence supporting or refuting the use of these approaches is summarized in relation to the American Academy of Neurology (AAN) guideline in the next section.

NUMBER-NEEDED-TO-TREAT ANALYSES AND TREATMENT GUIDELINES

Increasing emphasis is being placed on the translation of evidence-based medicine into clinical practice. Therefore, randomized placebo-controlled studies on neuropathic pain have been subjected to number-needed-to-treat analyses (NNT).[122] The NNT refers to the number of subjects that need to be treated to achieve a defined clinical response in a single patient. In the context of pain studies, a 50% or greater reduction in self-reports of pain is used as the defined response.[37] For studies that do not specifically use a 50% reduction as an outcome measure, excellent/good/moderate pain relief or no/slight pain intensity grades may be categorized as satisfying this degree of pain reduction.[41] NNT can be performed only on placebo-controlled studies, because a correction for placebo responders is included in the calculation. The formula is expressed as the reciprocal of the absolute risk reduction:

$$NNT = \frac{1}{[\text{response achieved}_{active}/\text{total}_{active}] - [\text{response achieved}_{placebo}/\text{total}_{placebo}]}$$

The 95% confidence interval (CI) for the NNT is obtained by taking the reciprocal value of the 95% CI as the absolute risk reduction. Although the NNT approach is only a coarse measure of a drug's effectiveness and does not account for study duration, it does inform on the rate and magnitude of the analgesic effect and allows for a reasonable comparison of different agents (**Table 3**).[32,76] Given the scarcity of head-to-head trials on neuropathic pain, the NNT can serve as a helpful guide in the choice of first-line and second-line agents. **Table 3** summarizes NNT data for various pharmacologic agents.[123,124] Based on these findings, tricyclic antidepressants are commonly recommended as first-line therapy for neuropathic pain.[37] Leading alternatives have been gabapentin, pregabalin, duloxetine, and tramadol.

A 2011 AAN evidence-based guideline, also endorsed by the American Association of Neuromuscular & Electrodiagnostic Medicine and the American Academy of

Table 3
NNT analysis for ≥50% pain relief

Pharmacologic Class	Neuropathic Pain[a]	Painful Diabetic Neuropathy[31]
Antidepressants, tricyclic antidepressants	2.6 (2.2–3.3)	3.0 (2.4–4.0) Balanced reuptake inhibitors[b] 2.0 (1.7–2.5) Noradrenergic reuptake inhibitors[c] 3.4 (2.3–6.6)
Antidepressants, SSRIs	6.7 (3.4–435)	6.7 (3.4–435) Paroxetine 2.9 Citalopram 7.7
Venlafaxine	5.2 (2.7–5.9)[56]	
Duloxetine 120 mg/d		4.9 (3.6–7.6)[124]
Pregabalin 300 mg/d		6.0 (4.2–10.4)[124]
Pregabalin 600 mg/d		4.0 (3.3–5.3)[124]
Gabapentin	3.7 (2.4–8.3)	3.7 (2.4–8.3)
Carbamazepine	3.3 (2.0–9.4)	3.3 (2.0–9.4)
Phenytoin	2.1 (1.5–3.6)	2.1 (1.5–3.6)
Tramadol	3.4 (2.3–6.4)	3.1
Oxycodone	2.5 (1.6–5.1)[100]	
Capsaicin	5.9 (3.8–13)	5.9 (3.8–13)
Mexiletine	10 (3.0 to infinity)	10 (3.0 to infinity)
Levodopa	3.4 (1.5 to infinity)	3.4 (1.5 to infinity)
Dextromethorphan	1.9 (1.1–3.7)	1.9 (1.1–3.7)

Values in parentheses are 95% confidence intervals.
[a] Composite analysis that combined studies with different causes of neuropathic pain.[37]
[b] Balanced reuptake inhibition of both serotonin and norepinephrine (amitriptyline, imipramine, colmipramine).
[c] Includes desipramine and maprotiline.

Physical Medicine and Rehabilitation, on the treatment of painful diabetic neuropathy, gave level A evidence for pregabalin as effective therapy.[125] Amitriptyline, capsaicin, duloxetine, gabapentin, isosorbide dinitrate spray, opioids (morphine sulfate, oxycodone controlled-release, tramadol), valproate, and venlafaxine all received level B evidence as probably effective. Level C recommendations were given for use of Lidoderm patches and adding venlafaxine to gabapentin. Doses for most of these agents can be found in **Table 4**.[123] Level B evidence was found to discourage the use of oxcarbazepine, lamotrigine, lacosamide, clonidine, pentoxyfylline, and mexiletine. Insufficient evidence (level U) was found to either support or refute the use of topiramate, vitamins, and α-lipoic acid.

Table 4
Pharmacologic therapy for neuropathic pain in peripheral neuropathy

Medication	Starting Dosage	Maintenance Dosages and Comments
First Line		
Gabapentin	100–300 mg tid	Increase by 300–400 mg increments every 5–7 d to 3600 mg qd divided in 3–4 doses
Tricyclic antidepressants	10–25 mg at qhs	Increase by 10–25 mg increments every 7 d to 100–150 mg at qhs. Titration can continue following blood levels (keep <500 ng/mL) and electrocardiogram
Tramadol	50 mg qd or bid	Increase by 50 mg increments every 5–7 d to a maximum of 100 mg qid
Duloxetine	30–60 mg qd	Increase by 30–60 mg increments up to 120 mg a day if daily 60-mg dose not effective
Pregabalin	50 mg tid	Increase to 100 mg tid. Can consider further titration to 200 mg tid
Second Line		
Carbamazepine	100–200 mg qd or bid	Increase by 100–200 mg every 7 d to 600 mg qd in divided doses. Careful titration can continue following blood levels. Extended-release forms can be given on a bid schedule
Bupropion SR	150 mg qd	After 1 wk, increase to 150 mg bid
Venlafaxine XR	75 mg qd	Increase by 75 mg increments every 7 d to 150–225 mg qd
Opiate analgesics	Varying doses. Initiate with short-acting agent qid, as needed	After 1–2 wk, replace with longer-acting agent on a qd or bid schedule. Careful titration is necessary, at times with supervision by a specialist in pain medicine
Topical Agents		
Capsaicin .075%	Apply tid or qid	Continue with starting dose. May be considered for first-line or adjunctive therapy
Lidoderm 5%	Apply half to 1 patch to affected region for 12 h in a 24-h period	Apply up to 3 patches per 24-h period

The 2011 AAN guideline also provided recommendations on nonpharmacologic approaches. Percutaneous electrical stimulation received a level B recommendation to be considered for treatment of painful diabetic neuropathy, based on 1 positive class I and 1 positive class II study. Electromagnetic field treatment, low-intensity lasers, and Reiki therapy were deemed probably not effective (level B).

GENERAL TREATMENT APPROACH

Pain management should begin with an effort to identify the cause of the neuropathy, as directed therapy may help alleviate the symptoms. Before the initiation of any therapy, the physician and patient should discuss the goals and expectations of treatment. It is important that the patient have a realistic view of therapy and understand that responses may vary from person to person, and that pain relief is rarely complete. Some physicians find it helpful to have patients monitor their pain level using simple rating scales that they can complete at home and bring to their appointment. Pharmacologic agents should be initiated at low doses, and titrated using small increments over several weeks until an adequate clinical response is observed or intolerable side effects appear.[5] Tolerance of agents with sedating profiles may be enhanced by starting the medication in a single bedtime dose. Slow titrations are especially important in elderly patients who are taking other medications for chronic medical illness.

Polypharmacy or multidimensional therapy may be considered when 1 drug provides partial relief but higher doses produce troublesome side effects. In this setting, a rational intervention would be to add a medication with a different mechanism of action or initiate a nonpharmacologic approach. Two common reasons for treatment failure in the neuropathic pain population are stopping titrations before effective dosing levels are reached and immediate initiation of polypharmacy.[5] A drug trial of at least 4 to 6 weeks is recommended before switching to or adding another medication.

Recommendations for first-line and second-line pharmacologic agents are provided in **Table 4**. These recommendations are based on the weight of evidence from randomized controlled trials, taking adverse effect risks into account. Other considerations when choosing between these agents include cost, underlying medical illness, and potential drug interactions. Although many patients with neuropathic pain are treated simultaneously with 2 or more of the agents listed, systematic evaluations of combination therapy are limited. As mentioned earlier, whether some medication classes are more effective than others in treating certain qualities of neuropathic pain has not been answered in convincing fashion.[31]

The future of neuropathic pain management is promising. Pharmacologic options continue to increase, and new agents are being investigated. Still, even current knowledge and available therapies seem underused. In a survey of 151 patients referred to a tertiary center, 25% had never received any of the conventional agents known to have efficacy for neuropathic pain.[126] More than 70% had never been prescribed anticonvulsants. Educational programs and raising awareness among health care professionals are of critical importance if advances in neuropathic pain management are to reach this large group of patients.

SUMMARY

Neuropathic pain is a common symptom and a major source of morbidity in patients with peripheral neuropathy. The mechanisms underlying the generation of neuropathic pain are not fully understood but likely involve a variety of pathophysiologic processes. Numerous clinical trials evaluating the efficacy of agents used in the treatment of neuropathic pain have been performed but are fraught with challenges and methodological shortcomings. Notwithstanding, there is good evidence for the use of tricyclic antidepressants, newer antidepressants (particularly serotonin-norepinephrine reuptake inhibitors), anticonvulsants, and several other medications in the treatment of neuropathic pain.

Case study

A 63 year-old woman developed numbness, tingling, and burning pain in her feet, progressing up to the ankles over 2 years. She has history of poorly controlled diabetes mellitus and depression. She denies any hand symptoms or limb weakness. She has been on gabapentin 600 mg PO tid with partial relief. Further increase of gabapentin was not tolerated due to side effects.

Examination showed normal strength, with decreased sensation to pinprick and light touch up to the ankles. Timed vibration was 5 seconds at the toes and proprioception was normal at the toes. Reflexes are normal in the arms and at the knees but ankle reflexes are absent. Gait was normal.

Laboratory studies including vitamin B12 level and thyroid studies were normal, and there was no serum monoclonal protein. Nerve conduction studies showed absent sural sensory responses, indicative of a sensory polyneuropathy.

Duloxetine was started at 30 mg once daily and was increased a week later to 60 mg once daily. This resulted in significant improvement of pain. No side effects were noted on the combination of gabapentin and cymbalta. On a subsequent clinic visit 6 months later, gabapentin was slowly tapered by 300 mg every 2 weeks until she was off gabapentin. Her neuropathic pain remained well controlled on duloxetine.

REFERENCES

1. International Association for the Study of Pain. Taxonomy. Available at: http://www.iasp-pain.org/AM/Template.cfm?Section=Pain_Defi.isplay.cfm&ContentID=1728. Accessed November 20, 2012.
2. Carter GT, Galer BS. Advances in the management of neuropathic pain. Phys Med Rehabil Clin North Am 2001;12:447–59.
3. Smith TE, Chong MS. Neuropathic pain. Hosp Med 2000;61:760–6.
4. Galer BS, Gianas A, Jensen MP. Painful diabetic polyneuropathy: epidemiology, pain description, and quality of life. Diabetes Res Clin Pract 2000;47:123–8.
5. Galer BS. Painful polyneuropathy. Neurol Clin 1998;16:791–811.
6. Periquet MI, Novak V, Collins MP, et al. Painful sensory neuropathy: prospective evaluation using skin biopsy. Neurology 2000;53:1641–7.
7. Lacomis D. Small-fiber neuropathy. Muscle Nerve 2002;26:173–88.
8. Wolfe GI, Baker NS, Amato AA, et al. Chronic cryptogenic sensory polyneuropathy: clinical and laboratory characteristics. Arch Neurol 1999;56:540–7.
9. Holland NR, Crawford TO, Hauer P, et al. Small-fiber sensory neuropathies: clinical course and neuropathology of idiopathic cases. Ann Neurol 1998;44:47–59.
10. Holland NR. Idiopathic painful sensory neuropathy. J Clin Neuromuscul Dis 2001;2:211–20.
11. Luciano CA, Russell JW, Banarjee TK, et al. Physiological characterization of neuropathy in Fabry disease. Muscle Nerve 2002;26:622–9.
12. Wolfe GI, Barohn RJ. Cryptogenic sensory and sensorimotor polyneuropathies. Semin Neurol 1998;18:105–11.

13. Simpson DM, McArthur JC, Olney R, et al. Lamotrigine for HIV-associated painful sensory neuropathies: a placebo-controlled trial. Neurology 2003;60:1508–14.
14. Woolf CJ, Mannion RJ. Neuropathic pain: aetiology, symptoms, mechanisms, and management. Lancet 1999;353:1959–64.
15. Ochoa J, Torebjork HE, Culp WJ, et al. Abnormal spontaneous activity in single sensory nerve fibres in humans. Muscle Nerve 1982;5:S74–7.
16. Devor M. The pathophysiology of damaged peripheral nerves. In: Wall PD, Melzack R, editors. Textbook of pain. Edinburgh (United Kingdom): Churchill Livingstone; 1994. p. 79–100.
17. Bennett G. The role of the sympathetic nervous system in painful peripheral neuropathy. Pain 1991;45:221–3.
18. Woolf CJ. Evidence for a central component of post-injury pain. Nature 1983; 306:686–8.
19. Gracely RH, Lynch SA, Bennett GJ. Painful neuropathy: altered central processing maintained dynamically by peripheral input. Pain 1992;51:175–94.
20. Besson JM. The neurobiology of pain. Lancet 1999;353:1610–5.
21. Galer BS. Neuropathic pain of peripheral origin: advances in pharmacologic treatment. Neurology 1995;45(Suppl 9):S17–25.
22. Backonja M, Beydoun A, Edwards KR, et al. Gabapentin for the symptomatic treatment of painful neuropathy in patients with diabetes mellitus. JAMA 1998; 280:1831–6.
23. Harati Y, Gooch C, Swenson M, et al. Double-blind randomized trial of tramadol for the treatment of the pain of diabetic neuropathy. Neurology 1998;50:1842–6.
24. Max MB, Lynch SA, Muir J, et al. Effects of desipramine, amitriptyline, and fluoxetine on pain in diabetic neuropathy. N Engl J Med 1992;326:1250–6.
25. Capsaicin Study Group. Treatment of painful diabetic neuropathy with topical capsaicin: a multicenter, double-blind, vehicle-controlled study. Arch Intern Med 1991;151:2225–9.
26. Sindrup SH, Gram LF, BrØsen K, et al. The selective serotonin reuptake inhibitor paroxetine is effective in the treatment of diabetic neuropathy symptoms. Pain 1990;42:135–44.
27. Kieburtz K, Simpson D, Yiannoutsos C, et al. A randomized trial of amitriptyline and mexiletine for painful neuropathy in HIV infection. Neurology 1998;51:1682–8.
28. Low PA, Opfer-Gehrking TL, Dyck PJ, et al. Double-blind placebo-controlled study of the application of capsaicin cream in chronic distal painful polyneuropathy. Pain 1995;62:163–8.
29. Eisenberg E, Lurie Y, Braker C, et al. Lamotrigine reduces painful diabetic neuropathy: a randomized, controlled study. Neurology 2001;57:505–9.
30. Semenchuk MR, Sherman S, Davis B. Double-blind, randomized trial of bupropion SR for the treatment of neuropathic pain. Neurology 2001;57:1583–8.
31. Sindrup SH, Jensen TS. Efficacy of pharmacological treatments of neuropathic pain: an update and effect related to mechanism of drug action. Pain 1999;83: 389–400.
32. Chong MS, Bajwa ZH. Diagnosis and treatment of neuropathic pain. J Pain Symptom Manage 2003;25:S4–11.
33. Melzack R. The short-form McGill Pain Questionnaire. Pain 1987;30:191–7.
34. Daut RL, Cleeland CS, Flanery RC. Development of the Wisconsin Brief Pain Questionnaire to assess pain in cancer and other diseases. Pain 1983;17:197–210.
35. Galer BS, Jensen MP. Development and preliminary validation of a pain measure specific to neuropathic pain: the Neuropathic Pain Scale. Neurology 1997;48: 332–8.

36. Calissi PT, Jaber LA. Peripheral diabetic neuropathy: current concepts of treatment. Ann Pharmacother 1995;29:769–77.
37. Sindrup SH, Jensen TS. Pharmacologic treatment of pain in polyneuropathy. Neurology 2000;55:915–20.
38. Vrethem M, Boivie J, Arnqvist H, et al. A comparison of amitriptyline and maprotiline in the treatment of painful polyneuropathy in diabetics and nondiabetics. Clin J Pain 1997;13:313–23.
39. Max MB, Kishore-Kumar R, Schafer SC, et al. Efficacy of desipramine in painful diabetic neuropathy: a placebo-controlled trial. Pain 1991;45:3–9.
40. Max MB, Culnane M, Schafer SC, et al. Amitriptyline relieves diabetic neuropathy pain in patients with normal or depressed mood. Neurology 1987;37:589–96.
41. McQuay HJ, Tramèr M, Nye BA, et al. A systematic review of antidepressants in neuropathic pain. Pain 1996;68:217–27.
42. Sindrup SH, Gram LF, Skjold T, et al. Clomipramine *vs* desipramine *vs* placebo in the treatment of diabetic neuropathy symptoms: a double-blind cross-over study. Br J Clin Pharmacol 1990;30:683–91.
43. Sindrup SH, Tuxen C, Gram LF, et al. Lack of effect of mianserin on the symptoms of diabetic neuropathy. Eur J Clin Pharmacol 1992;43:251–5.
44. Shlay JC, Chaloner K, Max MB, et al. Acupuncture and amitriptyline for pain due to HIV-related peripheral neuropathy: a randomized controlled trial. JAMA 1998;280:1590–5.
45. Kvinesdal B, Molin J, FrØland A, et al. Imipramine treatment of painful diabetic neuropathy. JAMA 1984;251:1727–30.
46. Wolfe GI, Barohn RJ. Painful peripheral neuropathy. Curr Treat Options Neurol 2002;4:177–88.
47. Sindrup SH, Bjerre U, Dejgaard A, et al. The selective serotonin reuptake inhibitor citalopram relieves the symptoms of diabetic neuropathy. Clin Pharmacol Ther 1992;52:547–52.
48. Brasch-Anderson C, Moller MU, Christiansen L, et al. A candidate gene study of serotonergic pathway genes and pain relief during treatment with escitalopram in patients with neuropathic pain shows significant association to serotonin receptor2C (HTR2C). Eur J Clin Pharmacol 2011;67(11):1131–7.
49. Goldstein DJ, Lu Y, Detke MJ, et al. Duloxetine vs. placebo in patients with painful diabetic neuropathy. Pain 2005;116:109–18.
50. Raskin J, Pritchett YL, Wang F, et al. A double-blind randomized multicenter trial comparing duloxetine with placebo in the management of diabetic peripheral neuropathic pain. Pain Med 2005;6:346–56.
51. Ascher JA, Cole JO, Colin JN, et al. Bupropion: a review of its mechanism of antidepressant activity. J Clin Psychiatry 1995;56:395–401.
52. Wolfe GI, Hotz SE, Barohn RJ. Treatment of painful peripheral neuropathy. J Clin Neuromuscul Dis 2002;4:50–9.
53. Holliday SM, Benfield P. Venlafaxine: a review of its pharmacology and therapeutic potential in depression. Drugs 1995;49:280–94.
54. Kunz NR, Goli V, Entsuah AR. Venlafaxine extended release in the treatment of pain associated with diabetic neuropathy [abstract]. Neurology 2000;54(Suppl 3):A441.
55. Simpson DA. Gabapentin and venlafaxine for the treatment of painful diabetic neuropathy. J Clin Neuromuscul Dis 2001;3:53–62.
56. Sindrup SH, Bach FW, Madsen C, et al. Venlafaxine versus imipramine in painful polyneuropathy: a randomized, controlled trial. Neurology 2003;60:1284–9.

57. Kuzniecky R, Ho S, Pan J, et al. Modulation of cerebral GABA by topiramate, lamotrigine, and gabapentin in healthy adults. Neurology 2002;58:368–72.
58. Petroff OA, Rothman DL, Behar KL, et al. The effect of gabapentin on brain gamma-aminobutyric acid in patients with epilepsy. Ann Neurol 1996;39: 95–9.
59. Taylor CP, Gee NS, Su TZ, et al. A summary of mechanistic hypotheses of gabapentin pharmacology. Epilepsy Res 1998;29:231–46.
60. Pandey CK, Bose N, Garg G, et al. Gabapentin for the treatment of pain in Guillain-Barré syndrome: a double-blinded, placebo-controlled, crossover study. Anesth Analg 2002;95:1719–23.
61. Serpell MG, Neuropathic Pain Study Group. Gabapentin in neuropathic pain syndromes: a randomised double-blind, placebo-controlled trial. Pain 2002; 99:557–66.
62. Pandey CK, Raza M, Tripathi M, et al. The comparative evaluation of gabapentin and carbamazepine for pain management in Guillain-Barré syndrome patients in the intensive care unit. Anesth Analg 2005;101:220–5.
63. Morello CM, Leckband SG, Stoner CP, et al. Randomized double-blind study comparing the efficacy of gabapentin with amitriptyline on diabetic peripheral neuropathy pain. Arch Intern Med 1999;159:1931–7.
64. Dallocchio C, Buffa C, Mazzarello P, et al. Gabapentin vs amitriptyline in painful diabetic neuropathic pain: an open-label pilot study. J Pain Symptom Manage 2000;20:280–5.
65. Backonja M, Glanzman RL. Gabapentin dosing for neuropathic pain: evidence from randomized, placebo-controlled clinical trials. Clin Ther 2003;25: 81–104.
66. Gorson K, Schott C, Herman R, et al. Gabapentin in the treatment of painful diabetic neuropathy: a placebo controlled, double blind, crossover trial. J Neurol Neurosurg Psychiatr 1999;66:251–2.
67. Leach MJ, Marden CM, Miller AA. Pharmacological studies on lamotrigine, a novel potential antiepileptic drug: II. Neurochemical studies on the mechanism of action. Epilepsia 1986;27:490–7.
68. McCleane G. 200 mg daily of lamotrigine has no analgesic effect in neuropathic pain: a randomized, double-blind, placebo-controlled trial. Pain 1999; 83:105–7.
69. Simpson DM, Olney R, McArthur JC, et al. A placebo-controlled trial of lamotrigine for painful HIV-associated neuropathy. Neurology 2000;54:2115–9.
70. Rao RD, Flynn PJ, Sloan JA, et al. Efficacy of lamotrigine in the management of chemotherapy-induced peripheral neuropathy: a phase 3 randomized, double-blind, placebo-controlled trial, N01C3. Cancer 2008;112(12):2802–8.
71. Edwards KR, Glantz MJ, Button J, et al. Efficacy and safety of topiramate in the treatment of painful diabetic neuropathy: a double-blind, placebo-controlled study [abstract]. Neurology 2000;54(Suppl):A81.
72. Thienel U, Neto W, Schwabe SK, et al. Topiramate in painful diabetic polyneuropathy: findings from three double-blind, placebo-controlled trials. Acta Neurol Scand 2004;110:221–31.
73. Raskin P, Donofrio PD, Rosenthal NR, et al. Topiramate vs placebo in painful diabetic neuropathy: analgesic and metabolic effects. Neurology 2004;63:865–73.
74. Backonja M. Use of anticonvulsants for treatment of neuropathic pain. Neurology 2002;59:S14–7.
75. Mendell JR, Sahenk Z. Painful sensory neuropathy. N Engl J Med 2003;348: 1243–55.

76. Rull JA, Quibrera R, González-Millán H, et al. Symptomatic treatment of peripheral diabetic neuropathy with carbamazepine (Tegretol): double blind crossover trial. Diabetologia 1969;5:215–8.

77. Wilton TD. Tegretol in the treatment of diabetic neuropathy. S Afr Med J 1974;48: 869–72.

78. May TW, Korn-Merker E, Rambeck B. Clinical pharmacokinetics of oxcarbazepine. Clin Pharmacokinet 2003;42:1023–42.

79. Pellock JM. Tricyclic anticonvulsants: safety and adverse effects. Epilepsy Behav 2002;3:S14–7.

80. Carrazana E, Mikoshiba I. Rationale and evidence for the use of oxcarbazepine in neuropathic pain. J Pain Symptom Manage 2003;25:S31–5.

81. Beydoun A, Shaibani A, Hopwood M, et al. Oxcarbazepine in painful diabetic neuropathy: results of a dose-ranging study. Acta Neurol Scand 2006;113: 395–404.

82. Grosskopf J, Mazzola J, Wan Y, et al. A randomized, placebo-controlled study of oxcarbazepine in painful diabetic neuropathy. Acta Neurol Scand 2006;114: 177–80.

83. Jensen TS. Anticonvulsants in neuropathic pain: rationale and clinical evidence. Eur J Pain 2002;6:61–8.

84. Kochar DK, Jain N, Agarwal RP, et al. Sodium valproate in the management of painful neuropathy in type 2 diabetes-a randomized placebo controlled study. Acta Neurol Scand 2002;106:248–52.

85. Rosenstock J, Tuchman M, LaMoreaux L, et al. Pregabalin for the treatment of painful diabetic peripheral neuropathy: a double-blind, placebo-controlled trial. Pain 2004;110:628–38.

86. Lesser H, Sharma U, LaMoreaux L, et al. Pregabalin relieves symptoms of painful diabetic neuropathy: a randomized controlled trial. Neurology 2004;63: 2104–10.

87. Richter RW, Portenoy R, Sharma U, et al. Relief of diabetic peripheral neuropathy with pregabalin: a randomized, placebo-controlled trial. J Pain 2005;6: 253–60.

88. Freynhagen R, Strojek K, Griesing T, et al. Efficacy of pregabalin in neuropathic pain evaluated in a 12-week, randomised, double-blind, multicentre, placebo-controlled trial of flexible- and fixed-dose regimens. Pain 2005;115:254–63.

89. Sharma U, Griesing T, Emir B, et al. Time to onset of neuropathic pain reduction: a retrospective analysis of data from nine controlled trials of pregabalin for painful diabetic peripheral neuropathy and postherpetic neuralgia. Am J Ther 2010; 17(6):577–85.

90. Errington AC, Stöhr T, Heers C, et al. The investigational anticonvulsant lacosamide selectively enhances slow inactivation of voltage-gated sodium channels. Mol Pharmacol 2008;73:157–69.

91. Ziegler D, Hidvegi T, Gurieva I, et al. Efficacy and safety of lacosamide in painful diabetic neuropathy. Diabetes Care 2010;33:839–41.

92. Shaibani A, Fares S, Selam JL, et al. Lacosamide in painful diabetic neuropathy: an 18-week double-blind placebo-controlled trial. J Pain 2009;10:818–28.

93. Wymer JP, Simpson J, Sen D, et al. Efficacy and safety of lacosamide in diabetic neuropathic pain: an 18-week double-blind placebo-controlled trial of fixed-dose regimens. Clin J Pain 2009;25:376–85.

94. Raffa RB, Friderichs E, Reimann W, et al. Opioid and nonopioid components independently contribute to the mechanism of action of tramadol, an "atypical" opioid analgesic. J Pharmacol Exp Ther 1992;260:275–85.

95. Richter W, Barth H, Flohe L, et al. Clinical investigation on the development of dependence during oral therapy with tramadol. Arzneimittelforschung 1985; 35:1742–4.

96. Sindrup SH, Andersen G, Madsen C, et al. Tramadol relieves pain and allodynia in polyneuropathy: a randomised, double-blind, controlled trial. Pain 1999;83: 85–90.

97. Harati Y, Gooch C, Swenson M, et al. Maintenance of long-term effectiveness of tramadol in treatment of the pain in diabetic neuropathy. J Diabetes Complications 2000;14:65–70.

98. Gimbel JS, Richards P, Portenoy RK. Controlled-release oxycodone for pain in diabetic neuropathy: a randomized controlled study. Neurology 2003;60:927–34.

99. Gilron I, Bailey JM, Dongsheng T, et al. Morphine, gabapentin, or their combination for neuropathic pain. N Engl J Med 2005;352:1324–34.

100. Watson CP, Babul N. Efficacy of oxycodone in neuropathic pain: a randomized trial in postherpetic neuralgia. Neurology 1998;50:1837–41.

101. Rowbotham MC, Twilling L, Davies PS, et al. Oral opioid therapy for chronic peripheral and central neuropathic pain. N Engl J Med 2003;348:1223–32.

102. Abrams DI, Jay CA, Shade SB, et al. Cannabis in painful HIV-associated sensory neuropathy. A randomized placebo-controlled trial. Neurology 2007; 68:515–21.

103. Oskarsson P, Ljunggren JG, Lins PE, et al. Efficacy and safety of mexiletine in the treatment of painful diabetic neuropathy. Diabetes Care 1997;20:1594–7.

104. Dejgård A, Petersen P, Kastrup J. Mexiletine for treatment of chronic painful diabetic neuropathy. Lancet 1988;1:9–11.

105. Stracke H, Meyer UE, Schumacher HE, et al. Mexiletine in the treatment of diabetic neuropathy. Diabetes Care 1992;15:1550–5.

106. Nishiyama K, Sakuta M. Mexiletine for painful alcoholic neuropathy. Intern Med 1995;34:577–9.

107. Kemper CA, Kent G, Burton S, et al. Mexiletine for HIV-infected patients with painful peripheral neuropathy: a double-blind, placebo-controlled, crossover treatment trial. J Acquir Immune Defic Syndr Hum Retrovirol 1998;19:367–72.

108. Tandan R, Lewis GA, Krusinski PB, et al. Topical capsaicin in painful diabetic neuropathy. Diabetes Care 1992;15:8–14.

109. Scheffler NM, Sheitel PL, Lipton MN. Treatment of painful diabetic neuropathy with capsaicin 0.075-percent. J Am Podiatr Med Assoc 1991;81:288–93.

110. Capsaicin Study Group. Effect of treatment with capsaicin on daily activities of patients with painful diabetic neuropathy. Diabetes Care 1991;15:159–65.

111. Paice JA, Ferrans CE, Lashley FR, et al. Topical capsaicin in the management of HIV-associated peripheral neuropathy. J Pain Symptom Manage 2000;19: 45–52.

112. Nolano M, Simone DA, Wendelschafer-Crabb G, et al. Topical capsaicin in humans: parallel loss of epidermal fibers and pain sensation. Pain 1999;81: 135–45.

113. Fitzgerald M. Capsaicin and sensory neurons: a review. Pain 1983;15:109–30.

114. Simpson DM, Brown S, Tobias J, et al. Controlled trial of high-concentration capsaicin patch for treatment of painful HIV neuropathy. Neurology 2008;70: 2305–13.

115. Clifford DB, Simpson DM, Brown S, et al. A randomized, double-blind, controlled study of NGX-4010, a capsaicin 8% dermal patch, for the treatment of painful HIV-associated distal sensory polyneuropathy. J Acquir Immune Defic Syndr 2012;59(2):126–33.

116. Ertas M, Sagduyu A, Arac N, et al. Use of levodopa to relieve pain from painful symmetrical diabetic polyneuropathy. Pain 1998;75:257–9.
117. Nelson KA, Park KM, Robinovitz E, et al. High-dose oral dextromethorphan versus placebo in painful diabetic neuropathy and postherpetic neuralgia. Neurology 1997;48:1212–8.
118. Sang CN, Booher S, Gilron I, et al. Dextromethorphan and memantine in painful diabetic neuropathy and postherpetic neuralgia: efficacy and dose-response trials. Anesthesiology 2002;96:1053–61.
119. Yuan RY, Sheu JJ, Yu JM, et al. Botulinum toxin for diabetic neuropathic pain. A randomized double-blind crossover trial. Neurology 2009;72:1473–8.
120. Valensi P, Le Devehat C, Richard JL, et al. A multicenter, double-blind, safety study of QR-333 for the treatment of symptomatic diabetic peripheral neuropathy: a preliminary report. J Diabetes Complications 2005;19:247–53.
121. Ziegler D, Ametov A, Barinov A, et al. Oral treatment with α-lipoic acid improves symptomatic diabetic polyneuropathy: the SYDNEY 2 trial. Diabetes Care 2006; 29:2365–70.
122. Cook RJ, Sackett DL. The number needed to treat: a clinically useful measure of treatment effect. BMJ 1995;310:452–4.
123. Wolfe GI, Trivedi JR. Painful peripheral neuropathy and its nonsurgical treatment. Muscle Nerve 2004;30:3–19.
124. Rutkove SB. A 52-year-old woman with disabling peripheral neuropathy: review of diabetic polyneuropathy. JAMA 2009;302:1451–8.
125. Bril V, England J, Franklin GM, et al. Evidence-based guideline: treatment of painful peripheral neuropathy. Neurology 2011;76:1758–65.
126. Gilron I, Bailey J, Weaver DF, et al. Patients' attitudes and prior treatments in neuropathic pain: a pilot study. Pain Res Manag 2002;7:199–203.

Entrapment Neuropathies

William David Arnold, MD*, Bakri H. Elsheikh, MBBS

KEYWORDS

- Compression neuropathy • Entrapment neuropathy • Nerve imaging
- Electrodiagnostic testing

KEY POINTS

- Clinical history and physical examination are usually sufficient to establish the diagnosis of entrapment neuropathy.
- Electrodiagnostic testing is helpful in confirming the diagnosis, determining severity, and excluding mimicking conditions.
- Peripheral nerve imaging technologies including ultrasonography, and magnetic resonance imaging may provide additional information particularly in atypical cases.
- In most cases of entrapment neuropathy, conservative management is effective.
- Sometimes surgical release is necessary for good treatment outcomes.

INTRODUCTION: GENERAL CONCEPTS

Compression neuropathy describes a heterogeneous group of focal neuropathy syndromes related to peripheral nerve compression resulting in pain, paresthesia, and loss of function of that nerve. The term entrapment neuropathy, although frequently used interchangeably with compression neuropathy, describes a subset of compression neuropathy related to chronic compression. Acute or chronic compression-related injury may occur in essentially any peripheral nerve, but certain considerations such as anatomic course, superficial location, or adjacent fibrous or osseous structures may predispose certain nerves to intrinsic or extrinsic compression-related injury. Mechanical pressure leads to associated ischemia and edema of the compressed nerve. Acute compression leads to focal demyelination, and if compression is sufficiently prolonged Wallerian-like axonal degeneration will occur. The clinical presentations of specific compression or entrapment syndromes depend on factors such as chronicity, location, severity, and mechanism of involvement of a particular nerve (**Fig. 1**).

Disclosures: None.
Department of Neurology, Division of Neuromuscular Medicine, The Ohio State University, 395 West 12th Avenue, Columbus, OH 43210, USA
* Corresponding author.
E-mail address: William.Arnold@osumc.edu

Neurol Clin 31 (2013) 405–424
http://dx.doi.org/10.1016/j.ncl.2013.01.002
0733-8619/13/$ – see front matter © 2013 Elsevier Inc. All rights reserved.

neurologic.theclinics.com

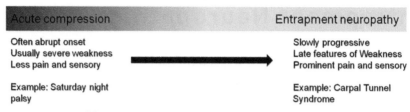

Fig. 1. Continuum of focal compression–related neuropathies.

The expected electrodiagnostic (Edx) findings include focal slowing of action-potential propagation (prolonged latency or slowed conduction velocity) across the site of compression consistent with a pathophysiology of focal demyelination. Edx parameters of amplitude loss are more indicative of severity and are helpful for prognosis.[1,2] Edx is particularly helpful in excluding the possibility of underlying generalized neuropathic process. Other multifocal neuropathic processes unrelated to peripheral nerve compression that may mimic entrapment neuropathy include peripheral nerve vasculitis or multifocal variants of immune-mediated neuropathy, such as Lewis-Sumner syndrome (multifocal acquired demyelinating sensory and motor neuropathy or MADSAM).[3]

In cases of acute or subacute compression-related neuropathy such as Saturday night palsy (radial neuropathy at the spiral groove), treatment may be simply be supportive, and improvement is expected over time without intervention. In other cases of chronic compression or entrapment neuropathy, such as carpal tunnel syndrome, symptoms may continue to progress despite modification of activities and avoidance of provocative activities. Such cases often require more aggressive intervention. The management of peripheral nerve entrapment syndromes depends on multiple factors including the chronicity and severity of symptoms, the underlying mechanism, and associated predisposing factors. Understanding the underlying mechanism of injury and the associated natural history is a fundamental aspect of designing an appropriate treatment plan. Coexistent systemic medical conditions may predispose an individual for the development of entrapment neuropathy. Such conditions may include, but are not limited to, endocrinologic disorders (diabetes, hypothyroidism, and acromegaly), the presence of a generalized neuropathy, rapid weight loss, and focal or generalized edema. Treatment of any possible predisposing systemic conditions should be optimized before considering aggressive treatment for entrapment neuropathy, such as surgical release.

DIAGNOSTIC APPROACH TO AND MANAGEMENT OF UPPER LIMB FOCAL NEUROPATHIES
Median Nerve

Anatomy
The median nerve is formed from fibers of the ventral roots of spinal nerves C5-T1. The fibers of C5-C7 travel within the lateral cord of the brachial plexus to merge with fibers traveling within the medial cord from the ventral roots of spinal nerves C8 and T1. The median nerve supplies no significant motor or sensory branches above the elbow. Within the forearm the median nerve provides motor innervation to all of the flexor muscles, excluding flexor carpi ulnaris and the fascicles of flexor digitorum profundus, to the ring and small fingers. Direct motor branches innervate the pronator teres, flexor carpi radialis, and flexor digitorum sublimis muscles. The anterior interosseous, a major branch of the median nerve within the forearm and thus spared in carpal tunnel

syndrome, supplies motor innervation to flexor digitorum profundus to digits 2 and 3, flexor pollicis longus, and pronator quadratus.

Before passing under the transverse carpal ligament and through the carpal tunnel, the palmar cutaneous nerve branches from the median nerve to supply sensation over the thenar eminence. As a consequence the sensation over the thenar eminence is always spared in carpal tunnel syndrome. Within the hand, the median nerve and its branches supply sensory innervation of the lateral portion of the hand and the palmar surface of the thumb, index, middle and lateral half of the ring finger, and motor innervation to abductor pollicis brevis, opponens pollicis, superficial head of the flexor pollicis brevis, and the first and second lumbrical muscles. The thenar compartment muscles including abductor pollicis brevis, opponens pollicis, and the superficial head of flexor pollicis brevis are innervated by the recurrent motor branch. The recurrent motor branch usually branches from the median nerve prior to the carpal tunnel, but travels along with the median nerve under the transcarpal ligament.[4] Because of this, the recurrent motor branch may rarely be selectively or more severely involved in comparison with the main median nerve during compression at the carpal tunnel, leading to motor-predominant presentation.

Median neuropathy
Carpal tunnel syndrome (CTS) is the clinical diagnosis that describes the constellation of symptoms associated with median nerve entrapment at the wrist. CTS is attributed to chronic compression of the median nerve within the carpal tunnel. It is a common clinical problem and the most common entrapment neuropathy, with an estimated prevalence of 2% in men and 3% in women.[5] Compression of the median nerve within the carpal tunnel leads to inhibition of axonal transport and reduction of epineurial blood flow, leading to intraneural edema, myelin thinning, and eventual nerve-fiber degeneration and fibrosis.[6–8]

Most CTS is idiopathic, with no specific predisposing condition identified. Systemic predisposing conditions include diabetes, pregnancy, thyroid disorders, chronic kidney disease, acromegaly, and obesity. Underlying peripheral neuropathy may also contribute to the development of CTS, particularly certain types of neuropathy, including hereditary neuropathy with predisposition to pressure palsies and familial amyloidosis related to transthyretin mutation. A family history of carpal tunnel may be present in up to 30% cases.[9,10] There are numerous studies suggesting that CTS is a cumulative trauma disorder, but studies also argue that body habitus, diabetes, age, and other factors influence work-related CTS.[11–13] Although a common misconception, there does not seem to be a clear association between keyboard use and the pathogenesis of CTS.[14]

Patients with CTS usually present with predominantly sensory features of distal median nerve dysfunction including pain, numbness, and tingling affecting the thumb, index, and middle fingers. These symptoms are typically intermittent early in the course of disease, and nocturnal worsening of symptoms or worsening symptoms with activity of the hands are common. Classically the sensory examination will demonstrate impairment of the distal medial distribution but spare the palm. Frequently, particularly early in the course of disease, the physical examination may be normal. Around 50% of patients with defined carpal tunnel will have a normal examination, and even with quantitative sensory testing around 20% of patients with defined carpal tunnel syndrome will have normal sensory findings.[15] Provocative maneuvers such as the Tinel or Phalen are often positive, but lack sensitivity and specificity.[16] The sensitivity and specificity of the Phalen test are 75% and 47%, respectively.[16] A positive Phalen test may be a negative prognostic indicator.[1] Pain may be a prominent feature in CTS, and it is not uncommon for patients to report symptoms of pain or numbness outside of the median distribution with numbness of the "whole hand," and pain radiating proximally to the forearm and elbow. Infrequently some patients do report associated referred pain to the shoulder. Motor findings involving the distal median innervated muscles may be seen in CTS, but significant weakness or atrophy is usually only seen in severe or very chronic cases. Patients will often complain of weakness or specifically "dropping" objects, which is usually due to sensory and proprioceptive defects rather than weakness; true weakness is not usually an early or prominent feature.

The overwhelming majority of median neuropathy occurs at the wrist within the carpal tunnel. Rarely proximal median neuropathy may occur, and mimic CTS. These cases can usually be distinguished by weakness of proximal median innervated muscles and the presence of sensory loss in the palmar aspect of the hand. Entrapment syndromes of the proximal median nerve have been described that are related to compression by the ligament of Struthers, biceps brachii aponeurosis, pronator teres muscle, and flexor digitorum superficialis muscle. Pronator syndrome is an ill-defined entrapment syndrome involving compression of the median nerve as it passes between the pronator teres muscle. Symptoms include aching pain in the forearm associated with sensory and/or motor deficits in the distribution of the proximal median nerve. Anterior interosseous syndrome describes symptoms of deep aching pain in the forearm followed by weakness in anterior interosseous-innervated muscles. There are numerous case reports in the literature describing a compressive cause in anterior interosseous syndrome, but care should be taken when attributing anterior interosseous neuropathy to compression, particularly in cases with an abrupt onset. There is significant overlap between anterior interosseous syndrome related to chronic compression and neuralgic amyotrophy (also known as Parsonage-Turner syndrome or idiopathic brachial plexus neuropathy).[17] Symptoms of slowly progressive pain localized to only the forearm associated with deficits in only the distribution of the anterior interosseous nerve may suggest chronic compression. Conversely, an abrupt onset of severe pain or weakness is usually less likely related to anterior interosseous nerve entrapment or compression.

Diagnostic modalities CTS is usually diagnosed on a clinical basis or in combination with Edx testing. Edx testing provides additional benefits of defining severity and excluding coexistent or mimicking conditions. There are numerous Edx techniques that may be used to confirm median neuropathy at the wrist. The role of such testing is to confirm or exclude demyelination of the median nerve at the carpal tunnel. Although dependent on choice of technique, Edx testing has an approximate sensitivity of 85% and specificity of 95% in detecting median neuropathy at the wrist in the setting of defined CTS.[18] Edx findings may be used to characterize the severity of median neuropathy at the wrist (**Table 1**).[1] Although it may be helpful to use this classification to guide treatment strategies, severity of symptoms often do not correlate closely with Edx findings. Standard median nerve conduction studies are usually

Table 1	
Electrodiagnostic grading of median neuropathy at the wrist	
Mild	Demyelination apparent on only sensory responses
Moderate	Demyelination on sensory and motor responses Axon loss on sensory response
Severe	No sensory response Motor axon loss may be apparent

normal in proximal median nerve entrapment syndromes, but the needle-electrode examination may show features of motor axon loss.

Ultrasound imaging is a rapidly advancing area of the assessment of focal neuropathies, and there has been progress recently in the diagnosis of CTS.[19] Although peripheral nerve ultrasound testing is not yet universally available and Edx testing remains the gold standard for compressive neuropathy, ultrasonography does offer several potential advantages including less pain than with Edx tests, structural assessment of the involved nerve and surrounding structures, and cost efficiency. Other diagnostic imaging modalities such as magnetic resonance imaging (MRI) or plain radiographs may also be helpful in select cases. There is no role for universal laboratory screening for associated systemic disorders in patients diagnosed with CTS, unless other systemic signs are evident by history or examination.

Therapeutic strategy The treatment strategies used in CTS are the best defined of all entrapment neuropathies, but despite this there continues to be a lack of complete understanding of the natural history of CTS. Up to 20% of patients with CTS will spontaneously improve without any intervention.[1] To determine the best treatment strategy, factors such as severity and duration of symptoms and the impact on the patient's function should be considered. Although Edx testing will often not correlate with symptom severity, Edx grading can be helpful in guiding treatment strategies. For most patients with mild or moderate median neuropathy on nerve conduction studies, a trial of conservative treatment should be attempted before aggressive strategies (**Fig. 2**). If significant median nerve injury is evident, early surgical intervention should

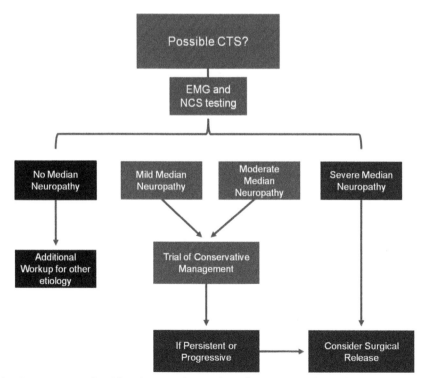

Fig. 2. Treatment algorithm for carpal tunnel syndrome using electrodiagnostic severity grading.

be considered to prevent further injury. Despite a lack of data to support or refute whether activity modification will modify the natural history of CTS, avoiding aggravating activities is reasonable and may be recommended. Wrist splints are an appropriate first-line treatment in all patients, excluding those with severe median neuropathy. Splints can be effective in up to 60% of patients and do not involve any risk.[20] Splints should be designed to maintain neutral wrist position and worn at night. There is no additional benefit derived from custom-designed splints or from daytime wear. Other conservative treatments (**Table 2**) such as injected steroids are effective and provide established, but usually temporary, relief.[21–23]

If a trial of conservative treatment is not effective, surgical intervention may be considered. Surgical intervention is the only definitive treatment in CTS that has been shown to provide lasting relief. Thus patient preference should weigh heavily on the decision to pursue surgery. In patients with persistent or severe CTS, surgical intervention using open or endoscopic techniques should be considered.[24,25] Surgical release is a safe and effective treatment. Although uncommon, failure to improve may occur because of persistent median nerve injury not reversible by decompression in severe or chronic cases, misdiagnosis, incomplete correction of compressive lesion, or delayed recurrent compression caused by local fibrosis.

CTS in certain clinical settings requires special consideration when determining the best management strategy. In untreated thyroid disease, pregnancy, or acromegaly, all of which may predispose or exacerbate symptoms of CTS, a trial of conservative management should be attempted while the underlying systemic condition is treated before proceeding with aggressive treatment measures.[26–28] Peripheral neuropathy is a risk factor for the development of CTS, but in cases of typical CTS superimposed on neuropathy, management should be similar to that for isolated CTS.[29] Hereditary neuropathy with predisposition to pressure palsy (HNPP) is an uncommon but important example of a generalized susceptibility of peripheral nerve compression that deserves special consideration in the management of entrapment neuropathy. HNPP is related to a PMP22 deletion, or rarely a point mutation, on chromosome 17p11.2-12 that usually leads to recurrent peripheral nerve compression syndromes at common sites of entrapment, with or without an underlying generalized neuropathy. In such individuals conservative management with ergonomic and activity modification is appropriate in most cases, but rarely cautious surgical intervention may be helpful in avoiding additional nerve compromise.[30,31]

Determining the most appropriate treatment of proximal median nerve compression syndromes is more challenging because of ill-defined syndromes. For pronator syndrome, conservative management includes avoidance of exacerbating activities and injection of the pronator teres muscle with local anesthetic agents and corticosteroids. Surgical intervention with pronator release should only be considered for severe, persistent symptoms in patients with a definite diagnosis.

Ulnar Nerve

Anatomy

The ulnar nerve originates from the lower trunk and medial cord of the brachial plexus. It is formed by sensory and motor axon contributions from the ventral roots of spinal nerves C8 and T1. The ulnar nerve supplies no sensory or motor innervation above the elbow. Within the forearm the ulnar nerve innervates the flexor carpi ulnaris and flexor digitorum profundus to digits 4 and 5. There are 2 sensory branches of the ulnar nerve that occur within the forearm. The palmar cutaneous nerve, which supplies sensation to the hypothenar region, leaves the ulnar nerve at the mid forearm and passes superficial to the Guyon canal. The dorsal ulnar cutaneous sensory nerve branches in the

Table 2
Treatment options for carpal tunnel syndrome

Type of Intervention	Delivery	Mechanism	Benefit	Risks
Nonsurgical				
Neutral wrist splints	Nighttime wear for at least 6 wk, indefinite if effective	Limit increased pressure within the carpal tunnel	Short-term benefit	Minimal
Injected corticosteroids	10–20 mg methylprednisolone or 10–20 mg triamcinolone acetonide	Reduced swelling within the carpal tunnel	Short-term benefit	Worsening symptoms, inadvertent median nerve injection, or infection
Oral corticosteroids	Prednisone 20 mg daily × 7 d, then 10 mg daily × 7 d	Reduced swelling within the carpal tunnel	Short-term benefit; less effective than injection	Systemic side effects
Ultrasound	Various treatment protocols	Increased cell permeability to promote healing	Mixed results; sustained therapy potentially more beneficial	Minimal
Surgical				
Carpal tunnel release	Open or endoscopic	Reduced pressure within the carpal tunnel	Definitive treatment-only treatment effective long term	Injury to vital structures, infection, persistent or worsening pain

distal forearm to supply the dorsal aspect of the medial hand, medial aspect of the fourth digit finger, and the dorsal aspect of the fifth digit. Entering the hand, the ulnar nerve passes through the Guyon canal and splits into 2 terminal branches. The superficial terminal branch supplies motor innervation to palmaris brevis and sensation to the distal medial palm and the palmar surfaces of the small finger, and the medial half of the ring finger. The deep terminal branch is a pure motor branch supplying motor innervation to the hypothenar, interossei, the third and fourth lumbrical, and adductor pollicis muscles.

Ulnar neuropathy

Ulnar nerve compression most commonly occurs in the region of the elbow, and ulnar neuropathy at the elbow (UNE) is the second most common entrapment neuropathy. Because of anatomic factors, UNE may occur in the setting of chronic entrapment or acute compression.

UNE usually occurs at the condylar groove and less frequently within the cubital tunnel. Compression at the condylar groove frequently occurs because of the superficial location and minimal protection of the ulnar nerve at this site. With compression at the cubital tunnel, known as cubital tunnel syndrome, the ulnar nerve is usually compressed 1.5 to 3 cm distal to the epicondyle. Tardy ulnar palsy, first described in 1878, involves the development of ulnar neuropathy owing to structural changes at the elbow following a remote fracture of the distal humerus.[32] UNE may occur more acutely in relation to trauma or positioning, and it is the most common focal neuropathy reported during general anesthesia for surgery.[33]

Less commonly, the ulnar nerve may also be compressed at the wrist. Ulnar neuropathy at the wrist (UNW) is usually classified according to which of the distal branches are involved.[34] Type I involves compression proximal to the Guyon canal leading to involvement of the superficial sensory, hypothenar motor, and deep motor branches. Type II involves compression within the canal, with involvement of only the superficial sensory branch. Type III involves compression distal to the superficial sensory branch, with compression of the hypothenar and the deep motor branch. Type IV involves compression distal to the superficial sensory and hypothenar motor branches, and involves only the deep motor branch. Type V involves compression of the deep motor branch just proximal to the branches to the adductor pollicis and first dorsal interosseous muscles.

Typically UNE is associated with sensory loss and paresthesia, initially intermittent, of the medial hand, dorsal and palmar aspects, and the medial half of the fourth and the fifth digit. In mild or early UNE, similar to CTS, the sensory examination may be normal. Patients may complain of an ache-like pain at the elbow, and will often self-report a Tinel phenomenon of the ulnar nerve at the elbow in the region of the ulnar groove. If UNE is severe, motor axon loss may occur and lead to weakness of all ulnar innervated muscles usually affecting the distal muscles more severely.[35] Occasionally some patients with UNE will lack prominent sensory symptoms, and present with significant weakness and atrophy. Whether or not sensation of the dorsal medial hand is involved can help localize ulnar neuropathy (always spared in UNW), but some patients with definite UNE will have sparing of sensation of the dorsal hand. This presentation can lead to significant diagnostic confusion, and has been attributed to relative sparing of dorsal ulnar cutaneous nerve fascicles versus a recently described anatomic variant in which the dorsal ulnar cutaneous nerve travels with the superficial radial nerve.[36]

There are several special tests or signs that have been described for the diagnosis of ulnar neuropathy. Though useful, these only supplement the detailed examination of individual muscles of the upper limb in the patient with a suspected peripheral nerve injury or entrapment.

The Wartenberg sign is an abduction of the fifth digit caused by weakness of the third palmar interosseous muscle (**Fig. 3**A). The Froment sign is a classically described sign of weakness of adductor pollicis, flexor pollicis brevis, and first dorsal interosseous muscles leading to functional substitution of flexor pollicis longus (**Fig. 3**B). The ulnar claw hand, or Duchenne sign, is the clawing of the fourth and fifth digits. It is worth mentioning that the ulnar claw hand may be confused with the hand of benediction seen in a severe proximal median nerve injury. In the hand of benediction, the thumb, index, and middle fingers fail to flex when the patient tries to make a fist, but by contrast, the ring and small finger fail to fully extend in the patient with an ulnar claw hand.

Diagnostic modalities Edx studies are the diagnostic test of choice in ulnar neuropathy. Most patients with ulnar neuropathy should undergo testing to confirm the presence of ulnar neuropathy, determine the severity, and to exclude other mimicking conditions, in particular disorders such as C8 radiculopathy or lower trunk/medial cord brachial plexopathy. The diagnostic sensitivity of Edx in ulnar neuropathy is approximately 80%. Similar to the median nerve, ultrasonography may be used to image the ulnar nerve to identify evidence of compression and occasionally identify the structural lesion predisposing to the development of neuropathy. While Edx continues to be the gold standard of diagnosis for ulnar neuropathy, ultrasonography may occasionally confirm cases with normal Edx results.[37] Other imaging modalities should also be used in cases with clinically apparent malalignment or a history of traumatic osseous injury (tardy ulnar palsy).

Therapeutic strategy All patients with ulnar neuropathy should be educated regarding the basic path of the ulnar nerve at the elbow and wrist, and should be instructed on ways to avoid excessive pressure or compression on the ulnar nerve. Treatment strategies are broadly grouped into either conservative (aimed at reducing mechanical pressure on the nerve) or surgical intervention. Most patients with UNE will improve

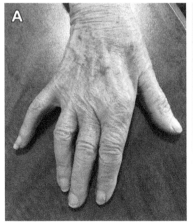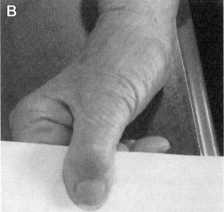

Fig. 3. Wartenberg sign (*A*) and Froment sign (*B*) during active thumb adduction in a patient with ulnar neuropathy at the elbow, as well as significant intrinsic hand weakness and atrophy.

with only conservative measures.[38,39] Conservative treatment measures include life-style modification to avoid increased pressure on the ulnar nerve, wearing external padding to reduce pressure at the elbow, and sleeping with straight elbows with or without the assistance of splinting.

Initial conservative therapeutic measures are appropriate for patients with mild (manual muscle testing of intrinsic hand muscles equal to grade 4 or greater) or no weakness, unless there is evidence for a structural abnormality at the elbow.[40] Patients with weakness evident on examination, even if mild, should be followed closely for signs of progression. Surgical intervention should be considered in patients who experience progression of weakness despite conservative management. Initial surgical management should be considered for patients with significant motor weakness or patients with persistent or progressive symptoms despite conservative treatment. One important exception is the patient who presents with an abrupt onset of UNE associated with findings of prominent ulnar motor conduction block (>50%) on Edx testing, in which case conservative management may be reasonable.[41] If necessary, there is a variety of surgical approaches beyond the scope of this article that may be used for ulnar neuropathy at the elbow, including medial epicondylectomy, cubital tunnel decompression, and ulnar nerve transposition. In general, the most minimal surgical approach that will address any structural or anatomic concerns should be used.

True entrapment neuropathy of UNW is uncommon; usually UNW occurs in the setting of acute or subacute compression. Typically patients will be able to describe an antecedent trauma preceding the onset of numbness or motor symptoms. Ulnar neuropathy at the wrist is also known as cyclist's palsy, owing to the incidence of UNW in cyclists in relation to trauma at the wrist from the handlebars. Occasionally a structural lesion (ie, ganglion cyst) may predispose an individual to the development of true ulnar nerve entrapment at the wrist and, if no clear history of trauma can be identified, evaluation for a structural lesion should be considered. Surgery is not indicated in most cases of UNW if there is no clear structural compression of the nerve.

Radial Nerve

Anatomy

The radial nerve originates from the posterior cord of the brachial plexus and is formed from fibers of the ventral roots of spinal nerves C5-T1. It provides motor innervation of the dorsal arm muscles (triceps brachii and anconeus) and muscles of the extensor compartment of the forearm as well as sensory innervation of the dorsal aspects of the thumb, index, and middle fingers and the dorsal lateral portion of the hand. There are several potential sites of compression along the path of the radial nerve, including compression at the intermuscular septum between the triceps and brachialis muscles at the level of the spiral groove (radial nerve), at the ligament of Frohse (posterior interosseous or deep radial nerve), between the heads of the supinator muscle (posterior interosseous), and under the edge of the brachioradialis muscle (superficial sensory branch of the radial nerve).

Radial neuropathy

Radial neuropathy is the third most common neuropathy of the upper limb. Whereas true entrapment of the radial nerve is very rare, subacute or acute compression of the radial nerve is more common. Acute compression at the spiral groove, the so-called Saturday night palsy, is the most common presentation of radial neuropathy. As the name implies, patients usually awaken with symptoms of weakness in radial innervated muscles sparing the triceps, sensory changes in the distribution of the radial nerve, and sometimes pain at the site of compression. Saturday night palsy is not, strictly speaking, an entrapment neuropathy but rather an acute or subacute compression neuropathy. In most cases this is a self-limited process with a good prognosis.[42–44]

Other focal compression–related radial neuropathies may occur at the elbow, forearm, and wrist. Syndromes involving the posterior interosseous nerve at the elbow include posterior interosseous nerve syndrome or radial tunnel syndrome, which are often considered the same entity. Radial tunnel syndrome is distinguished by the distinct lack of weakness. Of importance is that neuralgic amyotrophy has a particular predilection for the posterior interosseous nerve, and the clinical presentation of neuralgic amyotrophy and posterior interosseous nerve syndrome have significant overlap. The clinical presentation of posterior interosseous nerve syndrome may be associated with severe weakness, but cheiralgia paresthetica or Wartenberg syndrome describes the clinical syndrome of numbness and pain at the dorsal lateral hand and thumb, index, and middle fingers, associated with compression of the superficial radial nerve at the lateral wrist. This condition is usually the result of extrinsic compression such as an overly tight wristwatch or handcuffs. Thus the syndrome is sometimes referred to as handcuff palsy or wristwatch palsy.

Diagnostic modalities Diagnosis and localization can often be determined on a clinical basis alone. Edx testing is usually used to confirm the diagnosis of radial neuropathy and the location of injury while excluding mimicking conditions, in particular C7 radiculopathy, posterior cord plexopathy, or other less common disorders with predilection to radial nerve involvement such as multifocal motor neuropathy with conduction block. In addition to routine screening, Edx testing protocols usually involve electromyography (EMG) of radial innervated muscles and nerve-conduction study assessment of the radial sensory and motor nerve responses. In radial neuropathy at the spiral groove, features of neuropraxia are usually prominent, with conduction block and focal slowing at the site of compression. The radial sensory amplitude is often preserved, consistent with less prominent axonal loss. Most patients will have features of some axonal loss on needle-electrode examination, but this does not necessarily portend a poor prognosis.[43] Testing of nonradial nerves and nonradial innervated muscles should be performed to exclude a more generalized process. Ultrasonography has shown promise in focal neuropathies of the radial nerve attributable to compression, entrapment, and trauma.[45]

Therapeutic strategy Treatment of radial neuropathy is usually conservative, and surgical intervention is infrequently indicated or necessary (**Table 3**). After a neuropraxic injury typical of simple compression, essentially all patients will have complete recovery although some patients may not recover for up to 6 months. For a radial neuropathy at the spiral groove, supportive bracing of the wrist and finger extensors is helpful. For high radial neuropathies, bracing with static wrist extension with dynamic finger extension of the proximal phalanges will increase a patient's functional ability until nerve recovery.

Short-term immobilization to limit elbow extension, pronation of the forearm, and wrist flexion are appropriate for radial tunnel syndrome. Local steroid injection carefully directed to the site of local tenderness may be helpful.[46] Surgery is controversial and is rarely indicated. It may be helpful in select cases, but suboptimal outcomes are common with surgical intervention.[47] In posterior interosseous nerve syndrome a wrist-extension brace is appropriate if weakness is severe. Cheiralgia paresthetica

Table 3
Sites of radial nerve compression

Nerve/Site	Syndrome(s)	Mechanism	Treatment
Radial nerve at the spiral groove	Saturday night palsy	Usually extrinsic compression at the spiral groove, often during sleep or sedation	Supportive: wrist and finger extension bracing
Posterior interosseous (PIN)	PIN syndrome Radial tunnel syndrome	Poorly defined and controversial syndromes Arcade of Frohse, supinator muscle, and tendinous margin of extensor carpi radialis brevis	Avoidance of provoking activities Local steroid injection if persistent Rarely surgical release
Superficial radial sensory at the lateral wrist	Wartenberg syndrome (cheiralgia paresthetica)	Usually extrinsic compression	Supportive, remove external compression Local steroid injection if persistent Rarely neurolysis

usually responds to conservative treatment with removal of external compression. Occasionally local steroid injection dorsal to the first extensor compartment may be needed. Neurolysis of the superficial radial nerve is rarely indicated, but may be helpful in up to 80% of patients with symptoms that persist despite conservative management.[48]

DIAGNOSTIC APPROACH TO AND MANAGEMENT OF LOWER LIMB FOCAL NEUROPATHIES
Lateral Femoral Cutaneous Nerve (Lateral Cutaneous Nerve of the Thigh)

Anatomy
The lateral femoral cutaneous (LFC) nerve is a pure sensory nerve that arises from the dorsal divisions of the ventral primary rami of the L2-L3 spinal nerves. The nerve penetrates the psoas muscle and emerges along its lateral border, travels along the lateral aspect of the pelvis, and passes under the inguinal ligament approximately 1 cm medial to the anterior superior iliac spine to enter the thigh.[49] It supplies sensation to the skin over the anterior and lateral portion of the thigh.

Meralgia paresthetica
Meralgia paresthetica (MP), a Greek word denoting thigh pain, refers to the syndrome of numbness, paresthesia, and pain associated with LFC mononeuropathy. It occurs more frequently than previously proposed, with an incidence of 36.2 per 100,000 patient-years in a recent United States population–based study.[50] The incidence is highest in obese patients in their fourth to sixth decades; mean age at diagnosis is 50 years, with no gender predilection. The adjusted incidence among diabetic is 7-fold greater in comparison with the general population.[40]

MP is usually caused by compression of the LFC nerve as it passes under the lateral portion of the inguinal ligament. The condition is often idiopathic; however, described predisposing factors related to compression may include a large abdomen (pregnancy, obesity, or ascites), external compression from tight clothing or belts, or prolonged positioning (lithotomy positioning, cycling, or prolonged hip extension).[51] Other mechanisms of injury have been described, including injury during local surgery such as hip surgery, aortofemoral bypass, and cesarean section; direct trauma related to seat-belt injury; and malignant invasion.[52] Rarely, proximal injury in the pelvis related to psoas hemorrhage or other abnormalities is described.

Typically patients present with pain, numbness, and paresthesia in the lateral and or anterior aspect of the thigh. The distribution of symptoms may vary between patients, but the lateral aspect of the thigh is solely involved in the majority.[52] The pain onset is generally subacute and bears no relation to positioning, standing, or walking.[50] MP is usually unilateral, although bilateral presentation is occasionally described. The LFC nerve is a purely sensory nerve,[53] so no motor signs or symptoms are present. Early during MP or in patients with mild symptoms, examination may be normal. With increasing severity, sensory loss is present and may involve all or only part of the classically described distribution of the LFC nerve. Despite the reduced sensation, there is often skin hypersensitivity to touch. Otherwise the neurologic examination is normal. Reflexes, most importantly the patellar reflex, remain intact. Motor muscle weakness is characteristically absent, and if present other mimicking conditions such as upper lumbar radiculopathy, lumbar plexopathy, or femoral neuropathy are more likely.[54]

Diagnostic modalities The diagnosis of MP is usually a clinical one, supported by the characteristic distribution of pain and sensory changes on examination and the absence of motor or reflex abnormalities. Diagnostic investigations are, as a rule, only necessary in atypical cases. In this instance, imaging studies, EMG, and nerve conduction studies are helpful in excluding mimicking conditions. Nerve conduction studies to confirm LFC neuropathy can be unreliably present in healthy individuals, and are increasingly difficult to perform in the obese patient. However, a recent study using ultrasound-guided electrode placement in LFC sensory nerve studies revealed higher yield with less interside variability, including in obese subjects.[55] Diagnostic injections at the common site of entrapment can be helpful in confirming the diagnosis if clear relief of symptoms is provided. Imaging modalities may include MRI and ultrasonography.

Therapeutic strategy The symptoms of MP usually improve spontaneously within weeks to months. Therefore, conservative treatment should be encouraged. Conservative treatments should include removing sources of extrinsic compression such as compressive clothing or provocative postures. Weight loss should be encouraged in obese patients. In patients with persistent symptoms, neuropathic pain medications may be helpful for symptomatic management. In cases that do not respond with time and to conservative measures, steroid injection and surgery are considerations. A Cochrane review concluded that despite the lack of randomized controlled trials, there are high-quality observational studies reporting comparable high improvement rates for MP following local injection of corticosteroid and surgical interventions (either nerve decompression or neurectomy).[56]

Infiltration with local anesthetic and steroids may provide temporary relief and can be repeated at intervals. The use of ultrasound guidance is helpful.[57] Surgery is usually a last resort and is rarely needed for patients with severe refractory symptoms who are not responding to the aforementioned measures. Surgical interventions (decompression or sectioning) are reported to be effective in about 76% to 80% of cases.

Tibial Nerve

Anatomy

The tibial nerve, composed of L4, L5, S1, and S2 nerve roots, courses through the lumbosacral plexus and through the thigh within the sciatic nerve, along with the peroneal component. The sciatic nerve divides into the peroneal and tibial nerves proximal to the popliteal fossa. In the thigh, the tibial component of the sciatic nerve supplies all the hamstrings' muscles and half of the adductor magnus. In the popliteal fossa, it gives a medial sural cutaneous branch to form the sural nerve with contribution from the lateral sural cutaneous branch of the peroneal nerve. In the leg, the tibial nerve travels within the posterior compartment of the leg innervating all of the posterior compartment muscles. At the ankle, it gives a calcaneal branch and passes posterior to the medial malleolus through the tarsal tunnel, dividing into the medial and lateral plantar nerves.

Tarsal tunnel syndrome

Tarsal tunnel is a rare syndrome related to compression of the tibial nerve at the level of the tarsal tunnel. Despite the agreement on its existence, there is controversy regarding its prevalence. The tarsal tunnel is a fibro-osseous space, formed by the flexor retinaculum posterior and distal to the medial malleolus. The contents of the tarsal tunnel include the tibial nerve; posterior tibial artery and vein; and the tendons from the tibialis posterior, flexor digitorum longus, and flexor hallucis longus muscles. Contributing factors of tarsal tunnel syndrome include ankle sprain and fracture; tight-fitting footwear and other biomechanical issues such as joint hypermobility; and space-occupying lesions. In some cases it is idiopathic.

Symptoms of tarsal tunnel syndrome may include ankle pain and associated numbness, tingling, burning, and pain in the sole of the foot. The symptoms commonly worsen with weight bearing and at night. The presentation of tarsal tunnel syndrome may be variable; the entire tibial nerve may be involved, or there may be selective involvement of either the lateral or medial plantar branches. Findings on examination are typically few. The development of weakness or atrophy of the intrinsic foot muscles usually goes unnoticed because of its minimal functional implications. However, careful examination and comparison with the other foot, if findings are unilateral, can be helpful. Decreased sensation usually involves the sole of the foot sparing the heel, which is supplied by the calcaneal branch. There may be tenderness behind the medial malleolus and a positive Tinel sign over the tarsal tunnel.[58]

Diagnostic modalities Tarsal tunnel syndrome should be differentiated from other mimicking conditions including other neuropathic processes such as small fiber peripheral neuropathy or radiculopathy, particularly S1 radiculopathy.[59] Common musculoskeletal mimicking conditions include posterior tibial tendon dysfunction, plantar fasciitis, and plantar callosities. Tarsal tunnel syndrome is typically a clinical diagnosis supported by Edx findings. Nerve conduction studies may help to localize the lesion and to exclude mimicking conditions.[60–62] Imaging studies provide information helpful in excluding structural or space-occupying lesions.[63,64] Diagnosis is reasonably secured if a patient has typical foot pain and paresthesia, and a Tinel sign at the tarsal tunnel, and if classic Edx findings are present.[65]

Therapeutic strategy Individuals without a contributing structural or space-occupying lesion may respond adequately to conservative management, which may include nonsteroidal anti-inflammatories, neuropathic pain medications, activity modification, physical therapy, and biomechanical modification with shoes, inserts, or orthoses.[66]

Surgery is reserved for individuals with a definite diagnosis who have been resistant to conservative strategies.

Proximal tibial neuropathy
Entrapment of the tibial nerve proximal to the tarsal tunnel is rare. However, association with a Baker cyst, popliteal artery aneurysm, nerve sheath tumor and other mass lesions, and direct trauma has been described. In addition to the sensory loss at the sole of the foot, lateral-leg patients commonly present with weakness of the plantar flexion and inversion. Edx studies and imaging help to establish the diagnosis and identify the structural cause. Surgery is usually indicated in this setting for resection of the mass lesion.

Peroneal (Fibular) Nerve

Anatomy
The peroneal nerve is composed of the L4, L5, and S1 nerve roots, and travels through the lumbosacral plexus into the sciatic nerve alongside the tibial nerve component. The peroneal and tibial components of the sciatic nerve are divided by a connective tissue sheath, and proximal to the popliteal fossa the sciatic nerve separates into the peroneal and tibial nerves. In the thigh, the peroneal component of the sciatic nerve innervates only one muscle proximal to the knee, the short head of the biceps. After the peroneal nerve separate from the sciatic nerve it gives off the lateral cutaneous nerve of the calf, in the popliteal fossa, supplying sensation of the lateral upper leg. Thereafter, it travels around the fibular head and separates into the superficial and deep peroneal nerves. The superficial branch innervates the ankle everters and continues as the superficial peroneal sensory nerve supplying the lateral aspects of the lower leg and foot. The deep peroneal nerve runs into the anterior leg compartment and innervates the ankle dorsiflexors and toe extensors, and its terminal branch supplies sensation to the first dorsal web space.

Common peroneal neuropathy at the fibular head
Peroneal neuropathy at the fibular head is the most common compression mononeuropathy to affect the lower limbs. The superficial location of the nerve as it travels laterally around the fibular head makes it susceptible to compression. The mechanism of injury is typically related to external compression of the nerve against the fibula, in contrast to compression occurring between anatomic structures. Compression can occur with improper positioning during surgery, habitual leg crossing, squatting, tight-fitting casts, and compressive stockings. Other possible causes of common peroneal neuropathy may include Baker cyst, other mass lesions, tumors, knee surgeries, and direct trauma. Loss of fat pad surrounding the nerve at the fibular head is proposed to increase the risk of compression in patients with thin body habitus or following significant weight loss. Furthermore, common peroneal neuropathy can occur in association with noncompressive causes such as diabetes and vasculitis. In patients with common peroneal neuropathy, the deep peroneal fascicle is usually more affected than the superficial fascicle. Moreover, isolated deep peroneal injury is described in the setting of knee surgery, trauma, and anterior compartment syndrome.

Patients usually present with tripping, difficulty negotiating curbs, or gait change related to foot drop. Overall sensory symptoms tend to be minimal, with pain reported in 17%[67]; it is bilateral in 10% of patients.[67] A complete lesion of common peroneal neuropathy produces weakness in toe extension, foot eversion, and ankle dorsiflexion associated with sensory loss on the anterior lateral surface of the lower leg and dorsum of the foot. With a lesion at the fibular head there is sparing of the proximal anterior lateral leg related to the preserved lateral cutaneous nerve of the calf, which branches in the lateral popliteal fossa. A positive Tinel sign at the fibular head may be seen.

Diagnostic modalities Common peroneal neuropathy should be differentiated from mimicking conditions, mainly L5 radiculopathy, but other mimicking conditions may include sciatic neuropathy, motor neuron disease, and lumbosacral plexopathy. Preservation of ankle inversion is a feature of peroneal neuropathy that helps to distinguish it from L5 radiculopathy. Edx studies help to establish the diagnosis and exclude mimickers.[68] Imaging using ultrasonography or MRI helps as an adjunct to Edx studies and, most importantly, to identify patients with intraneural ganglia of the nerve,[69–71] which is a treatable but underreported cause of common peroneal neuropathy[72] caused by dissection of the synovial fluid along the nerve resulting from superior tibio-fibular joint capsular disruption.

Therapeutic strategy Patients usually respond to conservative treatment with avoidance of precipitating factors. In patients with severe foot drop, use of an ankle-foot orthosis should be considered for improvement of gait. Surgical treatment of peroneal intraneural ganglia has been associated with halted progression of neuropathy and improved clinical outcomes.

Peroneal neuropathy at the ankle

Deep peroneal nerve entrapment is sometimes referred to as anterior tarsal tunnel syndrome. There is disagreement regarding the use of this term, owing to the lack of a clearly defined fibro-osseous tunnel. Deep peroneal nerve compression may be acute, as in a traumatic injury, or related to chronic external pressure such as in relation to ill-fitting footwear. Patients present with pain on the dorsum of the foot and numbness in the first dorsal web. Diagnosis can be established by Edx studies. Treatment is usually conservative.

SUMMARY

Entrapment neuropathy is a frequent clinical problem with a significant impact on society. Effective management relies on a precise diagnosis and consideration of the underlying process when designing the treatment plan. In most cases of compressive neuropathies, such as radial neuropathy at the spiral groove or peroneal neuropathy at the fibular head, removal of the offending compression and supportive care is sufficient. However, in chronic compression (entrapment) more aggressive management and sometimes surgical release may be necessary for good treatment outcomes.

Case study

A 65-year-old woman presented with a 3-month history of right-hand numbness, grip weakness, and vague elbow pain. Examination demonstrated diminished sensation of the medial hand and fourth and fifth digits, and weakness in the ulnar innervated muscles associated with intrinsic hand muscle atrophy. Froment and Wartenberg signs were evident (see **Fig. 3**). There were no signs of malalignment of the elbow or subluxation of the ulnar nerve.

Electrodiagnostic testing confirmed UNE. The patient opted for initial conservative management including avoiding extrinsic compression of the ulnar nerve and a nocturnal splinting to encourage straight arm posture. Despite these measures, the patient experienced progressive symptoms of weakness. Surgical consultation was recommended. The patient underwent a medial epicondylectomy, and experienced resolution of pain and partial improvement in sensory loss and weakness.

REFERENCES

1. Padua L, Padua R, Aprile I, et al, Italian CTS Study Group. Multiperspective follow-up of untreated carpal tunnel syndrome: a multicenter study. Neurology 2001;56(11):1459–66.
2. Bland JD. Treatment of carpal tunnel syndrome. Muscle Nerve 2007;36(2): 167–71.
3. Saperstein DS, Katz JS, Amato AA, et al. Clinical spectrum of chronic acquired demyelinating polyneuropathies. Muscle Nerve 2001;24(3):311–24.
4. Kozin SH. The anatomy of the recurrent branch of the median nerve. J Hand Surg Am 1998;23(5):852–8.
5. Atroshi I, Gummesson C, Johnsson R, et al. Prevalence of carpal tunnel syndrome in a general population. JAMA 1999;282(2):153–8.
6. Keir PJ, Rempel DM. Pathomechanics of peripheral nerve loading. Evidence in carpal tunnel syndrome. J Hand Ther 2005;18(2):259–69.
7. Mackinnon SE, Dellon AL, Hudson AR, et al. Chronic nerve compression—an experimental model in the rat. Ann Plast Surg 1984;13(2):112–20.
8. Mackinnon SE, Dellon AL, Hudson AR, et al. Chronic human nerve compression—a histological assessment. Neuropathol Appl Neurobiol 1986;12(6):547–65.
9. Hess H, Baumann F. On the familial occurrence of bilateral carpal tunnel syndrome. Zeitschrift fur Orthopadie und Ihre Grenzgebiete 1969;106(3):565–9 [in German].
10. Elstner M, Bettecken T, Wasner M, et al. Familial carpal tunnel syndrome: further evidence for a genetic contribution. Clin Genet 2006;69(2):179–82.
11. Centers for Disease Control (CDC). Occupational disease surveillance: carpal tunnel syndrome. MMWR Morb Mortal Wkly Rep 1989;38(28):485–9.
12. Schnetzler KA. Acute carpal tunnel syndrome. J Am Acad Orthop Surg 2008; 16(5):276–82.
13. Atcheson SG, Ward JR, Lowe W. Concurrent medical disease in work-related carpal tunnel syndrome. Arch Intern Med 1998;158(14):1506–12.
14. Palmer KT, Harris EC, Coggon D. Carpal tunnel syndrome and its relation to occupation: a systematic literature review. Occup Med 2007;57(1):57–66.
15. Borg K, Lindblom U. Diagnostic value of quantitative sensory testing (QST) in carpal tunnel syndrome. Acta Neurol Scand 1988;78(6):537–41.
16. Katz JN, Larson MG, Sabra A. The carpal tunnel syndrome: diagnostic utility of the history and physical examination findings. Ann Intern Med 1990;112:321–7.
17. Kara M, Emlakcioglu E, Kaymak B, et al. Brachial neuritis mimicking severe anterior interosseous syndrome. Acta Reumatol Port 2010;35(1):114–5.
18. Jablecki CK, Andary MT, Floeter MK, et al. Practice parameter: electrodiagnostic studies in carpal tunnel syndrome. Report of the American Association of Electrodiagnostic Medicine, American Academy of Neurology, and the American Academy of Physical Medicine and Rehabilitation. Neurology 2002;58(11): 1589–92.
19. Cartwright MS, Hobson-Webb LD, Boon AJ, et al. Evidence-based guideline: neuromuscular ultrasound for the diagnosis of carpal tunnel syndrome. Muscle Nerve 2012;46(2):287–93.
20. Gerritsen AA, de Vet HC, Scholten RJ, et al. Splinting vs surgery in the treatment of carpal tunnel syndrome: a randomized controlled trial. JAMA 2002;288(10): 1245–51.
21. Herskovitz S, Berger AR, Lipton RB. Low-dose, short-term oral prednisone in the treatment of carpal tunnel syndrome. Neurology 1995;45(10):1923–5.

22. Marshall S, Tardif G, Ashworth N. Local corticosteroid injection for carpal tunnel syndrome. Cochrane Database Syst Rev 2002;(4):CD001554.
23. O'Connor D, Marshall S, Massy-Westropp N. Non-surgical treatment (other than steroid injection) for carpal tunnel syndrome. Cochrane Database Syst Rev 2003;(1):CD003219.
24. Katz JN, Keller RB, Simmons BP, et al. Maine carpal tunnel study: outcomes of operative and nonoperative therapy for carpal tunnel syndrome in a community-based cohort [Erratum appears in J Hand Surg [Am] 1999;24(1):201]. J Hand Surg Am 1998;23(4):697–710.
25. Korthals-de Bos IB, Gerritsen AA, van Tulder MW, et al. Surgery is more cost-effective than splinting for carpal tunnel syndrome in the Netherlands: results of an economic evaluation alongside a randomized controlled trial. BMC Musculoskelet Disord 2006;7:86.
26. Ablove RH, Ablove TS. Prevalence of carpal tunnel syndrome in pregnant women. WMJ 2009;108(4):194–6.
27. Jenkins PJ, Sohaib SA, Akker S, et al. The pathology of median neuropathy in acromegaly. Ann Intern Med 2000;133(3):197–201.
28. Purnell DC, Daly DD, Lipscomb PR. Carpal-tunnel syndrome associated with myxedema. Arch Intern Med 1961;108:751–6.
29. Morgenlander JC, Lynch JR, Sanders DB. Surgical treatment of carpal tunnel syndrome in patients with peripheral neuropathy. Neurology 1997;49(4):1159–63.
30. Taggart TF, Allen TR. Surgical treatment of a tomaculous neuropathy. J R Coll Surg Edinb 2001;46(4):240–1.
31. Grossman M, Feinberg J, DiCarlo E, et al. Hereditary neuropathy with liability to pressure palsies: case report and discussion. HSS J 2007;3(2):208–12.
32. Gay JR, Love JG. Diagnosis and treatment of tardy paralysis of the ulnar nerve. J Bone Joint Surg Am 1947;29:1087.
33. Alvine FG, Schurrer ME. Postoperative ulnar-nerve palsy. Are there predisposing factors? J Bone Joint Surg Am 1987;69(2):255–9.
34. Kothari MJ. Ulnar neuropathy at the wrist. Neurol Clin 1999;17(3):463–76.
35. Stewart JD. The variable clinical manifestations of ulnar neuropathies at the elbow. J Neurol Neurosurg Psychiatry 1987;50(3):252–8.
36. Leis AA, Wells KJ. Radial nerve cutaneous innervation to the ulnar dorsum of the hand. Clin Neurophysiol 2008;119(3):662–6.
37. Yoon JS, Walker FO, Cartwright MS. Ulnar neuropathy with normal electrodiagnosis and abnormal nerve ultrasound. Arch Phys Med Rehabil 2010;91(2):318–20.
38. Eisen A, Danon J. The mild cubital tunnel syndrome. Its natural history and indications for surgical intervention. Neurology 1974;24(7):608–13.
39. Padua L, Caliandro P, La Torre G, et al. Treatment for ulnar neuropathy at the elbow [Protocol]. Cochrane Database Syst Rev 2009;(1).1. http://dx.doi.org/10.1002/14651858.CD006839.
40. Stewart JE. Focal peripheral neuropathies. 4th edition. West Vancouver (Canada): JBJ Publishing; 2010.
41. Dunselman HH, Visser LH. The clinical, electrophysiological and prognostic heterogeneity of ulnar neuropathy at the elbow. J Neurol Neurosurg Psychiatry 2008;79(12):1364–7.
42. Sunderland S. Traumatic injures of peripheral nerves—simple compression injuries of the radial nerve. Brain 1945;68:56–72.
43. Arnold WD, Krishna VR, Freimer M, et al. Prognosis of acute compressive radial neuropathy. Muscle Nerve 2012;45(6):893–4.

44. Brown WF, Watson BV. AAEM case report #27: acute retrohumeral radial neuropathies. Muscle Nerve 1993;16(7):706–11.
45. Lo YL, Fook-Chong S, Leoh TH, et al. Rapid ultrasonographic diagnosis of radial entrapment neuropathy at the spiral groove. J Neurol Sci 2008;271(1–2):75–9.
46. Sarhadi NS, Korday SN, Bainbridge LC. Radial tunnel syndrome: diagnosis and management. J Hand Surg Br 1998;23(5):617–9.
47. Sotereanos DG, Varitimidis SE, Giannakopoulos PN, et al. Results of surgical treatment for radial tunnel syndrome. J Hand Surg Am 1999;24(3):566–70.
48. Stahl S, Kaufman T. Cheiralgia paresthetica—entrapment of the superficial branch of the radial nerve: a report of 15 cases. Eur J Plast Surg 1997;20(2):57–9.
49. de Ridder VA, de Lange S, Popta JV. Anatomical variations of the lateral femoral cutaneous nerve and the consequences for surgery. J Orthop Trauma 1999; 13(3):207–11.
50. Parisi TJ, Mandrekar J, Dyck PJ, et al. Meralgia paresthetica: relation to obesity, advanced age, and diabetes mellitus. Neurology 2011;77(16):1538–42.
51. Deal CL, Canoso JJ. Meralgia paresthetica and large abdomens. Ann Intern Med 1982;96(6 Pt 1):787–8.
52. Seror P, Seror R. Meralgia paresthetica: clinical and electrophysiological diagnosis in 120 cases. Muscle Nerve 2006;33(5):650–4.
53. Slobbe AM, Bohnen AM, Bernsen RM, et al. Incidence rates and determinants in meralgia paresthetica in general practice. J Neurol 2004;251(3):294–7.
54. Amrami KK, Felmlee JP, Spinner RJ. MRI of peripheral nerves. Neurosurg Clin N Am 2008;19(4):559–72.
55. Boon AJ, Bailey PW, Smith J, et al. Utility of ultrasound-guided surface electrode placement in lateral femoral cutaneous nerve conduction studies. Muscle Nerve 2011;44(4):525–30.
56. Khalil N, Nicotra A, Rakowicz W. Treatment for meralgia paraesthetica. Cochrane Database Syst Rev 2008;(3):CD004159.
57. Hurdle MF, Weingarten TN, Crisostomo RA, et al. Ultrasound-guided blockade of the lateral femoral cutaneous nerve: technical description and review of 10 cases. Arch Phys Med Rehabil 2007;88(10):1362–4.
58. Oh SJ, Meyer RD. Entrapment neuropathies of the tibial (posterior tibial) nerve. Neurol Clin 1999;17(3):593–615.
59. Fantino O, Coillard JY, Borne J, et al. Ultrasound of the tarsal tunnel: normal and pathological imaging features. J Radiol 2011;92(12):1072–80 [in French].
60. Patel AT, Gaines K, Malamut R, et al. Usefulness of electrodiagnostic techniques in the evaluation of suspected tarsal tunnel syndrome: an evidence-based review. Muscle Nerve 2005;32(2):236–40.
61. Toussaint CP, Perry Iii EC, Pisansky MT, et al. What's new in the diagnosis and treatment of peripheral nerve entrapment neuropathies. Neurol Clin 2010;28(4): 979–1004.
62. Galardi G, Amadio S, Maderna L, et al. Electrophysiologic studies in tarsal tunnel syndrome. Diagnostic reliability of motor distal latency, mixed nerve and sensory nerve conduction studies. Am J Phys Med Rehabil 1994;73(3):193–8.
63. Lopez-Ben R. Imaging of nerve entrapment in the foot and ankle. Foot Ankle Clin 2011;16(2):213–24.
64. Allen JM, Greer BJ, Sorge DG, et al. MR imaging of neuropathies of the leg, ankle, and foot. Magn Reson Imaging Clin N Am 2008;16(1):117–31.
65. Lau JT, Daniels TR. Tarsal tunnel syndrome: a review of the literature. Foot Ankle Int 1999;20(3):201–9.

66. Campbell WW, Landau ME. Controversial entrapment neuropathies. Neurosurg Clin N Am 2008;19(4):597–608.
67. BK. Peroneal neuropathy. Neurol Clin 1999;17(3):567–91.
68. Marciniak C, Armon C, Wilson J, et al. Practice parameter: utility of electrodiagnostic techniques in evaluating patients with suspected peroneal neuropathy: an evidence-based review. Muscle Nerve 2005;31(4):520–7.
69. Weig SG, Waite RJ, McAvoy K. MRI in unexplained mononeuropathy. Pediatr Neurol 2000;22(4):314–7.
70. Lo YI F, Fook-Chong S, Leoh TH, et al. High-resolution ultrasound as a diagnostic adjunct in common peroneal neuropathy. Arch Neurol 2007;64(12):1798–800.
71. Visser LH. High-resolution sonography of the common peroneal nerve: detection of intraneural ganglia. Neurology 2006;67(8):1473–5.
72. Young NP, Sorenson EJ, Spinner RJ, et al. Clinical and electrodiagnostic correlates of peroneal intraneural ganglia. Neurology 2009;72(5):447–52.

Diabetic Neuropathy Part 1
Overview and Symmetric Phenotypes

Mamatha Pasnoor, MD[a],*, Mazen M. Dimachkie, MD[a],
Patricia Kluding, PT, PhD[b], Richard J. Barohn, MD[a]

KEYWORDS

- Diabetic neuropathy • Diabetes mellitus • Pathogenesis

KEY POINTS

- Diabetic neuropathy is the most common type of neuropathy.
- Various types of neuropathies are associated with diabetes mellitus.
- Metabolic, vascular, inflammatory, and immune theories have been suggested for pathogenesis.
- Axonal and demyelination can be seen on electrophysiology and pathology.
- Treatment is mainly aimed at glycemic control and neuropathic pain management.

INTRODUCTION

Diabetes mellitus (DM) has 4 major complications: neuropathy, retinopathy, nephropathy, and vasculopathy. The various neuropathies associated with DM can clinically be divided into symmetric and asymmetric (focal and multifocal) forms (**Box 1**).[1] In addition, clinicians need to be aware of diabetic muscle infarction, a muscle disorder that can occur in diabetic patients. A practical approach to the diagnosis and management of diabetic symmetric neuropathies is discussed in this article.

EPIDEMIOLOGY

The estimated prevalence of DM in the United States in individuals 40 to 74 years old is 12% if only fasting blood sugar (FBS) criteria are used, but 14% if both FBS and glucose tolerance testing (GTT) criteria are used.[2] It is estimated that about half the adults with diabetes in the United States are undiagnosed.[3] If the population is considered, including children, DM has been reported to occur in 1% to 4%.[4] In

[a] Department of Neurology, University of Kansas Medical Center, Kansas City, KS, USA;
[b] Department of Physical Therapy and Rehabilitation Science, University of Kansas Medical Center, Kansas City, KS, USA
* Corresponding author.
E-mail address: mpasnoor@kumc.edu

Neurol Clin 31 (2013) 425–445
http://dx.doi.org/10.1016/j.ncl.2013.02.004   **neurologic.theclinics.com**

Box 1
Clinical classification of diabetic neuropathies

I. Symmetric polyneuropathies:

Fixed deficits:

    Distal sensory polyneuropathy (DSPN)

    Variants

        Acute, severe DSPN in early-onset diabetes

        Pseudosyringomyelic neuropathy

        Pseudotabetic neuropathy

    Autonomic neuropathy

Episodic symptoms:

    Diabetic neuropathic cachexia

    Hyperglycemic neuropathy

    Treatment-induced diabetic neuropathy

II. Asymmetric/focal and multifocal diabetic neuropathies:

Diabetic lumbosacral radiculoplexopathy (Bruns-Garland syndrome, diabetic amyotrophy, proximal diabetic neuropathy)

Truncal neuropathies (thoracic radiculopathy)

Cranial neuropathies

Limb mononeuropathies

---

the Rochester, Minnesota, population-based study, 1.3% of the population had DM.[4] According to the 2011 US Centers for Disease Control and Prevention National Diabetes Fact Sheet, diabetes affects 25.8 million Americans or 8.3% of the US population. That estimate includes 7 million undiagnosed cases. Among US residents aged 65 years and older, 10.9 million, or 26.9%, had diabetes in 2010. In 2005 to 2008, based on fasting glucose or hemoglobin A1c (HgbA1c) levels, 35% of US adults aged 20 years or older and 50% of adults aged 65 years or older had prediabetes, yielding an estimated 79 million American adults aged 20 years or older with prediabetes. Almost 30% of people with diabetes aged 40 years or older have impaired sensation in the feet.[5]

Approximately two-thirds of patients with insulin-dependent DM (IDDM) and non-IDDM (NIDDM) had subclinical or clinical evidence of a peripheral neuropathy. Roughly half of the diabetics had a symmetric polyneuropathy, a quarter had carpal tunnel syndrome, about 5% had autonomic neuropathy, and 1% had asymmetric proximal neuropathy. The occurrence of neuropathy correlates with the duration of DM, poor glycemic control, and with the presence of retinopathy and nephropathy.[4,6–11] In the study by Picart,[8] 7.5% of patients had neuropathy at the time of diagnosis, and, after 20 years of DM, 50% had neuropathy. Partanen and colleagues[9] showed that after 10 years of follow-up the percentage of diabetics with neuropathy increased from 8% at baseline to 42%.

DM Diagnostic Criteria

The American Diabetes Association (ADA) issued diagnostic criteria for DM in 1997,[2] with follow-up in 2003[12] and 2010.[13] The diagnosis is based on one of 4 abnormalities:

HgbA1c, fasting plasma glucose (FPG), random increased glucose with symptoms, or abnormal oral glucose tolerance test (OGTT) as follows:

1. HgbA1c greater than or equal to 6.5%. The test should be performed in a laboratory using a method certified by the National Standardization Program (NGSP) and standardized to the Diabetes Control and Complications (DCCT) assay.
2. FPG greater than or equal to 126 mg/dL (7.0 mmol/L) on repeat testing. Fasting is defined as no caloric intake for at least 8 hours.
3. Two-hour plasma glucose greater than or equal to 200 mg/dL (11.1 mmol/L) during an oral GTT. The test should be performed as described by the World Health Organization, using a glucose load containing the equivalent of 75 g anhydrous glucose dissolved in water.
4. In a patient with classic symptoms of hyperglycemia or hyperglycemic crisis, a random glucose greater than or equal to 200 mg/dL (11.1 mmol/L).

In the absence of unequivocal hyperglycemia, criteria 1 to 3 should be confirmed by repeat testing.

In evaluating a patient with a neuropathy, it is not sufficient to stop with the FBS in excluding DM. Although the new criteria allow for the use of HgbA1c as sufficient to diagnose DM, we still usually recommend OGTT in patients who are evaluated for neuropathy to consider DM as a potential cause.

Pathogenesis of Diabetic Neuropathy

The pathologic basis for diabetic neuropathy remains controversial in spite of the research efforts. There is evidence that both vascular and metabolic derangements may be responsible for peripheral nerve disorders in diabetes.[14–21] An overview of these mechanisms is helpful in approaching the different clinical presentations of diabetic neuropathies and in understanding the various experimental therapeutic trials. A simplified pathophysiologic scheme would primarily attribute the focal and multifocal neuropathies to a vascular basis, and the symmetric polyneuropathies to a metabolic disorder. However, we think that there is a spectrum of possible pathophysiologic cause of various diabetic neuropathies and evidence for either vascular or metabolic dysfunction is not restricted to a particular neuropathy (**Fig. 1**).[22–26]

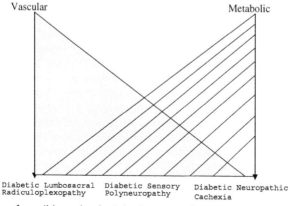

Fig. 1. Spectrum of possible pathophysiologic causes of various diabetic neuropathies.

Metabolic pathogenesis

Experimental models of acute, severe hyperglycemia can produce reduction in nerve conduction velocity and axonal shrinkage.[27] Glucose and myoinositol share a structural similarity and hyperglycemia may reduce myoinositol uptake in diabetic nerves. This reduction secondarily impairs the function of membrane-bound sodium/potassium ATPase, which can cause axoglial changes and alterations of conduction velocity.[28] However, in nerves from diabetic patients, endoneurial myoinositol was not decreased and, in 2 clinical trials, there was no benefit to patients from myoinositol supplementation.[29–32]

Another popular mechanism is an alteration of polyol metabolism. Persistent hyperglycemia activates the enzyme aldose reductase, thereby converting glucose to the polyol, sorbitol, and ultimately to fructose. Sorbitol, a compound with a degree of impermeability, accumulates in the nerve creating a hypertonic condition and subsequent water accumulation.

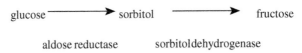

The accumulation of sorbitol and fructose increases the distance between capillaries, producing endoneurial hypoxia and oxidative stress. Aldose reductase inhibitors in animal models decrease sorbitol concentration in the sciatic nerve and restore conduction velocities to normal. In addition, protection from sorbitol increase in experimental diabetes using aldose reductase inhibitors prevents the loss of myoinositol from the nerve, which may connect 2 possible pathogenic mechanisms.[33]

Alterations of fatty acid metabolism can result from chronic hyperglycemia. In experimental diabetes there is a deficiency of gamma-linolenic acid that could lead to abnormalities in endoneurial blood flow through secondary deficiencies in arachidonic acid and prostaglandins.[34] This finding has led to clinical trials of diets enriched in linolenic acid.[35,36]

Chronic hyperglycemia increases glycosylation of proteins.[37–39] Glycation products can accumulate in tissues, producing microvascular disease by direct deposition on endothelial cell membranes or the generation of reactive oxygen species, which adds to oxidative stress.[40] Aminoguanidine, an inhibitor of advanced glycation, has been used in experimental animal models of diabetes and is currently being studied in humans.[41]

Vascular pathogenesis

It has been postulated that hypoxia or ischemia is involved in diabetic polyneuropathy.[16,42–47] The ultrastructural studies of Dyck and colleagues[44–46] have shown that the increase in basement membrane area and endothelial cell degeneration is associated with severity of polyneuropathy. On a more macroscopic level, the study of the distribution of fiber loss in diabetic nerves also suggests a vascular disorder.[20,48–50] In the study by Dyck and colleagues,[50] the multifocal pattern of fiber loss could still be identified in the sural nerve. Johnson and colleagues[20] identified changes in the perineurium and surrounding epineurium that resembled those seen in peripheral nerve vasculitis. Although these ultrastructural vessel changes could account for these ischemic morphologic features, there is evidence that chronic hyperglycemia may produce hypoxia or frank ischemia.[47,51,52]

Autopsy material from patients with diabetic cranial third nerve palsy reveals central fascicular injury suggesting ischemia.[53–55] Even diabetic patients who never experienced third nerve palsy show microfasciculation on autopsy compared with controls.[56] An autopsy study in diabetic asymmetric proximal lower extremity neuropathy by Raff and colleagues[57,58] showed ischemic infarcts of the proximal major nerve trunks of the leg and lumbosacral plexus with multiple areas of decreased myelinated fiber density at these levels. Said and colleagues[59,60] biopsied the cutaneous nerve of the thigh in patients with this disorder and showed asymmetric fasicular loss in some patients. In a study of sural nerve biopsies from patients with diabetic lumbosacral radiculoplexopathy, there was multifocal variability in nerve fiber density with nonrandom fiber loss between and within fascicles.[61] In the Mayo Clinic series of Pascoe and colleagues[62] in 6 biopsied patients with diabetic proximal neuropathy, a multifocal distribution of fiber loss was noted in 3 sural nerve specimens. In a recent Mayo Clinic series, changes suggesting ischemia were found in the most of 33 nerve biopsies with diabetic radiculoplexus neuropathy.[63]

Local sural nerve blood flow in patients with mild diabetic polyneuropathy was assessed using laser Doppler flowmetry.[64] Patients with peripheral nerve vasculitis who showed abnormal sural nerve blood flow served as controls. No relationship was found between sural nerve blood flow and the presence or development of distal symmetric neuropathy. One study showed that activation of the complement pathway and formation of the membrane attack complex could injure blood vessels and adversely affect the circulation in the endoneurium.[65]

Immunologic/inflammatory pathogenesis
An immune-mediated pathogenesis has recently been advocated in some cases of diabetic neuropathy.[66] In a study of proximal asymmetric neuropathy that showed asymmetric nerve fiber loss, an additional feature was lymphocytic epineurial inflammation resembling vasculitis. Krendel and colleagues[67] found similar perivascular inflammation in 7 of 10 patients with asymmetric lumbosacral neuropathy. In a Mayo Clinic study of diabetic proximal neuropathy, 2 out of 6 sural nerve biopsies showed perivascular mononuclear inflammatory infiltrates.[62] Younger and colleagues[68] biopsied 20 patients with diabetic neuropathy, 6 with distal symmetric and 14 with asymmetric neuropathy. Seven patients had epineurial vessel inflammation on routine paraffin sections, 2 with distal symmetric and 5 with asymmetric neuropathy. With immunohistochemistry, the number of patients with T-cell microvasculitis increased to 12 (60% of biopsied patients) with the inflammatory cells being predominantly CD8+ T cells. The presence of tumor necrosis factor, interleukin-6, interleukin-1β, interleukin-1α, and C5b-9 in several specimens further led the investigators to suggest an immune-mediated pathogenesis of the neuropathy.

In the Mayo large series of patients with diabetic radiculoplexus neuropathy, perivascular mononuclear cells were found in all 33 biopsied patients, most of whom also showed changes of ischemia.[63]

Pathology and Pathophysiology

Axonal degeneration or segmental demyelination
There has been some debate regarding whether the primary lesion in diabetic neuropathy is the axon or Schwann cell/myelin. Ballin and Thomas[69] identified onion bulbs and teased nerve fiber, suggesting recurrent demyelination, and Vital[70,71] reported both segmental demyelination and axonal degeneration. Dyck and colleagues[50] showed that the changes of axonal degeneration and regeneration were more frequent than those of segmental demyelination and remyelination, and, in the setting of multifocal fiber loss, they concluded that axonal degeneration was the primary process. Studies by Said and coleagues[72,73] of the sural nerves of patients with prominent small-fiber sensory loss found pathologic evidence for axonal degeneration, as

well as both primary and secondary segmental demyelination. Therefore, if a sural nerve biopsy is obtained from a typical patient with distal symmetric diabetic neuropathy, a broad spectrum of axonal and myelin pathologic changes can be expected. For this reason, the sural nerve biopsy is often not helpful in diabetic neuropathy in attempting to determine whether the underlying process is axonal degeneration or demyelination/remyelination.

The electrophysiologic studies can similarly show evidence of axonal degeneration and demyelination. An early and characteristic feature of diabetic neuropathy is prolonged distal latencies and F waves, slow conduction velocity, and reduced amplitude of potentials.[7,74–76] Behse and colleagues[77] thought that the conduction velocity slowing was from loss of large fibers. However, another reason for slow conduction velocity may be a functional alteration at nodes of Ranvier.[16] Although frank conduction block and temporal dispersion are usually not found in diabetic neuropathies, the degree of latency and velocity abnormalities can be so severe that so-called demyelinating electrophysiologic criteria may be met.[78] Krendel and colleagues[67] found that demyelinating electrophysiologic criteria were met in 6 of 21 patients with proximal diabetic neuropathy. In the Mayo Clinic series of Pascoe and colleagues,[62] 28 of 42 patients with proximal diabetic neuropathy were classified as axonal and 14 as demyelinating. Temporal dispersion was noted in 14 patients, and conduction block in 2 patients. However, the patients with these demyelinating findings invariably had axonal features as well.

Finding electrophysiologic changes that fulfill demyelinating criteria superimposed on axonal degeneration in a diabetic patient needs to be interpreted with caution. Chronic inflammatory demyelinating polyneuropathy (CIDP) can develop in diabetic patients,[79–81] but these cases are not thought to be related to the underlying diabetes. In support of the lack of association, a recent Olmstead County epidemiologic study identified DM in 4% of 23 CIDP cases and in 12% of matched controls.[82] Electrophysiologic changes of demyelination in a diabetic patient with a symmetric distal or an asymmetric proximal neuropathy may not necessarily imply an immune-mediated neuropathy that will respond to immunosuppressive therapy. In cases of marked demyelination, correlation with the clinical pattern and temporal profile are essential to distinguish CIDP from distal symmetric peripheral polyneuropathy and avoid unnecessary therapies. Jaradeh and colleagues[83] presented 15 patients with progressive polyradiculoneuropathy in diabetes with presentation similar to CIDP. Electrophysiology was predominantly axonal, and cerebrospinal fluid showed increased protein in 14 and oligoconal bands in 5. Sural nerve biopsy performed in 14 patients showed fiber loss, segmental demyelination, inflammatory infiltrates, and onion bulbs. All patients had benefit with immunomodulating therapy.[83]

TYPES OF DIABETIC NEUROPATHIES
Symmetric Neuropathies

Symmetric neuropathies with fixed deficits
DSPN DSPN is the most common form of diabetic neuropathy. This is primarily a length-dependent sensory neuropathy, and significant distal weakness is uncommon. However, as with cryptogenic distal sensory neuropathy, there is usually electrophysiologic evidence for subclinical motor involvement. The clinical and electrophysiologic findings in both cryptogenic and diabetic distal sensory and sensorimotor neuropathy are similar.[84] However, because diabetic patients are often monitored closely before they develop symptoms of neuropathy, the earliest signs of neuropathy may be decreased distal vibration, touch, and pin sensation and ankle

reflex loss on examination. The first symptoms are usually decreased feeling or tingling in the toes. Dysesthesias, usually burning pain, may develop, although most diabetic patients with a distal sensory neuropathy do not complain of significant discomfort. In a population of 382 insulin-treated diabetic subjects, 41 (10.7%) had painful symptoms.[85] In a 2-phase cross-sectional descriptive study of patients with type 2 diabetes (postal survey followed by neurologic history and examination) up to 27% of diabetic patients experienced neuropathic pain or mixed pain resulting in a significant negative effect on quality of life.[86] Sensory symptoms can eventually progress up the ankles and knees and to the fingers, hands, and forearms. If sensory loss extends to the elbows, patients can then develop a symmetric midline truncal wedge-shaped area of sensory loss.[87]

Although there may be atrophy and weakness of the toe extensor and flexor muscles, significant distal ankle weakness is uncommon. If profound distal upper and lower extremity weakness is present in a diabetic patient, an evaluation for other causes of neuropathy is warranted.

Progression of DSPN is usually slow. In the Rochester Diabetic Neuropathy Study, none of the 380 diabetic patients had polyneuropathy that was disabling even when followed for many years.[4] An exception to this rule is the unusual cases of severe sensory and autonomic neuropathy that can occur in the first several after the onset of type 1 diabetes.[73] It is not known why some patients develop this unusually severe form of neuropathy in the early stages of the disease and there is no relationship between the neuropathy and hyperglycemia or the initiation of insulin therapy.

Several examination scales have been developed to establish neuropathy.[88,89] Most of these focus primarily on large-fiber function. The Utah Early Neuropathy Scale was shown to be a sensitive clinical measure of sensory and small-fiber neuropathy.[90] England and colleagues[91,92] recently established the American Academy of Neurology practice parameters for evaluation of distal symmetric polyneuropathy (DSP).[93] In routine clinical practice, documenting an abnormal sensory, reflex, and occasionally a motor examination is sufficient to diagnose neuropathy in a diabetic patient with appropriate symptoms. The use of monofilaments to assess touch-pressure sensation has become important as well as the Rydell-Seifert semiquantitative tuning fork.[94]

Depending on the clinical context, it may be appropriate to perform screening blood tests for other causes of neuropathy (complete blood count, chem 20, vitamin B_{12} level, Venereal Disease Research Laboratory test, serum immunofixation). Equipment for detecting sensory loss, such as computerized quantitative sensory testing, and both simple and complex grading systems have been developed for assessing diabetic neuropathy, and are primarily useful in the context of entering patients in research protocols; they are not needed clinically in most patients.[95,96] Skin biopsies have become a tool to diagnose small-fiber neuropathy in patients with normal electrodiagnostic testing.[84,88]

If severe foot ulcers and neurogenic arthropathies develop, this is often labeled pseudosyringomyelic diabetic neuropathy. There is a selective loss of pain fibers resulting in impaired cutaneous and deep pain and temperature sensation.[72,97] Severe proprioceptive loss is uncommon, but occasionally this can occur when there is prominent large-fiber involvement. These patients develop sensory ataxia and autonomic manifestations with impotence, bladder atony, and pupillary changes and thus have been called the pseudotabetic form of diabetic neuropathy. However, severe proprioception deficits and ataxia are uncommon in diabetes, and when present should lead to a search for other potential causes (syphilis, vitamin B_{12} deficiency, paraneoplastic or Sjogren syndrome sensory neuronopathy, CIDP). However, we think that the pseudosyringomyelic, pseudotabetic, and the early-onset neuropathy described by

Said and colleagues[73] are all severe variants of diabetic DSPN and probably not distinct forms of neuropathy.

Treatment of DSPN

Glucose control In general, patients with strict control of blood glucose have fewer diabetic neuropathy complications.[10,11,98] Several studies have shown that tight glucose control with aggressive insulin therapy can reduce the risk for development of neuropathy.[7,99,100] The DCCT trial convincingly showed that intensive insulin therapy with an insulin pump or 3 or more daily injections is more effective than conventional therapy in reducing neuropathy.[99] Neuropathy occurred in only 5% of intensively treated patients compared with 13% of those conventionally treated. Overall neuropathy was reduced by 64% over 5 years in the intensively treated group. In a follow-up 13 to 14 years after DCCT closeout, the prevalence of neuropathy increased from 9% to 25% in the former intensive and from 17% to 35% in the former conventional treatment groups ($P<.001$), and the incidence of neuropathy remained lower among former intensive treatment subjects.[101] This finding supports the importance and benefits of early intensive insulin treatment in reducing the risk of neuropathy, even more than a decade later.

Other experimental approaches Many different approaches to treat diabetic neuropathy and the other complications of diabetes have been attempted, but in general there has been little success. Several of these experimental approaches were described and referenced earlier. Despite numerous trials of various aldose reductase inhibitors, none have been shown to prevent neuropathy or the progression of deficits.[11,102–104]

In streptozotocin-induced diabetic rats, treatment with alpha-lipoic acid improved nerve blood flow and improved conduction velocity. Alpha-lipoic acid (also known as thioctic acid) may act as an antioxidant free-radical scavenger, and it may inhibit nonenzymatic glycation.[85,86,105,106] A placebo-controlled trial using intravenous alpha-lipoic acid reduced neuropathic symptoms in diabetic patients.[107] In a 5-week randomized controlled trial of oral alpha-lipoic acid 600, 1200, or 1800 mg daily, there was a 50% pain reduction as measured by the Total Symptom Score, including stabbing and burning pain, across all doses, which was statistically significant compared with the placebo response (32%, $P<.05$).[108] A more recent study suggested that 4-year treatment with oral alpha-lipoic acid 600 mg once daily in mild to moderate distal symmetric neuropathy did not influence the primary composite end point of Neuropathy Impairment Score of the Lower Limbs and 7 neurophysiologic tests.[109] Besides being well tolerated, the investigators suggested a clinically meaningful improvement and prevention of progression of neuropathic impairment, but these results have yet to be duplicated by other investigators. Oral alpha-lipoic acid can be obtained in health-food stores, and should be started at 300 mg daily and increased to as much as 600 mg twice a day.

There has recently been interest in nerve growth factor (NGF) therapy as a treatment of diabetic neuropathy.[110] In experimental animal models of diabetes, there is some evidence for decreased NGF expression in various target tissues, and NGF treatment in these models prevented the manifestations of neuropathy.[111–115] In humans with diabetic neuropathy, NGF levels are reduced in skin biopsy specimens.[116] In a phase II placebo-controlled trial of subcutaneous NGF in 250 patients with diabetic neuropathy, the only end point that reached statistical significance was the patient's overall global symptom assessment that they felt improved. There was a trend toward improvement in quantitative cold detection thresholds and in the small-fiber sensory components of neuropathy impairment score. However, in the larger phase III trial, there was no benefit in the NGF group on any end point.

Symptomatic treatment If a patient's with diabetic neuropathy does not complain of pain, symptomatic treatment is of no value and is not necessary. Symptoms of numbness and tingling should not be treated.

The most frequently used oral drugs for the symptomatic treatment of diabetic and nondiabetic painful neuropathy are the tricyclic antidepressants, carbamazepine, gabapentin, mexiletene, and, more recently, pregabalin and cymbalta.[117–125] All physicians have their own preferences for first-line, second-line, and third-line drugs. Our preference and the doses are listed in **Table 1**. For further information on the treatment refer to the article by Jaya Trivedi and colleagues elsewhere in this issue. Recent evidence-based guidelines for treatment of pain in diabetic neuropathy were published by the American Academy of Neurology.[93] According to this, pregabalin is established as effective and should be offered for relief of Diabetic Polyneuropathy (DPN). Venlafaxine, duloxetine, amitriptyline, gabapentin, valproate, opioids (morphine sulfate, tramadol, and oxycodone controlled release), and capsaicin are probably effective and should be considered for treatment of PDN.[123] Other treatments have less robust evidence or the evidence is negative.[124] Effective treatments for DPN are available, but many have side effects that limit their usefulness, and few studies have sufficient information on treatment effects on function and quality of life. For further review of neuropathic pain management, the reader is referred to the article elsewhere in this issue.

Topical therapy with capsaicin and lidocaine creams can be tried.[126,127] In our experience, few patients respond to these modalities and the creams are difficult to use because they need to be applied several times a day. Lidoderm patches may be effective, but they are expensive and cumbersome to apply to the soles of both feet.[128,129] Transcutaneous nerve stimulation is occasionally helpful. An unusual alternative-medicine approach to painful neuropathies with magnetic inserts has received some attention.[130] A blinded controlled crossover study reported benefit with magnet therapy.[131] A larger multicenter study of repetitive and cumulative exposure to low-frequency pulsed electromagnetic fields in 225 subjects with painful diabetic neuropathy did not show any effect on pain reduction.[132] It did show in a subgroup of 27 subjects who completed serial biopsies that 29% of magnet-treated subjects had an increase in distal leg ENFD of at least 0.5 standard deviations, whereas none did in the sham group ($P = .04$).

Exercise therapy is being investigated as another treatment modality. A small pilot study reported improvements in neuropathic pain and symptoms as well as cutaneous nerve fiber branching on proximal skin biopsy following a 10-week supervised exercise program in 17 patients with diabetic peripheral neuropathy. These findings are particularly promising given the short duration of the intervention, but need to be validated by comparison with a control group in future studies.[133]

Autonomic neuropathy Autonomic manifestations can affect cardiovascular, genito-urinary, or gastrointestinal organ systems so that patients develop orthostasis, tachycardia/tachyarrhythmias, gastroparesis, impotence, bladder atony, or impotence. Other autonomic manifestations include profuse nocturnal or postprandial sweating and abnormal pupillary light responses. The nerve fibers that mediate sweating undergo distal damage. One electrophysiologic technique for evaluating these nerve fibers is to test for sympathetic skin responses.[123] Diabetic diarrhea and incontinence are rare but can be disabling. Gastrointestinal autonomic dysfunction is assessed with various radiographic techniques, but the easiest is to show the abnormally slow

Table 1
Pharmacologic therapy for neuropathic pain

Therapy	Route	Oral Starting Doses	Maintenance Doses
First Line			
Tricyclic antidepressants	Oral	10–25 mg at bedtime	Increase by increments of 10–25 mg to 100–150 mg at bedtime
Gabapentin (Neurontin)	Oral	300 mg tid	Increase by increments of 300–400 mg to 2400–6000 mg daily divided in 3–4 doses
Tramadol (Ultram)	Oral	50 mg bid or tid	Increase by 50-mg increments to a maximum of 100 mg qid
Duloxetine (Cymabalta)	Oral	30 mg/d	Increase by increments of 30–60 mg up to 120 mg/d
Pregabalin (Lyrica)	Oral	50 mg tid	Increase to 300 mg/d
Second Line			
Venlafaxine XR (Effexor)	Oral	37.5–75 mg once a day	Increase by 75-mg increments to 150–225 mg a day
Valproate	Oral	250 mg bid to tid	Increase by 250-mg increments up to 1500 mg/d
Carbamazepine	Oral	200 mg bid	Increase by 200-mg increments to 200–400 mg 3 to 4 times a day; follow drug levels on doses greater than 600 mg/d
Oxcarbazepine (Trileptal)	Oral	150–300 mg bid	Increase by 300-mg increments to 600–1200 mg 2 times a day
Lamotrigine (Lamictal)	Oral	25 mg once a day or bid	Increase by 25-mg increments weekly to 100–200 mg bid
Topiramate (Topamax)	Oral	25–50 mg at bedtime	Increase by 50-mg increments weekly to 200 mg bid
Third Line			
Bupropion SR (Welbutrin)	Oral	150 mg/d	After 1 week, increase to 150 mg twice a day
Tiagabine hydrochloride (Gabitril)	Oral	4 mg/d	Increase to 4–12 mg bid
Keppra (Levetiracetam)	Oral	250 mg at bedtime	Increase by increments of 250–500 mg to 1500 mg 2 times a day
Zonisamide (Zonegran)	Oral	100 mg at bedtime	Increase by 100-mg increments to 400–600 mg at bedtime
Mexiletine	Oral	200 mg once a day	Increase by 200-mg increments to a maximum of 200 mg tid
Phenytoin	Oral	200 mg at bedtime	Increase by 100-mg increments to 300–400 mg daily divided in 1–2 doses, following drug levels
Newer Drugs			
Savella	Oral	12.5 mg at bedtime × 1 d	12.5 mg bid × 2 d then 25 mg bid × 4 d, then stay on 50 mg bid. May increase up to 100 mg bid

(continued on next page)

Table 1
(continued)

| Therapy | Oral | | |
	Route	Starting Doses	Maintenance Doses
Vimpat	Oral	50 mg by mouth bid	In 1 wk, go to 100 mg bid. May increase up to 200 mg bid
Topical Agents			
Over the Counter			
Capsaicin 0.075%	Topical	Apply to affected region tid to qid	Continue with starting dose
Salicylate 10%–15%	Topical	Apply to affected region tid to qid	Continue with starting dose
Menthol 16%/ camphor 3% (+/−)	Topical	Apply to affected region tid to qid	Continue with starting dose
By Prescription			
Lidocaine 2.5%/ prilocaine 2.5%	Topical	Apply to affected region tid to qid	Continue with starting dose
Lidocaine patch 5%	Topical	Apply over adjacent, intact skin	Increase up to 3 patches worn for 12 h of 24-h period
Doxepin 5% (Zolopan)	Topical	Apply to affected region bid	Continue with starting dose
Diclofenac sodium gel (Voltaren Gel 1%)	Topical	Apply to affected region tid to qid	Continue with starting dose
By Prescription: Only at Compounding Pharmacies			
Ketoprofen 5%/ amitriptyline 2%/ tetracaine 1%	Topical[a]	Apply to affected region bid	Increase up to a schedule of qid
Ketoprofen 10%/ cyclobenzaprine 1%/ lidocaine 5%	Topical[a]	Apply to affected region bid	Increase up to a schedule of qid
Ketamine 5%/ amitriptyline 4%/ gabapentin 4%	Topical[a]	Apply to affected region bid	Increase up to a schedule of tid
Carbamazepine 5%/ lidocaine 5%	Topical[a]	Apply to affected region bid	Increase up to a schedule of qid
Amitriptyline 2%/ lioresal 2%	Topical[a]	Apply to affected region tid to qid	Continue with starting dose

[a] Must be compounded by pharmacy (to locate your local compounding pharmacy, call the International Academy of Compounding Pharmacists, 1-800-927-4227).

passage of barium through the gut.[134] Impotence is the most common clinical manifestation of autonomic neuropathy, affecting more than 50% of men with diabetes.

Treatment Orthostatic symptoms can be treated with fludrocortisone (0.1 mg twice a day), the nonsteroidal antiinflammatory agents ibuprofen and indomethacin, and the oral sympathomimetic agent midodrine.[105–107,135–137] Midodrine (ProAmatine) is an alpha-adrenoreceptor agonist that increases blood pressure by producing arterial and venous constriction. The recommended dose is 10 mg 3 times daily. Pharmacotherapy can be tried for delayed gastric emptying (metoclopramide; erythromycin)[138,139] and diarrhea (clonidine).[140] Impotence can be treated with oral phosphodieterase-5 inhibitors such as sildenafil (Viagra)[141] and, less commonly, with injectable (phentolamine/papervine) drug therapy or penile prosthesis.[142,143]

Symmetric neuropathies with episodic symptoms

Diabetic neuropathic cachexia Diabetic neuropathic cachexia is an uncommon syndrome initially described by Ellenberg[144] in 1974 in which patients develop profound weight loss, a symmetric sensory peripheral neuropathy, and painful dysesthesias over the limbs and trunk, without associated weakness.[144–149] Unlike other symmetric neuropathies caused by diabetes, diabetic neuropathic cachexia is reversible over a period of weeks to months. Most reported patients have been men, usually in the sixth or seventh decades of life, but there have been 2 cases described in women. All cases initially show a precipitous weight loss of up to 60% of total body weight, leading at times to an incorrect suspicion of an underlying cancer. Patients may experience intense contact hypersensitivity and may also describe intermittent stabbing or shooting pains. The pain tends to be worse at night or during periods of relaxation. The presence of proximal or truncal symmetric dysesthesias associated with profound weight loss should be clinical clues that support the diagnosis of diabetic neuropathic cachexia rather than the more common DSPN of diabetes. Patients may also experience depression, anorexia, and impotence. Sensory impairment associated with diabetic neuropathic cachexia is generally minimal, by contrast with the severity of the patient's complaints of pain, and in some cases may not be clinically detectable. Some reports describe associated muscle atrophy and weakness, whereas others have reported normal strength.

Diabetic neuropathic cachexia can occur in patients with both type 1 and type 2 diabetes. There is a lack of correlation with other microvascular complications of diabetes such as nephropathy or retinopathy. Most cases are associated with poor glucose control. Some of these cases have been associated with malabsorption.[150]

Treatment of diabetic neuropathic cachexia can be difficult and strict diabetic control is usually necessary. The usual drugs to treat neuropathic pain can be tried, but they are often unsuccessful and the temporary use of narcotics is often needed. The prognosis is usually good, and patients typically recover their baseline weight with resolution of the painful sensory symptoms within 1 year. A residual sensorimotor neuropathy is common. Recurrent diabetic neuropathic cachexia has also been reported (**Fig. 2**).[138]

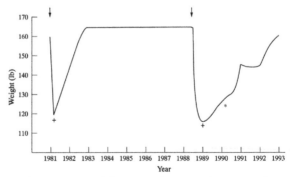

Fig. 2. Patient's weight over time and the onset of neuropathic pain and initiation of diabetic therapy. +, initiation of oral hypoglycemic; *, initiation of insulin; ↓, onset of pain. (*From* Jackson CE, Barohn RJ. Diabetic neuropathic cachexia: report of a recurrent case. J Neurol Neurosurg Psychiatry 1998;64:786; with permission.)

The eventual resolution of diabetic neuropathic cachexia with concomitant weight gain and the lack of correlation with other microvascular complications of diabetes suggest a primarily dysmetabolic process (see **Fig. 1**). However, the pathophysiologic basis of the disorder remains unknown.

Other possible transient symmetric sensory neuropathies Other cases of transient distal sensory paresthesias and pain have been alleged to be caused by hyperglycemia (hyperglycemic neuropathy) or insulin neuritis following the institution of insulin.[97,151,152] The insulin neuritis is usually characterized by acute severe pain, peripheral nerve degeneration, and autonomic dysfunction after intensive glycemic control, which often parallels worsening retinopathy and resolves in weeks or months.[153] Clinical features and objective measures of neuropathy can improve in these patients despite a prolonged history of poor glucose control.[151] So-called hyperglycemic neuropathy may occur at the time of diagnosis or may follow an episode of ketotic coma, and the symptoms rapidly subside once the diabetes is controlled.

Llewelyn and colleagues[152] reported similar symptoms within 6 weeks of establishing good diabetic control with insulin, and pain persisted for 4 to 5 months.[125] It is still unclear whether these are distinct peripheral neuropathy entities.

Case study

A 42-year-old man developed numbness and tingling in the toes, progressing up to the ankles over 2 years. He describes burning pain in his feet, mainly at night. He recently started noticing symptoms of numbness and tingling in distal fingers. He denies any weakness. He was recently diagnosed with diabetes.

Examination showed normal strength, with decreased pinprick and light touch sensations to the ankles and distal fingers. Timed vibration is 0 seconds at the toes, 10 seconds at the ankles, and proprioception is normal at the toes. Reflexes are normal in the arms and at the knees but ankle reflexes are absent. Gait is normal.

Routine neuropathy laboratory studies were unremarkable except for mild increase of HgbA1c 6.0%, and 2-hour glucose tolerance test showed a 2-hour glucose of 250 mg/dL. Electrodiagnostic testing showed absent sural sensory responses and decreased peroneal and tibial motor amplitudes, showing evidence of moderate axonal sensorimotor polyneuropathy.

He was started on gabapentin with initial improvement of pain. Over the next 2 years there was progression of pain with mild worsening of weakness distally. Duloxetine was later started because of worsening of the pain. He also developed diabetic retinopathy and diabetic medications had to be adjusted because of worsening blood sugar control.

REFERENCES

1. Barohn RJ. Diabetic neuropathy. 2nd edition. Decision Making in Pain Management; 2006. p. 82–3.
2. The Expert Committee on the Diagnosis and Classification of Diabetes Mellitus. Report of the Expert Committee on the Diagnosis and Classification of Diabetes Mellitus. Diabetes Care 1997;20:1183–97.
3. Harris MI, Hadden WC, Knowler WC, et al. Prevalence of diabetes and impaired glucose tolerance and plasma glucose levels in the U.S. population ages 20-74. Diabetes 1987;36:523–34.
4. Dyck PH, Kratz KM, Karnes JL, et al. The prevalence by staged severity of various types of diabetic neuropathy, retinopathy, and nephropathy in a

population-based cohort: the Rochester Diabetic Neuropathy Study. Neurology 1993;43:817–24.

5. Centers for Disease Control and Prevention. National fact sheet, 2011. Atlanta (GA): CDC, USHHS; 2011. Available at: http://www.cdc.gov/diabetes/pubs/pdf/ndfs_2011. Accessed December 1, 2012.

6. Melton LJ, Dyck PJ. Clinical features of the diabetic neuropathies: Epidemiology. In: Dyck PJ, Thomas PK, Asbury AK, et al, editors. Diabetic neuropathy. Philadelphia: WB Saunders; 1987. p. 27–35.

7. Diabetes Control and Complications Trial. Effect of intensive diabetes treatment on nerve conduction in the Diabetes Control and Complications Trial. Ann Neurol 1995;38:869–80.

8. Picart J. Diabetes mellitus and its degenerative complications: a prospective study of 4,400 patients observed between 1947 and 1973. Diabetes Care 1978;1:168–88, 252–63.

9. Partanen J, Kiskanen L, Lehtinen J, et al. Natural history of peripheral neuropathy in patients with non-insulin-dependent diabetes mellitus. N Engl J Med 1995;333:89–94.

10. Nathan DM. Long-term complications of diabetes mellitus. N Engl J Med 1993;328:1676–85.

11. Clark CM, Lee DA. Prevention and treatment of the complications of diabetes mellitus. N Engl J Med 1995;332:1210–7.

12. Genuth S, Alberti KG, Bennett P, et al. Expert Committee on the Diagnosis and Classification of Diabetes Mellitus. Follow-up report on the diagnosis of diabetes mellitus. Diabetes Care 2003;26(11):3160.

13. American Diabetes Association. Diagnosis and classification of diabetes mellitus. Diabetes Care 2010;33(Suppl 1):S62.

14. Brown MJ, Asbury AK. Diabetic neuropathy. Ann Neurol 1984;15:2–12.

15. Low PA. Recent advances in the pathogenesis of diabetic neuropathy. Muscle Nerve 1987;10:121–8.

16. Dyck PJ, Giannini C. Pathologic alterations in the diabetic neuropathies of humans: a review. J Neuropathol Exp Neurol 1996;55:1181–93.

17. Sima AA. Pathological definition and evaluation of diabetic neuropathy and clinical correlations. Can J Neurol Sci 1994;21:S13–7.

18. Stevens MJ, Feldman EL, Greene DA. The aetiology of diabetic neuropathy: the combined roles of metabolic and vascular defects. Diabet Med 1995;12:566–79.

19. Thomas PK. Diabetic neuropathy: models, mechanism, and mayhem. Can J Neurol Sci 1992;19:1–7.

20. Johnson PC, Doll SC, Cromey DW. Pathogenesis of diabetic neuropathy. Ann Neurol 1986;19:450–7.

21. Dyck PJ, Thomas PK, Asbury AK, et al. Diabetic neuropathy. Philadelphia: WB Saunders; 1987.

22. Cameron N, Eaton SE, Cotter M, et al. Vascular factors and metabolic interactions in the pathogenesis of diabetic neuropathy. Diabetalogia 2001;44(11):1973–88.

23. Gries FA, Cameron NE, Low PA, et al, editors. Textbook of diabetic neuropathy. Stuttgart (Germany): Thieme; 2003.

24. Boulton AJ, Malik RA, Arezzo JC, et al. Diabetic somatic neuropathies. Diabetes Care 2004;27(6):1458–86.

25. Edwards JL, Vincent AM, Cheng HT, et al. Diabetic neuropathy: mechanisms to management. Pharmacol Ther 2008;120(1):1–34.

26. Vincent AM, Hinder LM, Pop-Busui R, et al. Hyperlipidemia: a new therapeutic target for diabetic neuropathy. J Peripher Nerv Syst 2009;14(4):257–67.

27. Dyck PJ, Lambert EH, Windebank AJ, et al. Acute hyperosmolar hyperglycemia causes axonal shrinkage and reduced nerve conduction velocity. Exp Neurol 1981;71:507–14.

28. Greene DA, Lattimer SA. Impaired rat sciatic nerve sodium-potassium adenosine triphosphatase in acute streptozotocin diabetes and its correction by dietary myo-inositol supplementation. J Clin Invest 1983;72:1058–63.

29. Dyck PJ, Sherman WR, Hallcher LM, et al. Human diabetic endoneurial sorbitol, fructose, and myo-inositol related to sural nerve morphometry. Ann Neurol 1980; 8:590–6.

30. Dyck PJ, Zimmerman BR, Vilen TH, et al. Nerve glucose, fructose, sorbitol, myo-inositol, and fiber degeneration and regeneration in diabetic neuropathy. N Engl J Med 1988;319:542–8.

31. Gregersen G, Bertelsen B, Harbo H. Oral supplementation of myoinositol: effects on peripheral nerve function in human diabetics and on the concentration in plasma, erythrocytes, urine and muscle tissue in human diabetics and normals. Acta Neurol Scand 1983;67:164–72.

32. Gregersen G, Borsting H, Theil P, et al. Myoinositol and function of peripheral nerves in human diabetics: a controlled clinical trial. Acta Neurol Scand 1978; 58:241–8.

33. Gillon KR, Hawthorne JN, Tomlinson DR. Myo-inositol and sorbitol metabolism in relation to peripheral nerve function in experimental diabetes in the rat: the effect of aldose reductase inhibition. Diabetologia 1983;25:365–71.

34. Horrobin DF. Essential fatty acids in the management of impaired nerve function in diabetes. Diabetes 1997;46(Suppl 2):S90–3.

35. Jamal GA, Carmichael H. the effect of gamma-linolenic acid on human diabetic polyneuropathy: a double-blind placebo-controlled trial. Diabet Med 1990;7: 319–23.

36. Keen H, Payan J, Allawi J, et al. Treatment of diabetic neuropathy with gamma-linolenic acid. Diabetes Care 1993;16:8–15.

37. Brownlee M. Advanced protein glycosylation in diabetes and aging. Annu Rev Med 1995;46:223–34.

38. Brownlee M, Cerami A, Vlassara H. Advanced glycosylation end products in tissue and the biochemical basis of diabetic complications. N Engl J Med 1988;318:1315–21.

39. Vlassara H. Recent progress in advanced glycation end products and diabetic complications. Diabetes 1997;46:S19–25.

40. Feldman EL, Russell JW, Sullivan KA, et al. New insights into the pathogenesis of diabetic neuropathy. Curr Opin Neurol 1999;12:553–63.

41. Soulis-Liparota T, Cooper M, Papazoglou D, et al. Retardation by amino-guanidine of development of albuminuria, mesangial expansion, and tissue fluorescence in streptozocin-induced diabetic rat. Diabetes 1991;40: 1328–34.

42. Williams E, Timperly WR, Ward JD, et al. Electron microscopic studies of vessels in diabetic peripheral neuropathy. J Clin Pathol 1980;33:462–70.

43. Malik RA, Newrick PG, Sharma AK, et al. Microangiopathy in human diabetic neuropathy: relationship between capillary abnormalities and the severity of neuropathy. Diabetologia 1989;32:92–102.

44. Yasuda H, Dyck PJ. Abnormalities of endoneurial microvessels and sural nerve pathology in diabetic neuropathy. Neurology 1987;37:20–8.

45. Giannini C, Dyck PJ. Ultrastructural morphometric features of human sural nerve endoneurial microvessels. J Neuropathol Exp Neurol 1993;52:361–9.

46. Giannini C, Dyck PJ. Ultrastructural morphometric abnormalities of sural nerve endoneurial microvessels in diabetes mellitus. Ann Neurol 1994;36:408–15.
47. Dyck PJ. Hypoxic neuropathy: does hypoxia play a role in diabetic neuropathy? The 1988 Robert Wartenberg Lecture. Neurology 1989;39:111–8.
48. Sugimura K, Dyck PJ. Multifocal fiber loss in proximal sciatic nerve in symmetric distal diabetic neuropathy. J Neurol Sci 1982;53:501–9.
49. Dyck PJ, Karnes JL, O'Brien P, et al. The spatial distribution of fiber loss in diabetic polyneuropathy suggests ischemia. Ann Neurol 1986;19:440–9.
50. Dyck PJ, Lais A, Karnes JL, et al. Fiber loss is primary and multifocal in sural nerves in diabetic polyneuropathy. Ann Neurol 1986;19:425–39.
51. Low PA, Tuck RR, Dyck PJ, et al. Prevention of some electrophysiologic and biochemical abnormalities with oxygen supplementation in experimental diabetic neuropathy. Proc Natl Acad Sci U S A 1984;81:6894–8.
52. Low PA, Schmelzer JD, Ward KK, et al. Experimental chronic hypoxic neuropathy: relevance to diabetic neuropathy. Am J Physiol 1986;251:E94–9.
53. Asbury AK, Aldredge H, Herschberg R, et al. Oculomotor palsy in diabetes mellitus: a clinicopathological study. Brain 1970;93:555–66.
54. Weber RB, Daroff RB, Mackey EA. Pathology of oculomotor nerve palsy in diabetics. Neurology 1970;20:835–8.
55. Dreyfus PM, Hakim S, Adams RD. Diabetic ophthalmoplegia. AMA Arch Neurol Psychiatry 1957;77:337–49.
56. Smith BE, Dyck PJ. Subclinical histopathological changes in the oculomotor nerve in diabetes mellitus. Ann Neurol 1992;32:376–85.
57. Raff M, Asbury AK. Ischemic mononeuropathy and mononeuropathy multiplex in diabetes mellitus. N Engl J Med 1968;279:17–22.
58. Raff MC, Sangalang V, Asbury AK. Ishemic mononeuropathy multiplex associated with diabetes mellitus. Arch Neurol 1968;18:487–99.
59. Said G, Goulon-Goeau C, Lacroix C, et al. Nerve biopsy findings in different patterns of proximal diabetic neuropathy. Ann Neurol 1994;35:559–69.
60. Said G, Elgrably F, Lacroix C, et al. Painful proximal diabetic neuropathy: inflammatory nerve lesions and spontaneous favorable outcome. Ann Neurol 1997;41:762–70.
61. Barohn RJ, Sahenk Z, Warmolts JR, et al. The Bruns-Garland syndrome (diabetic amyotrophy): revisited 100 years later. Arch Neurol 1991;48:1130–5.
62. Pascoe MK, Low PA, Windebank AJ, et al. Subacute diabetic proximal neuropathy. Mayo Clin Proc 1997;72:1123–32.
63. Dyck PJ, Novell JE, Dyck PJ. Microvasculitis and ischemia in diabetic lumbosacral radiculopexus neuropathy. Neurology 1999;53:2113–21.
64. Theriault M, Dort J, Sutherland G, et al. Local human sural nerve blood flow in diabetic and other polyneuropathies. Brain 1997;120:1131–8.
65. Rosoklija GB, Dwork AJ, Younger DS, et al. Local activation of the complement system in endoneurial microvessels of diabetic neuropathy. Acta Neuropathol 2000;99(1):55–62.
66. Dyck PJ, Windebank AJ. Diabetic and nondiabetic lumbosacral radiculoplexus neuropathies: new insights into pathophysiology and treatment. Muscle Nerve 2002;25(4):477–91.
67. Krendel DA, Costigan DA, Hopkins LC. Successful treatment of neuropathies in patients with diabetes mellitus. Arch Neurol 1995;52:1053–61.
68. Younger DS, Rosoklija G, Hays AP, et al. Diabetic peripheral neuropathy: a clinicopathologic and immunohistochemical analysis of sural nerve biopsies. Muscle Nerve 1996;19:722–7.

69. Ballin RH, Thomas PK. Hypertrophic changes in diabetic neuropathy. Acta Neuropathol 1968;11:93–102.
70. Vital C, Vallat JM, LeBlanc M, et al. Peripheral neuropathies caused by diabetes mellitus. Ultrastructural study of 12 biopsied cases. J Neurol Sci 1973;18: 381–98.
71. Vital C, LeBlanc M, Vallat JM, et al. Ultrastructural study of peripheral nerve in 16 diabetics without neuropathy. Comparisons with 16 diabetic neuropathies and 16 non-diabetic neuropathies. Acta Neuropathol 1974;30:63–72.
72. Said G, Slama G, Salva J. Progressive centripetal degeneration of axons in small fibre diabetic polyneuropathy. Brain 1983;106:791–807.
73. Said G, Goulon-Goeau C, Slama G, et al. Severe early-onset polyneuropathy in insulin-dependent diabetes mellitus. A clinical pathological study. N Engl J Med 1992;326:1257–63.
74. Dyck PJ, Karnes JL, Daube J, et al. Clinical and neuropathological criteria for the diagnosis and staging of diabetic polyneuropathy. Brain 1985;108:861–80.
75. Claus D, Mustafa C, Vogel W, et al. Assessment of diabetic neuropathy: definition of norm and discrimination of abnormal nerve function. Muscle Nerve 1993; 16:757–68.
76. Albers JW, Brown MB, Sima AA, et al. Nerve conduction measures in mild diabetic neuropathy in the Early Diabetes Intervention Trial: the effects of age, sex, type of diabetes, disease duration, and anthropometric factors. Tolrestat Study Group for the Early Diabetes Intervention Trial. Neurology 1996;46: 85–91.
77. Behse F, Buchthal F, Carlsen F. Nerve biopsy and conduction studies in diabetic neuropathy. J Neurol Neurosurg Psychiatry 1977;40:1072–82.
78. Ad Hoc Subcommittee of the American Academy of Neurology AIDS Task Force. Research criteria for diagnosis of chronic inflammatory demyelinating polyneuropathy (CIDP). Neurology 1991;41:617–8.
79. Cornblath DR, Drach DB, Griffin JW. Demyelinating motor neuropathy in patients with diabetic polyneuropathy [abstract]. Ann Neurol 1987;22:126S.
80. Stewart JD, McKelvey R, Durcan L, et al. Chronic inflammatory demyelinating polyneuropathy (CIDP) in diabetics. J Neurol Sci 1996;142:59–64.
81. Uncini A, De Angelis MV, Di Muzio A, et al. Chronic inflammatory demyelinating polyneuropathy in diabetics: motor conductions are important in the differential diagnosis with diabetic polyneuropathy. Clin Neurophysiol 1999; 110:705–11.
82. Laughlin RS, Dyck PJ, Melton LJ, et al. Incidence and prevalence of CIDP and the association of diabetes mellitus. Neurology 2009;73(1):39–45.
83. Jaradeh SS, Prieto TE, Lobeck LJ. Progressive polyradiculoneuropathy in diabetes: correlation of variables and clinical outcome after immunotherapy. J Neurol Neurosurg Psychiatry 1999;67(5):607–12.
84. Pasnoor M, Herbelin L, Johnson M, et al. Clinical electrophysiologic and skin biopsy findings in cryptogenic sensorimotor polyneuropathy compared to diabetic polyneuropathy and normal controls. Neurology 2009;72(Suppl 3): A217.
85. Boulton AJ, Knight G, Drury J, et al. The prevalence of symptomatic diabetic neuropathy in an insulin-treated population. Diabetes Care 1985;8: 125–8.
86. Davies M, Brophy S, Williams R, et al. The prevalence, severity, and impact of painful diabetic peripheral neuropathy in type 2 diabetes. Diabetes Care 2006;29(7):1518–22.

87. Waxman SG, Sabin TD. Diabetic truncal polyneuropathy. Arch Neurol 1981;38: 46–7.
88. Dyck PJ, Davies JL, Litchy WJ, et al. Longitudinal assessment of diabetic poly-neuropathy using a composite score in the Rochester Diabetic Neuropathy Study cohort. Neurology 1997;49:229–39.
89. Feldman E, Stevens MJ, Thomas PK, et al. A practical two-step quantitative clin-ical and electrophysiological assessment for the diagnosis and staging of dia-betic neuropathy. Diabetes Care 1994;17:1281–9.
90. Singleton JR, Bixby B, Russell JW, et al. The Utah Early Neuropathy Scale: a sensitive clinical scale for early sensory predominant neuropathy. J Peripher Nerv Syst 2008;13:218–27.
91. England JD, Gronseth GS, Franklin G, et al. Practice parameter: evaluation of distal symmetric polyneuropathy: role of laboratory and genetic testing (an evidence-based review). Report of the American Academy of Neurology, American Association of Neuromuscular and Electrodiagnostic Medicine, and American Academy of Physical Medicine and Rehabilitation. Neurology 2009; 72(2):185–92.
92. England JD, Gronseth GS, Franklin G, et al. Practice parameter: evaluation of distal symmetric polyneuropathy: role of autonomic testing, nerve biopsy, and skin biopsy (an evidence-based review). Report of the American Academy of Neurology, American Association of Neuromuscular and Electrodiagnostic Medicine, and American Academy of Physical Medicine and Rehabilitation. Neurology 2009;72(2):177–84.
93. Bril V, England J, Franklin GM, et al. Evidence-based guideline: treatment of painful diabetic neuropathy. Report of the American Academy of Neurology, the American Association of Neuromuscular and Electrodiagnostic Medicine, and the American Academy of Physical Medicine and Rehabilitation. Neurology 2011;76(20):1758–65.
94. Vinik AI, Mehrabyan A. Diabetic neuropathies. Med Clin North Am 2004;88(4): 947–99.
95. Dyck PJ, Karnes JL, O'Brien PC, et al. The Rochester Diabetic Neuropathy Study: reassessment of tests and criteria for diagnosis and staged severity. Neurology 1992;42:1164–70.
96. Peripheral Nerve Society. Diabetic polyneuropathy in controlled clinical trials: consensus report of the Peripheral Nerve Society. Ann Neurol 1995;38:478–82.
97. Thomas PK, Brown MJ. Diabetic polyneuropathy. In: Dyck PJ, Thomas PK, Asbury AK, et al, editors. Diabetic neuropathy. Philadelphia: WB Saunders; 1987. p. 56–65.
98. Service FJ, Rizza RA, Daube JR, et al. Near normoglycemia improved nerve conduction and vibration sensation in diabetic neuropathy. Diabetologia 1985; 28:722–7.
99. The Diabetes Control and Complication Trial Research Group. The effect of intensive treatment of diabetes on the development and progression of long-term complications in insulin-dependent diabetes mellitus. N Engl J Med 1993;329:977–86.
100. Warmolts JR, Mendell JR, O'Dorisio TM, et al. Comparison of the effects of continuous subcutaneous infusion and split-mixed injection of insulin on nerve function in type I diabetes mellitus. J Neurol Sci 1987;82:161–9.
101. Albers JW, Herman WH, Pop-Busui R, et al. Diabetes Control and Complications Trial/Epidemiology of Diabetes Interventions and Complications Research Group. Effect of prior intensive insulin treatment during the Diabetes Control

and Complications Trial (DCCT) on peripheral neuropathy in type 1 diabetes during the Epidemiology of Diabetes Interventions and Complications (EDIC) Study. Diabetes Care 2010;33(5):1090–6.

102. Lewin IG, O'Brien IA, Morgan MG, et al. Clinical and neurophysiological studies with the aldose reductase inhibitor, sorbinil, in symptomatic diabetic neuropathy. Diabetologia 1984;26:445–8.

103. Sundkvist G, Armstrong FM, Bradbury JE, et al. Peripheral and autonomic nerve function in 259 diabetic patients with peripheral neuropathy treated with ponalrestat (an aldose reductase inhibitor) or placebo for 18 months: United Kingdom/Scandinavian Ponalrestat Trial. J Diabet Complications 1992;6: 123–30.

104. Pfeifer MA, Schumer MP, Gelber DA. Aldose reductase inhibitors: the end of an era or the need for different trial designs? Diabetes 1997;46(Suppl 2):S82–9.

105. Packer L, Roy S, Sen CK. Alpha-lipoic acid: a metabolic antioxidant and potential redox modulator of transcription. Adv Pharmacol 1997;38:79–101.

106. Nagamatsu M, Nickander KK, Schmelzer JD, et al. Lipoic acid improves nerve blood flow, reduces oxidative stress, and improves distal nerve conduction in experimental diabetic neuropathy. Diabetes Care 1995;18:1160–7.

107. Ziegler D, Hanefeld M, Ruhnau KJ, et al. Treatment of symptomatic diabetic peripheral neuropathy with the anti-oxidant alpha-lipoic acid. A 3-week multicenter randomized controlled trial (ALADIN Study). Diabetologia 1995;38:1425–33.

108. Ziegler D, Ametov A, Barinov A, et al. Oral treatment with alpha-lipoic acid improves symptomatic diabetic polyneuropathy: the SYDNEY 2 trial. Diabetes Care 2006;29(11):2365–70.

109. Ziegler D, Low PA, Litchy WJ, et al. Efficacy and safety of antioxidant treatment with α-lipoic acid over 4 years in diabetic polyneuropathy: the NATHAN 1 trial. Diabetes Care 2011;34(9):2054–60.

110. Apfel SC, Kessler JA, Adornato BT, et al. Recombinant human nerve growth factor in the treatment of diabetic polyneuropathy. Neurology 1998;51:695–702.

111. Fernyhough P, Diemel LT, Brewster JW, et al. Altered neurotrophin mRNA levels in peripheral nerve and skeletal muscle of experimentally diabetic rats. J Neurochem 1995;64:1231–7.

112. Rodriquez-Pena A, Botana M, Gonzalez M, et al. Expression of neurotrophins and their receptors in sciatic nerve of experimentally diabetic rats. Neurosci Lett 1995;200:37–40.

113. Fernyhough P, Diemel LT, Trewster WJ, et al. Deficits in sciatic nerve neuropeptide content coincide with a reduction in target tissue nerve growth factor messenger RNA in streptozocin-diabetic rats: effects of insulin treatment. Neuroscience 1994;62:337–44.

114. Apfel SC, Arezzo JC, Brownlee M, et al. Nerve growth factor administration protects against experimental diabetic sensory neuropathy. Brain Res 1994; 634:7–12.

115. Hellweg R, Vavich G, Hartung HD, et al. Axonal transport of endogenous nerve growth factor (NGF) and NGF receptor in experimental diabetic neuropathy. Exp Neurol 1994;130:24–30.

116. Anand P, Terenghi G, Warner G, et al. The role of endogenous nerve growth factor in human diabetic neuropathy. Nat Med 1996;2:703–7.

117. Max MB, Lynch SA, Muir J, et al. Effects of desipramine, amitriptyline, and fluoxetine on pain in diabetic neuropathy. N Engl J Med 1992;326:1250–6.

118. Kvinesdal B, Molin J, Froland A, et al. Imipramine treatment of painful diabetic neuropathy. JAMA 1984;251:1727–30.

119. Mendel CM, Klein RF, Chappell DA, et al. A trial of amitriptyline and fluphenazine in the treatment of painful diabetic neuropathy. JAMA 1986;255:637–9.

120. Dejgard A, Petersen P, Kastrup J. Mexiletine for treatment of chronic painful diabetic neuropathy. Lancet 1988;1:9–11.

121. Backonja M, Beydoun A, Edwards KR, et al. Gabapentin for the symptomatic treatment of painful neuropathy in patients with diabetes mellitus: a randomized controlled trial. JAMA 1998;280:1831–6.

122. Rosenstock J, Tuchman M, LaMoreaux L, et al. Pregabalin for the treatment of painful diabetic peripheral neuropathy: a double-blind, placebo-controlled trial. Pain 2004;110:628–38.

123. Harati Y, Gooch C, Swenson M, et al. Double-blind randomized trial of tramadol for the treatment of the pain of diabetic neuropathy. Neurology 1998;50: 1842–6.

124. Nelson KA, Park KM, Robinovitz E, et al. High-dose oral dextromethorphan versus placebo in painful diabetic neuropathy and postherpetic neuralgia. Neurology 1997;48:1212–8.

125. Lesser H, Sharma U, LaMoreaux L, et al. Pregabalin relieves symptoms of painful diabetic neuropathy: a randomized controlled trial. Neurology 2004;63: 2104–10.

126. Ross DR, Varipara RJ. Treatment of painful diabetic neuropathy with topical capsaicin. N Engl J Med 1989;321:474–5.

127. The Capsaicin Study Group. Treatment of painful diabetic neuropathy with topical capsaicin: a multi-center, double-blind, vehicle controlled study. Arch Intern Med 1991;151:2225–9.

128. Rowbotham MC, Davies PS, Verkempnick C, et al. Lidocaine patch: a double-blind controlled study of a new treatment method for postherpetic neuralgia. Pain 1996;65(1):39–44.

129. Galer BS, Rowbotham MC, Pevander J, et al. Topical lidocaine patch relieves postherpetic neuralgia more effectively than a vehicle topical patch: results of an enriched enrollment study. Pain 1999;80(3):533–8.

130. Weintraub MI, Wolfe GI, Barohn RA, et al, Magnetic Research Group. Static magnetic field therapy for symptomatic diabetic neuropathy: a randomized, double-blind, placebo-controlled trial. Arch Phys Med Rehabil 2003;84(5): 736–46.

131. Weintraub MI. Magnetic bio-stimulation in painful diabetic peripheral neuropathy: a novel intervention - a randomized, double-placebo crossover study. Am J Pain Manag 1999;9:8–17.

132. Weintraub MI, Herrmann DN, Smith AG, et al. Pulsed electromagnetic fields to reduce diabetic neuropathic pain and stimulate neuronal repair: a randomized controlled trial. Arch Phys Med Rehabil 2009;90(7):1102–9.

133. Kluding PM, Pasnoor M, Singh R, et al. The effect of exercise on neuropathic symptoms, nerve function, and cutaneous innervation in people with diabetic peripheral neuropathy. J Diabet Complications 2012;26(5):424–9.

134. Malcolm A, Camilleri M. Treatment of diabetic gastroparesis and diarrhea. In: Dyck PJ, Thomas PK, editors. Diabetic neuropathy. 2nd edition. Philadelphia: WB Saunders; 1999. p. 517–29.

135. Robertson D, Davis TL. Recent advances in the treatment of orthostatic hypotension. Neurology 1995;45(Suppl 5):S26–32.

136. Jankovic J, Gilden JL, Hiner BC, et al. Neurogenic orthostatic hypotension: a double-blind placebo-controlled study with midodrine. Am J Med 1993;95: 34–48.

137. Low PA, Gilden JL, Freeman R, et al. Efficacy of midodrine vs placebo in neurogenic orthostatic hypotension. A randomized, double-blind multicenter study. JAMA 1997;227:1046–51.

138. Snape WJ Jr, Battle WM, Schwartz SS, et al. Metoclopramide to treat gastroparesis due to diabetes mellitus: a double-blind, controlled trial. Ann Intern Med 1982;96:444–6.

139. Janssens J, Peeters TL, Vantrappen G, et al. Improvement of gastric emptying in diabetic gastroparesis by erythromycin: preliminary studies. N Engl J Med 1990;332:1028–31.

140. Fedorak RN, Field M, Chang EB. Treatment of diabetic diarrhea with clonidine. Ann Intern Med 1985;102:197–9.

141. Goldstein I, Lue TF, Padma-Nathan H, et al. Oral sildenafil in the treatment of erectile dysfunction. N Engl J Med 1998;338:1397–404.

142. Gasser TC, Roach RM, Larsen EH, et al. Intracavernous self-injection with phentolamine and papaverine for the treatment of impotence. J Urol 1987;137: 678–80.

143. Scott FB, Fishman IJ, Light JK. An inflatable penile prosthesis for treatment of diabetic impotence. Ann Intern Med 1980;92:340–2.

144. Ellenberg M. Diabetic neuropathic cachexia. Diabetes 1974;23:418–23.

145. Jackson CE, Barohn RJ. Diabetic neuropathic cachexia: report of a recurrent case. J Neurol Neurosurg Psychiatry 1998;64:785–7.

146. Archer AG, Watkins PJ, Thomas PK, et al. The natural history of acute painful neuropathy in diabetes mellitus. J Neurol Neurosurg Psychiatry 1983;46:491–9.

147. Gade GN, Hofeldt FD, Treece GL. Diabetic neuropathic cachexia: beneficial response to combination therapy with amitriptyline and fluphenazine. JAMA 1980;243:1160–1.

148. Blau RH. Diabetic neuropathic cachexia: report of a woman with this syndrome and review of the literature. Arch Intern Med 1983;143:2011–2.

149. Wright DL, Shah JH. Diabetic neuropathic cachexia and hypothyroidism in a woman. Mol Med 1987;84:143–5.

150. D'Costa DF, Price DE, Burden AC. Diabetic neuropathic cachexia associated with malabsorption. Diabet Med 1992;9:203–5. http://dx.doi.org/10.1111/j.1464-5491.1992.tb01758.x.

151. Caravati CM. Insulin neuritis: a case report. Va Med Mon 1933;59:745–6.

152. Llewelyn JG, Thomas PK, Fonseca V, et al. Acute painful diabetic neuropathy precipitated by strict glycaemic control. Acta Neuropathol 1986;72:157–63.

153. Gibbons CH, Freeman R. Treatment-induced diabetic neuropathy: a reversible painful autonomic neuropathy. Ann Neurol 2010;67(4):534–41.

Diabetic Neuropathy Part 2
Proximal and Asymmetric Phenotypes

Mamatha Pasnoor, MD*, Mazen M. Dimachkie, MD,
Richard J. Barohn, MD

KEYWORDS

- Diabetic asymmetric neuropathies • Diabetic amyotrophy
- Focal diabetic neuropathy • Diabetic lumbosacral radiculoplexopathy
- Symmetric diabetic amyotrophy

KEY POINTS

- Diabetic neuropathy presents with varied manifestations, including proximal and asymmetric types.
- Except for entrapments, diabetic amyotrophy is the most common form of asymmetric diabetic neuropathy.
- Diabetic amyotrophy can present asymmetrically or symmetrically, with a rapid or insidious onset.
- Symmetric form of diabetic amyotrophy can be indistinguishable from chronic inflammatory demyelinating polyneuropathy.
- Treatment of diabetic amyotrophy with intravenous immunoglobulin or immunosuppressive drugs is controversial.
- Truncal radiculopathy can cause abdominal muscle weakness.
- Patients with diabetes can develop third, fourth, sixth, and seventh cranial nerve palsies.
- Patients with diabetes are more susceptible to compression mononeuropathies than those who are not diabetic.
- Muscle infarction can also be seen in diabetic individuals and is clinically distinct from diabetic amyotrophy.
- Treatment is mostly strict diabetic control and supportive in most of these conditions.

INTRODUCTION

Distal symmetric polyneuropathy is most common type of neuropathy associated with diabetes; however, many subtypes of diabetic neuropathies were defined even as early as in the 1800s.[1-4] Included in these descriptions are patients with proximal

Department of Neurology, University of Kansas Medical Center, 3599 Rainbow Boulevard, Mail-Stop 2012, Kansas City, KS 66160, USA
* Corresponding author.
E-mail address: mpasnoor@kumc.edu

Neurol Clin 31 (2013) 447–462
http://dx.doi.org/10.1016/j.ncl.2013.02.003   neurologic.theclinics.com
0733-8619/13/$ – see front matter © 2013 Elsevier Inc. All rights reserved.

diabetic neuropathy, truncal neuropathy, limb mononeuropathies, and cranial neurop-athies (**Box 1**). Bruns[5] focused further on the entity of proximal diabetic neuropathy. Various theories have been proposed for the pathogenesis of these neuropathies. Treatment in most cases is tight and stable glycemic control and pain management. A practical approach to the diagnosis and management of asymmetric and focal diabetic neuropathies is reviewed in this article.

ASYMMETRIC/FOCAL NEUROPATHIES
Diabetic Lumbosacral Radiculoplexopathy (Diabetic Amyotrophy, Bruns-Garland Syndrome, Proximal Diabetic Neuropathy)

The most common, and often misdiagnosed, multifocal asymmetric diabetic neurop-athy is the lumbosacral radiculoplexopathy syndrome (DLSRP).[6] This disorder has been referred to by many names, including proximal diabetic neuropathy, ischemic mononeuropathy multiplex, femoral or femoral-sciatic neuropathy, and most often, diabetic amyotrophy and the "Bruns-Garland syndrome," after the 2 physicians who first reported this entity.[5-21] Bruns[5] first described diabetic patients with asymmetric proximal weakness and pain in 1890. Later, Garland,[13] in the 1950s, used the term diabetic amyotrophy because of the muscle atrophy in the thighs. But this term can falsely imply that the primary lesion is on the muscle and therefore we use the term DLSRP.

Clinical presentation
DLSRP syndrome affects an older group of diabetic individuals, more frequently men, usually older than 50, but occasionally we have seen the syndrome in middle-aged diabetic individuals. Most patients have type 2 diabetes mellitus; however, this can occur even in individuals with type 1 diabetes. In a series of 27 patients reported by Coppack and Watkins,[22] 24 patients had type 2 diabetes mellitus and 3 had type 1 diabetes mellitus. The development of this neuropathy is often unrelated to glucose control or the duration of glucose intolerance. DLSRP can be the presenting manifes-tation leading to the initial diagnosis of diabetes.

This neuropathy begins with severe unilateral pain in the back, hip, or thigh, which subsequently spreads to the other side within weeks to months.[6,19,22] Patients are frequently misdiagnosed as having a compressive lumbosacral radiculopathy. Some patients undergo unnecessary lumbar surgery despite minor changes on lumbar magnetic resonance imaging (MRI) scan. Given the associated weight loss, patients are often suspected to have a pelvic tumor. Within days to weeks of the pain onset, patients develop weakness in typically proximal and, to a lesser extent, distal leg muscles.

Box 1
Clinical classification of asymmetric diabetic neuropathies

Asymmetric/Focal and Multifocal Diabetic Neuropathies:

Diabetic lumbosacral radiculoplexopathy (Bruns-Garland syndrome; diabetic amyotrophy; proximal diabetic neuropathy)

Truncal neuropathies (thoracic radiculopathy)

Cranial neuropathies

Limb mononeuropathies

On examination, there is weakness of hip flexors, adductors and extensors, knee flexors and extensors, and ankle dorsiflexors and plantar flexors of varying degree. Profound atrophy of the thigh and at times distal lower extremity muscles develops. Weakness usually encompasses multiple root or plexus levels and is rarely isolated to an individual root or peripheral nerve. Thus, in cases in which knee extension weakness is prominent and the possibility of a diabetic "femoral neuropathy" is considered, if one looks closely at other L2–L4 muscles either on the neurologic examination or with needle electromyography (EMG), the disease process can usually be found in these adjacent areas. Similarly, if there is a significant foot drop, there is also usually evidence of involvement in tibial or other L5 innervated muscles, and the process is actually not confined to the peroneal nerve. There is usually distal sensory loss, but this is often indistinguishable from the sensory abnormalities of distal symmetric polyneuropathy (DSPN), which often is present before the development of the radiculoplexopathy. Loss of knee and ankle reflexes is common.

Although the condition usually begins in one leg, spread to the other leg within weeks or months is rather frequent. The disorder worsens in a gradually progressive or stepwise manner. Cases have been documented in which there is worsening for 18 months.[6] Eventually, the process stabilizes and gradually improves, although the recovery may take many months. In many cases, some degree of permanent weakness may persist (**Fig. 1**).[6]

In about one-third of the cases, weakness spreads to proximal arm muscles and is attributed to cervicobrachial radiculoplexopathy.[11,19,23] Approximately 12% of patients develop thoracic radiculopathy, leading to radiating pain in the chest or abdomen and intercostal muscle weakness.[24,25] Respiratory weakness has also been described with this neuropathy.[26]

Diagnostic workup

Electrophysiologically, nerve conduction study findings may not differentiate DLSRP neuropathy from DSPN, except for an asymmetric reduction of the femoral compound muscle action potential amplitudes in unilateral cases. However, the needle EMG reveals abundant fibrillation potentials in weak proximal and distal leg muscles, as well as in the lumbosacral paraspinous muscles.[6] The cerebrospinal fluid (CSF) protein is often elevated, usually between 60 and 100 mg/dL, but occasionally as high as 400 mg/dL. The erythrocyte sedimentation rate may be elevated as well, but is usually less than 50 mm/h. MRI with gadolinium may show nerve root enhancement.[27]

Sural nerve biopsy is not essential to the diagnosis of DLSRP syndrome. When done to exclude mimics, it shows significant fiber loss, often in an asymmetric fashion within and between fascicles, resembling focal ischemia (**Fig. 2**).[6,9–11] An ischemic pathogenesis was documented by Raff and colleagues[7,8] in an autopsy study showing infarcts of proximal nerve trunks of the leg and lumbosacral plexus. Asymmetric fiber loss in sural nerve may support this theory; however, it should be remembered that even patients with typical DSPN may show this multifocal pattern at times. The presence of occasional thinly myelinated fibers on plastic-embedded sections or short, thin segments on teased nerve fiber preparations should not lead the physician to diagnose a demyelinating neuropathy, as these findings can be seen in DSPN as well. However, it should be emphasized that the electrophysiologic, biopsy, and laboratory features are often not particularly helpful, and the diagnoses of DLSRP is primarily clinically based on the history and neurologic examination.

There is probably a small subset of diabetic patients with amyotrophy who develop a painless, symmetric proximal neuropathy involving the lower extremities. Asbury,[21]

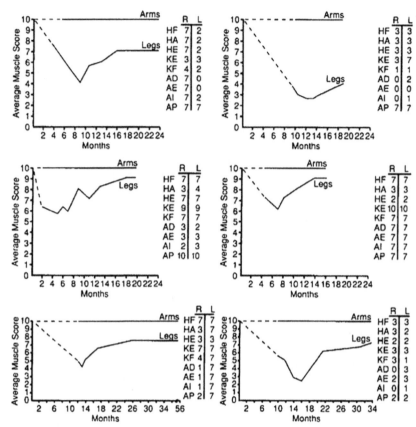

Fig. 1. Course of muscle strength in 6 patients showing progressive leg weakness. Broken lines represent the period before the initial evaluations. Solid lines represent the course during our serial examinations. The average muscle score, shown in the table adjacent to each graph, is based on a modified Medical Research Council scale expanded to a 10-point scale (see text). The scores for leg strength are those at the nadir of the illness. AD, ankle dorsiflexion; AE, ankle eversion; AL, ankle inversion; AP, ankle plantar flexion; HA, hip abduction; HE, hip extension; HF, hip flexion; KE, knee extension; KF, knee flexion; L, left; R, indicates right. (*From* Barohn RJ, Sahenk Z, Warmolts JR, et al. The Bruns-Garland syndrome (diabetic amyotrophy): revisited 100 years later. Arch Neurol 1991;48:1130–5; with permission.)

favoring the term proximal diabetic neuropathy, considered that there was a spectrum ranging from asymmetrical cases with a rapid onset to patients with symmetric proximal weakness of insidious onset. Chokroverty and colleagues[16,17] emphasized insidious bilateral onset of proximal weakness. Pascoe and colleagues[11] published a Mayo clinic series of 44 patients with symmetric proximal weakness that has a more restricted distribution and seems to be monophasic and self-limiting, differentiating from chronic inflammatory demyelinating neuropathy (CIDP). However, the symmetric presentation seems to be uncommon and tends to occur more often in young type 1 diabetic individuals who are having poor glycemic control. Therefore, we have divided the proximal diabetic amyotrophies (DAM) into 2 forms: DAM-1 and DAM-2 (**Table 1**).[28]

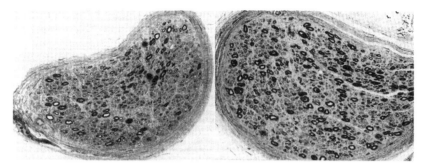

Fig. 2. Cross sections of sural nerve fascicles, 1-μm thick. Nonrandom fiber loss is more apparent and more severe in the left than in the right. (*From* Barohn RJ, Sahenk Z, Warmolts JR, et al. The Bruns-Garland syndrome (diabetic amyotrophy): revisited 100 years later. Arch Neurol 1991;48:1130–5; with permission.)

If asymmetric diabetic neuropathies occur in only about 1% of the diabetic population, we think the painless, symmetric form of diabetic amyotrophy (DAM-1) is even more uncommon. This form superficially resembles idiopathic CIDP. We believe that for every 10 to 20 patients with asymmetric/painful amyotrophy (DAM-2) seen at a tertiary care neuromuscular centers, only one DAM-1 patient will be seen. Whether or not the pathogenesis of DAM-1 is different from DAM-2 and is more in line with metabolic dysfunction is unknown.

Management
Treatment is centered around pain control and strict glycemic control. Both groups spontaneously improve over a period of months. Physical therapy can assist in improving functional mobility.

Controversy involving DLSRP is whether or not there is an immune-mediated pathogenesis component and if patients respond favorably to immunomodulating therapy. This concept was first introduced by Bradley and colleagues[29] in 1984 in their report of 6 patients with a painful lumbosacral plexopathy, elevated sedimentation rate, mild

Table 1
Diabetic amyotrophy: 2 presentations

	DAM-1	DAM-2
Type of DM	Type 1 >2	Type 2 >1
Onset in legs and progression	Bilateral/Insidious Chronic	Unilateral/Acute Stepwise/Goes to other leg
Distribution	Symmetric proximal	Asymmetric proximal and distal
Pain	No	Yes
Sensory symptoms	No	Yes
Poor DM control	Yes	Yes
Weight loss	Yes	Yes
Spontaneous improvement	Yes	Yes
Frequency	Very, very rare	Uncommon: ~1%
Spread to arm	Yes: ?Common	Yes: 10%

Abbreviations: DAM, diabetic amyotrophy; DM, diabetes mellitus.

perivascular inflammation on sural nerve biopsy, and asymmetric nerve fiber loss. Five were treated with immunosuppressive drugs (prednisone alone or prednisone and cyclophosphamide) and 4 improved or stopped progressing. They did not believe the diabetic individuals had typical DLSRP because "they continued to deteriorate and to have pain for several months despite careful control of the diabetes, and only began to improve following treatment with prednisone, although this therapy worsened their diabetes." Thus, Bradley and colleagues[29] felt the diabetes in their patients was incidental. Of course, others have also reported idiopathic lumbosacral plexitis in nondiabetic patients (analogous to idiopathic brachial plexitis).[30,31] Interestingly, in the earlier reports of idiopathic lumbosacral plexitis, patients improved spontaneously. Verma and Bradley[32] advocated the use of intravenous immunoglobulin (IVIG) for idiopathic lumbosacral plexitis.

Krendel and colleagues[33] (in 1995) reported their experience using immunotherapy in 21 patients with diabetic neuropathy. They divided their patients into 2 groups: Group A consisted of 15 patients who had "multifocal axonal inflammatory vasculopathy" and most of these patients seemed to correspond to what we described previously as DLSRP. Group B patients consisted of 6 diabetic individuals who had both arm and leg involvement, and although in 3 patients the process was asymmetric, the investigators stated this group had "demyelinating" neuropathy by electrophysiologic criteria. Group A patients had perivascular inflammation on nerve biopsy and group B patients had "onion bulbs" but no inflammation. All patients received some form of immunomodulatory therapy (15, IVIG; 13, prednisone; 5, cyclophosphamide; 3, plasma exchange; 1, azathioprine) in various combinations, and all improved. Krendel and colleagues'[33] conclusion was that there are 2 forms of immune-mediated neuropathy in diabetic patients that responds to treatment. Younger and colleagues[34] reported their experience finding evidence of inflammation in 20 patients with diabetic neuropathy: 4 had DSPN, 12 had "proximal diabetic neuropathy," and 4 had mononeuropathy multiplex. All patients with proximal diabetic neuropathy and mononeuropathy multiplex had asymmetric features and we would currently consider them as having DLSRP. As noted in the pathogenesis section see the article by Pasnoor and colleagues elsewhere in this issue, 12 of 20 had some evidence of inflammatory cells, including 2 with DSPN. Younger and colleagues treated 8 patients with IVIG (2 DSPN, 1mononeuropathy multiplex, 5 proximal diabetic neuropathy), all of whom had perivascular inflammation, and they reported that all improved.

In the Mayo Clinic group series by Pascoe and colleagues,[11] 3 of 9 patients undergoing sural nerve biopsy had a multifocal distribution of fiber loss, and 2 had perivascular mononuclear inflammatory infiltrates. Twelve were treated with IVIG, and 9 improved. Of the 29 untreated patients, 17 spontaneously improved. They concluded that the "efficacy of immunotherapy is unproven but such intervention may be considered in the severe progressive cases or ones associated with severe neuropathic pain."

The experience of the French group led by Gerard Said is important to note. In an article published in 1994, they reported inflammatory and ischemic lesions in nerve biopsy specimens of the intermediate cutaneous nerve of the thigh in patients with DLSRP.[9] Three patients with "severe and prolonged painful disability" improved dramatically with corticosteroid treatment. In a subsequent report in 1997 of 4 patients with DLSRP, Said and colleagues[10] described patients who had symptoms for 4, 6, 12, and 18 months before biopsy. Although all patients showed perivascular inflammation on nerve biopsy, to the investigators' surprise, all became pain free with subsequent improvement of their weakness shortly following the biopsy. They concluded that despite the treatment with prednisone they used in their initial article, that

DLSP "is self-limited and does not require the use of corticosteroids or immunomodulators." In a series by Dyck and colleagues,[35] all 33 patients with DLSRP had some evidence of microvasculitis on nerve biopsy, and nearly all improved spontaneously. A report by the group from Houston found 18 of 19 patients with DLSRP had substantial improvement without immunomodulating therapy.[36]

Despite many months of persistent symptoms or progression in some patients with DLSRP, eventually all patients spontaneously have resolution of pain and slow improvement of weakness (see **Fig. 1**).[6] Treatment with IVIG or other immunosuppressive drugs is controversial. In a prospective case series, 5 patients with severe pain received IVIG after having no response to symptomatic therapy for pain and corticosteroids.[37] Four had a decrease in pain. In contrast, Zochodne and colleagues[38] in 2003 reported a patient who developed DLSRP while on immunosuppressive regimen consisting of cyclosporine and myophenolate mofetil for an allograft cardiac transplant and 2 patients with DLSRP who did not respond to IVIG treatment, arguing that immunosuppressive therapy did not prevent onset of DLSRP. In our opinion, we do not believe IVIG should be used in patients with DLSRP. At this time, we are not convinced that this form of immunomodulating therapy is indicated. Perhaps this question can be resolved with a controlled trial, but such a trial will be difficult, as each center sees a handful of patients annually and it will be difficult to get the pharmaceutical industry and the Food and Drug Administration to support a large multi-center IVIG trial in this rare disorder.

On the other hand, the experience of Said and Bradley with the improvement of pain with prednisone should not be ignored. According to a recent Cochrane review of immunotherapy for diabetic amyotrophy (DA) only one completed controlled trial using IV methyprednisolone in DA was found.[39,40] High doses of corticosteroids may lead to improvement of severe pain in some patients with DLSRP, and this may be analogous to the improvement of neuropathic pain in patients who are believed to have reflex sympathetic dystrophy.[41,42] Perhaps breaking the pain syndrome in this manner may subsequently allow patients to begin moving their weak extremities easier. Presently, there is no convincing evidence from randomized trial to support any recommendation on the use of any immunotherapy treatment in DLSRP.[39]

We believe one should be cautious about jumping to the conclusion that finding mild perivascular inflammation on biopsy, or demyelination features on either electrophysiology or pathology suggest that DLSRP is a disease that is primarily immune-mediated and will respond to immunomodulating therapy. We cautioned previously about the danger of heavily relying on electrophysiologic evidence of demyelination on nerve conduction studies (NCS) of diabetic patients, as some will fulfill research electrophysiologic criteria for CIDP even though the clinical pattern does not correspond to CIDP, but actually is that of DLSRP. Similar caution should be used with data from nerve biopsies of patients with DLSRP in concluding these patients have either vasculitis or a demyelinating neuropathy. In routine clinical practice, we do not recommend either nerve biopsy or immunomodulating therapy in patients with typical DLSRP. Finally, we would also caution clinicians about splitting patients with otherwise typical DLSRP because of nerve root enhancement on lumbar MRI scan.[27] If other etiologies are excluded by CSF analysis, the mere finding of root enhancement on MRI in DLSRP should not necessarily lead to the initiation of immunomodulating therapy.

Other DLSRP caveats

Cervical brachial radiculoplexopathy Although cervical/brachial plexus involvement is uncommon, it does occur.[11,23] In the classic early Mayo Clinic series of "diabetic polyradiculopathy" reported by Bastron and Thomas[19] in 1981 of 105 patients, 81 had lower extremity involvement, 15 had upper extremity involvement, and 12 had thoracic/abdominal involvement. Obviously, a few patients had involvement of more than one region. As mentioned previously, in the Mayo Clinic series of Pascoe and colleagues,[11] all 44 patients had (by definition) leg weakness, and 12 of these also had arm weakness (7 bilateral, 5 unilateral). Occasionally, patients with DLSRP develop arm pain and weakness days to weeks after the initial leg symptoms.[43,44] The arm involvement is usually proximal and distal, similar to the pattern of weakness seen in the legs. Interestingly, the arm symptoms can begin or continue to progress after the leg symptoms have plateaued or begun to improve.

Thus, whereas cervical/brachial root and plexus involvement has not been emphasized a great deal in diabetic radiculoplexopathy, the clinician should be aware of this possibility. We do believe that in this setting, a more extensive workup probably is to exclude other disease entities. All of these patients should have a CSF examination for infectious and neoplastic diseases, and nerve biopsy is probably warranted to exclude true vasculitic neuropathy.

CIDP in diabetic patients Diabetic patients can develop typical CIDP but, as mentioned previously, there is no increased risk of CIDP in diabetic patients.[45–48] The clinical features of gradually progressive, usually painless, proximal and distal symmetric weakness and numbness in the arms and legs should be sufficient to distinguish CIDP from the typical symmetric and asymmetric diabetic neuropathies; however, the laboratory results in this setting may not be particularly helpful, especially the CSF protein. If there is an underlying diabetic DSPN on NCS and needle EMG, electrophysiologic results can also be relatively unhelpful unless clear-cut and ample features of an acquired, markedly demyelinating neuropathy are present. In addition, nerve biopsy in many diabetic neuropathies can show thinly myelinated fibers, and therefore we usually do not pursue nerve biopsy in this setting. Diagnosis is usually based on the clinical presentation and it is reasonable to proceed with immunomodulating therapy when CIDP is strongly suspected.

True mononeuritis multiplex in diabetes: does it exist? Finally, a comment should be made regarding "mononeuritis multiplex" in diabetic patients. We suspect that most of these patients have diabetic radiculoplexopathy, usually lumbosacral, but rarely cervical-brachial. It is uncommon for diabetic patients to develop a true mononeuritis multiplex in which individual distal peripheral nerves (eg, femoral, peroneal, tibial, ulnar, median or radial) are "picked-off" in a subacute or acute fashion. It is difficult to find good documentation of this in the literature. Although the early articles by Raff and colleagues[7,8] use the term "mononeuropathy multiplex," if one reads of clinical description of their 7 cases, they all had typical DLSRP with proximal and distal involvement not confined to an individual nerve. If a diabetic patient develops a true mononeuritis multiplex, the usual causes need to be pursued (vasculitis, infectious, and hereditary). We believe that if one wants to include diabetes mellitus in the differential diagnosis of true mononeuritis multiplex, it should be at the bottom of such a list.

OTHER ASYMMETRIC NEUROPATHIES
Truncal Radiculopathy

Another common focal form of diabetic radiculopathy involves isolated thoracic roots.[49–52] This is presumably a focal diabetic radiculopathy that is similar to DLSRP except for the location on the trunk, thorax, or abdomen.

Clinical presentation

Patients develop abrupt pain over days to weeks with severe dysesthesias in a dermatomal pattern. In some patients, the pain may not radiate entirely around the trunk in a full radicular pattern, but the symptoms and signs may occur in smaller, restricted regions that imply damage of the dorsal or ventral rami or their medial or lateral branches.[25] Multiple thoracic dermatomes can be involved. Although most cases are unilateral at onset, it can evolve bilaterally, much like DLSRP. In fact, in our experience, it is not uncommon during the evaluation of a patient with typical DLSRP to uncover that at some point over the preceding year or 2 the patient had an episode of truncal pain and dysesthesias, or was diagnosed with truncal "shingles" without a rash. Patients can occasionally develop weakness of the rectus abdominus muscles. Some patients may present with pseudohernia caused by weakening of the abdominal musculature.[49,53]

On the other hand, although most patients do not demonstrate obvious motor involvement, needle EMG can reveal abnormalities in the paraspinous or abdominal wall muscles.

Diagnostic workup

Nerve conductions may reveal abnormalities related to distal symmetric polyneuropathy. Needle EMG findings include fibrillations in the paraspinous or abdominal wall muscles.[51,54,55]

Management

Treatment is directed at symptomatic pain management, see the article by Pasnoor and colleagues elsewhere in this issue on DSPN, in this volume. Truncal radiculopathy should be distinguished from the wedge-shaped midline area of symmetric truncal sensory loss that can occur in advanced DSPN[50] and from rare discogenic thoracic radiculopathy.

Prognosis

The natural history is similar to DLSRP, with persistence of sensory symptoms for weeks to months, with gradual resolution.

Cranial Neuropathies

Diabetic patients can suddenly develop a unilateral third, fourth, sixth, or seventh cranial nerve palsy. The oculomotor nerve was found to be most frequently affected in one study by Greco and colleagues[56] looking at 61 patients with diabetic cranial nerve palsies. The hallmark of diabetic third nerve palsy is pupillary sparing in most cases.

Clinical presentation

Retro-orbital pain accompanies about half of the cases. Sparing of the pupil in diabetic third nerve palsies is due to sparing of axons at the periphery of the nerve involved in pupillary function. Pathologic evidence supports the concept that the process is probably attributable to an ischemic watershed phenomenon in the central part of the nerve.[57–60]

It has been suggested that patients with diabetes are more likely to develop a seventh cranial nerve palsy.[61] However, Bell palsy is a common event and it is difficult to substantiate if it is indeed more prevalent in diabetes.[62] It is interesting to note that in the Rochester Diabetic Neuropathy Study, neither cranial mononeuropathies nor truncal radiculopathies were more common in diabetic patients compared with control subjects.[63]

Diagnostic workup
Imaging studies may be necessary to rule out stroke in some cases; however, history alone without additional testing is sufficient in most of these patients.

Management and prognosis
The main risk factors for the development of cranial neuropathies are duration of diabetes and the patient's age.[64] Treatment should be mainly focused on management of diabetes.

Most patients make a full recovery, with some early evidence of improvement within 2 to 3 months.

Isolated Mononeuropathies

Clinical presentation
It is generally believed and established in studies that diabetic individuals are more susceptible to compression injuries compared with nondiabetic individuals.[65] This would include the median nerve at the carpal tunnel, ulnar nerve at the elbow, the peroneal (fibular) nerve at the fibular head, and perhaps the lateral cutaneous femoral nerve (meralgia paresthetica) at the hip. In the early study by Mulder and colleagues[66] in 103 cases of diabetes, 16 had mononeuropathies affecting 29 nerves as follows: common peroneal, 13; median nerve (carpal tunnel), 9; ulnar nerve, 5; lateral femoral cutaneous nerve, 1; and femoral nerve, 1, the latter being likely due to DLSRP. Meralgia paresthetica (mononeuropathy of the lateral femoral cutaneous nerve) is associated with diabetes mellitus irrespective of obesity and advanced age.[67]

In a study from Rochester, Minnesota, there was evidence that carpal tunnel syndrome is more common in diabetes mellitus than in the general population.[68] In another Rochester Diabetic Neuropathy Study, approximately one-quarter of patients had subclinical carpal tunnel syndrome on NCS, but only 7.7% were symptomatic.[63]

Diagnostic workup
Diagnosis is usually established with electrophysiologic testing; however, electrophysiologic diagnosis of carpal tunnel or other mononeuropathies is sometimes difficult in individuals with diabetic polyneuropathy. One study showed that segmental and comparative median nerve conduction tests in combination with standard nerve conduction resulted in more accurate diagnosis of carpal tunnel syndrome in patients with diabetic polyneuropathy.[69]

DIABETIC MUSCLE INFARCTION

In the context of discussing the various diabetic neuropathies, it is relevant to review another neuromuscular complication of diabetes in which the muscle itself is the target organ rather than the nerve. It is an underdiagnosed complication of long-standing diabetes.[70]

Clinical Presentation

Diabetic muscle infarction (DMI) begins with the abrupt onset of thigh pain, tenderness, and swelling.[71–76] Over a period of days, a firm mass develops in nearly half of cases. The muscles most frequently involved are the vastus lateralis and medialis, thigh adductors, and biceps femoris. Calf involvement is reported in up to 20% of cases and bilateral involvement in 8% of cases.[77] Compared with 130 cases, there are 5 case reports of DMI affecting muscles of the upper limb of patients, particularly in patients with type 2 diabetes with end-stage renal disease.[78] Edema from the swelling can extend to the knee and mimic a joint effusion.[70] DMI tends to occur in younger, poorly controlled diabetic patients with other end-organ complications. There are no associated systemic symptoms or signs indicative of infection and no skin discoloration suggesting cellulitis or thrombophlebitis. The painful mass persists for weeks, occasionally with exacerbation of symptoms, and then spontaneously resolves over weeks to several months. Contralateral involvement of the other thigh can occur, even after the initial episode resolves. Up to 50% of cases will recur, mostly involving previously unaffected muscle groups.[77]

Diagnostic Workup

Creatine kinase can be normal or modestly elevated. Needle EMG demonstrates fibrillation potentials in the involved muscles with a loss of voluntary motor unit potentials in the most affected areas. Remaining motor unit potentials may be brief and short, reflecting fragmentation of the motor unit. MRI scan of the limb muscle reveals increased signal on T2-weighted images in the involved thigh muscles, indicative of marked muscle edema extending into the perifascicular and subcutaneous tissues (**Fig. 3**).[72,73,79] Gadolinium contrast administration is contraindicated in those with renal impairment. Radionuclide imaging with Technetium-99 demonstrates radiopharmaceutical accumulation and muscle ultrasound shows hyperechoic signal in the mass.[73]

Biopsy of the region consists of large confluent areas of muscle necrosis and edema, with loss of the normal architectural pattern. A muscle biopsy is often not needed because it may prolong recovery and is indicated only when the presentation is atypical, response is poor, or diagnosis is uncertain. Biopsy, when performed,

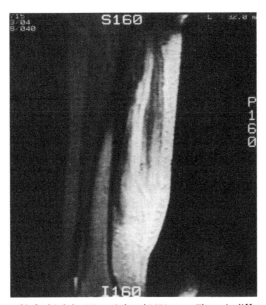

Fig. 3. Sagittal view of left thigh by T2-weighted MRI scan. There is diffuse high signal in the biceps femoris, semimembra-nosus, and semitendinosus muscles, whereas the bone and anterior compartment muscles appear normal. (*From* Barohn RJ, Kissel JT. Case-of-the-month: painful thigh mass in a young woman: diabetic muscle infarction. Muscle Nerve 1992;15:850–5; with permission.)

Table 2 DLSRP versus DMI	DLSRP	DMI
Pain	+	+
Focally tender	−	+
Swelling/mass	−	+
Progression	+	+
Bilaterally	+	+
Atrophy	+	−
Distal weakness	+	±
Sensory symptoms	±	−
MRI muscle	Normal	Abnormal
EMG	Neuropathic	Myopathic

Abbreviations: DLSRP, diabetic lumbosacral radiculoplexopathy; DMI, diabetic muscle infarction; EMG, electromyogram; MRI, magnetic resonance imaging; +, present; −, absent; ±, maybe present or absent.

shows pale muscle on gross examination and areas of muscle necrosis and edema surrounded by muscle fibers in various stages of degeneration and regeneration, with hyalinosis and thickening of arterioles.[71]

The differential diagnosis of DMI includes, in addition to DLSRP, infection (abscess, pyomyositis, necrotizing fasciitis), focal myositis, venous thrombosis, and tumor. Both DMI and DLSRP syndromes begin with the abrupt onset of lower extremity pain that can ultimately involve the opposite side. In DLSRP the pain is usually localized to the low back, hip, or buttocks with radiation into the thigh; whereas, in DMI, the pain is more focal and associated with swelling and a firm mass. Patients with DLSRP develop dramatic weakness and atrophy in proximal, and usually distal lower extremity muscles. Sensory symptoms (other than pain) do not result from DMI unless there is a prior distal symmetric polyneuropathy. Whereas the imaging studies of the thigh will be focally abnormal with swelling and infarction in DMI, they may show diffuse denervating changes and atrophy on T2 sequences of the hip, thigh, and leg muscles in DLSRP. The EMG in DLSRP is different in that it is characterized by widespread fibrillations in many muscles (usually including the paraspinous muscles), with long-duration, polyphasic motor unit potentials and decreased recruitment pattern. NCS may not be helpful in distinguishing the disorders, as both may show evidence of a distal symmetric polyneuropathy.

Although there are obvious differences between DMI and DLSRP (**Table 2**), the abrupt onset of both syndromes, and pathologic evidence for probable focal ischemia in the muscle (DMI) and nerve (DLSRP) supports the theory that both entities have a primary vascular microangiopathic etiology.

Management and Prognosis

The treatment of DMI is supportive. No evidence-based recommendations are available on management of this condition; however, a retrospective analysis supports conservative management with bed rest, leg elevation, and adequate analgesia. Activities should be avoided to avoid increasing the pain. There is no evidence to support the use of corticosteroids or surgery. Short-term prognosis is good, but the recurrence rate is high (40%), and recurrences may not affect the same muscle group.[80]

Case study

A 62-year-old diabetic man on an oral hypoglycemic treatment developed sudden severe pain that started in the lower back and radiated to the right leg. Within 3 days, he experienced weakness in the same leg. After 1 month, similar pain and weakness occurred in the left leg. Symptoms persisted for 4 months, during which time the patient had a 9-kg unintentional weight loss. Neurologic examination revealed asymmetric proximal and distal weakness in both legs. There was asymmetric atrophy of the quadriceps and hamstring muscles. A stocking pattern of loss of pinprick, light touch, and vibration sense was found. Tendon reflexes were absent at the ankles and trace at the knees bilaterally. Upper extremities had normal motor and sensory function.

At the time of initial evaluation, fasting glucose was mildly elevated (140 mg/dL), with a glycosylated hemoglobin of 7.5% and fasting blood sugar of 135 mg/dL. Peroneal motor conduction velocity was reduced at 36 m/s, and compound motor action potential was reduced at 300 μV. Tibial nerve conduction was 38 m/s, and sural potentials were absent. Median and ulnar nerve conduction velocities were normal. Bilateral femoral motor conduction studies showed an amplitude of 3 mV on left and 1 mV on right. An EMG revealed active denervation potentials in proximal (quadriceps, adductor longus, gluteus medius, and hamstrings), distal (gastrocnemius and anterior tibial), and lumbosacral paraspinal muscles bilaterally.

His recovery was protracted. Diabetes mellitus was managed by his primary care physician and he achieved better control of his diabetes. He required a right knee brace for ambulation and was treated with gabapentin (Neurontin) for pain control. Leg weakness progressed for 3 additional months before subsequent gradual improvement of strength. At the 6-month follow-up, the pain had almost resolved; however, he still had considerable residual weakness.

REFERENCES

1. Althaus J. On sclerosis of the spinal cord, including locomotor ataxy, spastic spinal paralysis and other system diseases of the spinal cord: their pathology, symptoms, diagnosis, and treatment. London (United Kingdom): Green & Company; 1885.
2. Leyden E. Entzundung der peripheren Nerven. Deut Militar Zeitsch 1887;17:49.
3. Auche M. Des alterations des nerfs périphériques. Arch Med Exp Anat Pathol 1890;2:635.
4. Pryce TD. On diabetic neuritis with a clinical and pathological description of three cases of diabetic pseudo-tabes. Brain 1893;16:416.
5. Bruns L. Ueber neuritische Lahmungen beim Diabetes mellitus. Berl Klin Wochensher 1980;27:509–15.
6. Barohn RJ, Sahenk Z, Warmolts JR, et al. The Bruns-Garland syndrome (diabetic amyotrophy): revisited 100 years later. Arch Neurol 1991;48:1130–5.
7. Raff M, Asbury AK. Ischemic mononeuropathy and mononeuropathy multiplex in diabetes mellitus. N Engl J Med 1968;279:17–22.
8. Raff MC, Sangalang V, Asbury AK. Ishemic mononeuropathy multiplex associated with diabetes mellitus. Arch Neurol 1968;18:487–99.
9. Said G, Goulon-Goeau C, Lacroix C, et al. Nerve biopsy findings in different patterns of proximal diabetic neuropathy. Ann Neurol 1994;35:559–69.
10. Said G, Elgrably F, Lacroix C, et al. Painful proximal diabetic neuropathy: inflammatory nerve lesions and spontaneous favorable outcome. Ann Neurol 1997;41: 762–70.
11. Pascoe MK, Low PA, Windebank AJ, et al. Subacute diabetic proximal neuropathy. Mayo Clin Proc 1997;72:1123–32.
12. Garland H, Taverner D. Diabetic myelopathy. Br Med J 1953;1:405–8.
13. Garland H. Diabetic amyotrophy. Br Med J 1955;2:1287–90.

14. Locke S, Lawrence DG, Legg MA. Diabetic amyotrophy. Am J Med 1963;34: 775–85.
15. Calverley JR, Mulder DW. Femoral neuropathy. Neurology 1960;10:963–7.
16. Chokroverty S, Reyes MG, Rubino FA, et al. The syndrome of diabetic amyotrophy. Ann Neurol 1977;2:181–94.
17. Chokroverty S. AAEE Case Report #13: diabetic amyotrophy. Muscle Nerve 1987; 10:679–84.
18. Subramony SH, Wilbourn AJ. Diabetic proximal neuropathy. J Neurol Sci 1982;53: 293–304.
19. Bastron JA, Thomas JE. Diabetic polyradiculopathy. Mayo Clin Proc 1981;56: 725–32.
20. Williams IR, Mayer RF. Subacute proximal diabetic neuropathy. Neurology 1976; 26:108–16.
21. Asbury AK. Proximal diabetic neuropathy. Ann Neurol 1977;2:179–80.
22. Coppack SW, Watkins PJ. The natural history of diabetic femoral neuropathy. Q J Med 1991;79(288):307–13.
23. Katz JS, Saperstein DS, Wolfe G, et al. Cervicobrachial involvement in diabetic radiculoplexopathy. Muscle Nerve 2001;24:794–8.
24. Streib EW, Sun SF, Paustian EF, et al. Diabetic thoracic radiculopathy: electrodiagnostic study. Muscle Nerve 1986;9:548–53.
25. Stewart JD. Diabetic truncal neuropathy: topography of the sensory deficit. Ann Neurol 1989;25:233–8.
26. Brannagan TH, Promisloff RA, McCluskey LF, et al. Proximal diabetic neuropathy presenting with respiratory weakness. J Neurol Neurosurg Psychiatry 1999;67: 539–41.
27. O'Neil BJ, Flanders AE, Escandon S, et al. Treatable lumbosacral polyradiculitis masquerading as diabetic amyotrophy. J Neurol Sci 1997;151:223–5.
28. Amato AA, Barohn RJ. Diabetic lumbosacral polyradiculoneuropathies. Curr Treat Options Neurol 2001;3(2):139–46.
29. Bradley WG, Chad D, Verghese JP, et al. Painful lumbosacral plexopathy with elevated erythrocyte sedimentation rate: a treatable inflammatory syndrome. Ann Neurol 1984;15:457–64.
30. Evans BA, Stevens JC, Dyck PJ. Lumbosacral plexus neuropathy. Neurology 1981;31:1327–30.
31. Sander JE, Sharp FR. Lumbosacral plexus neuritis. Neurology 1981;31:470–3.
32. Verma A, Bradley WG. High-dose intravenous immunoglobulin therapy in chronic progressive lumbosacral plexopathy. Neurology 1994;44:248–50.
33. Krendel DA, Costigan DA, Hopkins LC. Successful treatment of neuropathies in patients with diabetes mellitus. Arch Neurol 1995;52:1053–61.
34. Younger DS, Rosoklija G, Hays AP, et al. Diabetic peripheral neuropathy: a clinicopathologic and immunohistochemical analysis of sural nerve biopsies. Muscle Nerve 1996;19:722–7.
35. Dyck PJB, Novell JE, Dyck PJ. Microvasculitis and ischemia in diabetic lumbosacral radiculopexus neuropathy. Neurology 1999;53:2113–21.
36. Lovitt SM, Pleitez MY, Copeland KJ, et al. Proximal diabetic neuropathy improves spontaneously without expensive and dangerous treatment [abstract]. Neurology 2000;54:A212–3.
37. Tamburin S, Zanette G. Intravenous immunoglobulin for the treatment of diabetic lumbosacral radiculoplexus neuropathy. Pain Med 2009;10(8):1476–80.
38. Zochodne DW, Isaac D, Jones C. Failure of immunotherapy to prevent, arrest or reverse diabetic lumbosacral plexopathy. Acta Neurol Scand 2003;107(4):299–301.

39. Chan YC, Lo YL, Chan ES. Immunotherapy for diabetic amyotrophy. Cochrane Database Syst Rev 2012;(6):CD006521.
40. Dyck PJB, O'Brien P, Bosch EP, et al. The multi-center, double-blind controlled trial of IV methylprednisolone in diabetic lumbosacral radiculoplexus neuropathy. Neurology 2006;66(5 Suppl 2):A191.
41. Kozin F, Ryan LM, Carerra GF, et al. The reflex sympathetic dystrophy syndrome (RSDS). III. Scitigraphic studies, further evidence for the therapeutic efficacy of systemic corticosteroids, and proposed diagnostic criteria. Am J Med 1981;70: 23–30.
42. Barohn RJ. Reflex sympathetic dystrophy due to peripheral neuropathy and utility of the three-phase bone scan: case series and review. Adv an Clin Neurosci 1997;7:129–50.
43. Katz JS, Wolfe GI, Burns D, et al. Diabetic radiculoplexopathy with cervicobrachial involvement [abstract]. Neurology 2000;54:A367.
44. Riley DE, Shields RW. Diabetic amyotrophy with upper extremity involvement [abstract]. Neurology 1984;34(Suppl 1):216.
45. Cornblath DR, Drach DB, Griffin JW. Demyelinating motor neuropathy in patients with diabetic polyneuropathy [abstract]. Ann Neurol 1987;22:126S.
46. Stewart JD, McKelvey R, Durcan L, et al. Chronic inflammatory demyelinating polyneuropathy (CIDP) in diabetics. J Neurol Sci 1996;142:59–64.
47. Uncini A, De Angelis MV, Di Muzio A, et al. Chronic inflammatory demyelinating polyneuropathy in diabetics: motor conductions are important in the differential diagnosis with diabetic polyneuropathy. Clin Neurophysiol 1999;110:705–11.
48. Laughlin RS, Dyck PJ, Melton LJ, et al. Incidence and prevalence of CIDP and the association of diabetes mellitus. Neurology 2009;73(1):39–45.
49. Chiu HK, Trence DL. Diabetic neuropathy, the great masquerader: truncal neuropathy manifesting as abdominal pseudohernia. Endocr Pract 2006;12(3): 281–3.
50. Waxman SG, Sabin TD. Diabetic truncal polyneuropathy. Arch Neurol 1981;38: 46–7.
51. Sun SF, Streib EW. Diabetic thoracoabdominal neuropathy: clinical and electrodiagnostic features. Ann Neurol 1981;9:75–9.
52. Longstretch GF, Newcomer AD. Abdominal pain caused by diabetic radiculopatly. Ann Intern Med 1977;86:166–86.
53. Parry GJ, Floberg J. Diabetic truncal neuropathy presenting as abdominal hernia. Neurology 1989;39:1488–90.
54. Boulton AM, Angus E, Ayyar DR. Diabetic thoracic polyradiculopathy presenting as an abdominal swelling. Br Med J (Clin Res Ed) 1984;289:798–9.
55. Kikta DG, Breuer AC, Wilbourn AJ. Thoracic root pain in diabetes: the spectrum of clinical and electromyographic findings. Ann Neurol 1982;11:80–5.
56. Greco D, Gambina F, Pisciotta M, et al. Clinical characteristics and associated comorbidities in diabetic patients with cranial nerve palsies. J Endocrinol Invest 2012;35(2):146–9.
57. Asbury AK, Aldredge H, Herschberg R, et al. Oculomotor palsy in diabetes mellitus: a clinicopathological study. Brain 1970;93:555–66.
58. Weber RB, Daroff RB, Mackey EA. Pathology of oculomotor nerve palsy in diabetics. Neurology 1970;20:835–8.
59. Dreyfus PM, Hakim S, Adams RD. Diabetic ophthalmoplegia. AMA Arch Neurol Psychiatry 1957;77:337–49.
60. Smith BE, Dyck PJ. Subclinical histopathological changes in the oculomotor nerve in diabetes mellitus. Ann Neurol 1992;32:376–85.

61. Korczyn AD. Bell's palsy and diabetes mellitus. Lancet 1971;1:108–9.
62. Aminoff MJ, Miller AL. The prevalence of diabetes mellitus inpatients with Bell's palsy. Acta Neurol Scand 1972;48:381–4.
63. Dyck PH, Kratz KM, Karnes JL, et al. The prevalence by staged severity of various types of diabetic neuropathy, retinopathy, and nephropathy in a population-based cohort: the Rochester diabetic neuropathy study. Neurology 1993;43: 817–24.
64. Ostrić M, Vrca A, Kolak I, et al. Cranial nerve lesion in diabetic patients. Coll Antropol 2011;35(Suppl 2):131–6.
65. Wilbourn AJ. Diabetic entrapment and compression neuropathies. In: Dyck PJ, Thomas PK, editors. Diabetic neuropathy. 2nd edition. Philadelphia: WB Saunders; 1999. p. 481–508.
66. Mulder DW, Lambert EH, Bastrom JA, et al. The neuropathies associated with diabetes mellitus; a clinical and electromyographic study of 103 unselected diabetic patients. Neurology 1961;11:275–84.
67. Parisi TJ, Mandrekar J, Dyck PJ, et al. Meralgia paresthetica: relation to obesity, advanced age, and diabetes mellitus. Neurology 2011;77(16):1538–42.
68. Stevens JC, Sun S, Beard CM, et al. Carpal tunnel syndrome in Rochester, Minnesota, 1961–1980. Neurology 1988;38:134–8.
69. Gazioglu S, Boz C, Cakmak VA. Electrodiagnosis of carpal tunnel syndrome in patients with diabetic polyneuropathy. Clin Neurophysiol 2011;122(7):1463–9.
70. Trujillo-Santos AJ. Diabetes muscle infarction: an underdiagnosed complication of long-standing diabetes. Diabetes Care 2003;26:211–5.
71. Angervall L, Stener B. Tumoriform focal muscle degeneration in two diabetic patients. Diabetologica 1965;1:39–42.
72. Barohn RJ, Kissel JT. Case-of-the-month: painful thigh mass in a young woman: diabetic muscle infarction. Muscle Nerve 1992;15:850–5.
73. Barohn RJ, Bazan C, Timmons JH, et al. Bilateral diabetic thigh muscle infarction. J Neuroimaging 1994;4:43–4.
74. Banker B, Chester S. Infarction of the thigh muscle in the diabetic patient. Neurology 1973;23:667–77.
75. Chester S, Banker B. Focal infarction of muscle in diabetes. Diabetes Care 1986; 9:623–30.
76. Singer S, Rosenberg AE. Case records of the MGH Weekly clinicopathological exercises. Case 29-1997. A 54-year-old diabetic woman with pain and swelling of the leg. N Engl J Med 1997;337(12):839–45.
77. Mathew A, Reddy IS, Archibald C. Diabetic muscle infarction. Emerg Med J 2007; 24(7):513–4.
78. Joshi R, Reen B, Sheehan H. Upper extremity diabetic muscle infarction in three patients with end-stage renal disease: a case series and review. J Clin Rheumatol 2009;15(2):81–4.
79. Jelinek JS, Murphey MD, Aboulafia AJ, et al. Muscle infarction in patients with diabetes mellitus: MR imaging findings. Radiology 1999;211:241–7.
80. Kapur S, McKendry RJ. Treatment and outcomes of diabetic muscle infarction. J Clin Rheumatol 2005;11:8–12.

Cryptogenic Sensory Polyneuropathy

Mamatha Pasnoor, MD[a],*, Mazen M. Dimachkie, MD[b],
Richard J. Barohn, MD[a]

KEYWORDS

- Idiopathic neuropathy • Chronic sensory/sensorimotor polyneuropathy
- Polyneuropathy • Neuropathic pain

KEY POINTS

- Cyrptogenic or idiopathic sensory polyneuropathy is a common type of neuropathy seen in patients usually older than 50 years.
- Symptoms and signs are predominantly sensory while motor manifestations are usually mild or absent.
- Extensive evaluation usually does not reveal any identifiable abnormalities on laboratory testing. In up to one-third of cases, electrophysiologic testing is normal. Skin biopsy may be helpful in this subgroup.
- Management is focused on patient reassurance, treatment of the neuropathic pain, and rehabilitative care.

INTRODUCTION

Acquired chronic sensory and sensorimotor polyneuropathies (CSPNs) are common in middle and late adulthood, with an estimated prevalence of more than 3%.[1] The majority of acquired neuropathies are secondary to readily identifiable causes, such as diabetes, alcohol abuse, or iatrogenic causes, specifically medications. However, once known causes are excluded, a sizable minority of acquired neuropathies remains idiopathic, referred to in this article as CSPN. Although prior reports describing CSPN have used other terms such as idiopathic neuropathy or small-fiber sensory peripheral neuropathy, the term CSPN is preferred by the authors. The diagnostic criteria for CSPN have been established by Wolfe and colleagues[2] and are used by many physicians (**Box 1**). In earlier series, the cryptogenic group was thought to comprise as much as 50% to 70% of polyneuropathy (PN) cases (**Table 1**).[3–5] These studies,

[a] Department of Neurology, University of Kansas Medical Center, 3599 Rainbow Boulevard, Kansas City, KS 66160, USA; [b] Department of Neurology, University of Kansas Medical Center, 3599 Rainbow Boulevard, Kansas City, KS 66160, USA
* Corresponding author. University of Kansas Medical Center, 3599 Rainbow Boulevard, Mail-stop 2012, Kansas City, KS 66160.
E-mail address: mpasnoor@kumc.edu

Neurol Clin 31 (2013) 463–476
http://dx.doi.org/10.1016/j.ncl.2013.01.008
0733-8619/13/$ – see front matter © 2013 Elsevier Inc. All rights reserved.
neurologic.theclinics.com

Box 1
Diagnostic criteria for CSPN

Inclusion Criteria

- Symptoms

  - Loss of sensation (numbness) or altered sensation (tingling/paresthesia/dysesthesia or pain beginning in the distal extremities (usually with onset in feet before hands)

  - Symptoms present for at least 3 months

  - No symptoms of weakness

  - Symptoms of gait unsteadiness and autonomic dysfunction are allowable

- Signs

  - Sensory signs are present in a symmetric fashion in distal limbs and may include any of the following: loss of vibration, proprioception, light touch, pain (pinprick), or temperature

  - Hyporeflexia or areflexia may be present but is not required, even at the ankles

  - Minimal weakness or atrophy is allowable in muscles supplying movement to the fingers and toes

- Laboratory Studies

  - Electrophysiology: sensory and motor NCS and needle EMG are often, but not invariably, abnormal; when abnormal, findings indicate a primarily axonal PN

  - Quantitative sensory tests: vibration and temperature thresholds are often, but not invariably, abnormal

  - Other studies: if NCS/EMG and QST are normal, other studies including skin-punch biopsy to measure epidermal nerve-fiber density and autonomic studies, including sudomotor tests (quantitative sudomotor axon reflex test, silastic imprint testing, sympathetic skin response) and vasomotor tests (heart rate variability to deep breathing, Valsalva ratio), may provide evidence of peripheral nerve dysfunction

  - Blood and urine tests: these should be normal or negative; a monoclonal protein by serum protein electrophoresis and/or immunofixation electrophoresis is allowable in patients with MGUS

Exclusion Criteria

- Any identifiable metabolic, toxic, infectious, systemic, or hereditary disorder known to cause PN

- NCS abnormalities consistent with demyelination

- If a monoclonal gammopathy is present, the presence of an underlying lymphoproliferative disorder, malignancy, or amyloidosis

- Weakness on examination other than mild toes and/or finger weakness

Abbreviations: CSPN, cryptogenic sensory polyneuropathy; EMG, electromyography; MGUS, monoclonal gammopathy of uncertain significance; NCS, nerve conduction studies; PN, polyneuropathy; QST, quantitative sensory testing.
Adapted from Wolfe GI, Baker NS, Amato AA, et al. Chronic cryptogenic sensory polyneuropathy: clinical and laboratory characteristics. Arch Neurol 1999;56(5):540–7.

---

however, were largely based on younger groups of inpatients, many of whom presented with severe weakness resembling acute or chronic inflammatory demyelinating PN.[3] Later studies have revised the frequency of CSPN downward to 10% to 35%, with most estimates clustered in the range 10% to 25%.[2,6–12] One recent study, which included testing for impaired glucose tolerance and celiac disease in patients with

Table 1 Studies of polyneuropathy patients with percentages of idiopathic cases		
Authors,[Ref.] Year	Polyneuropathy Patients	Idiopathic Patients
Prineas,[23] 1970	278	107 (38%)
Dyck et al,[16] 1981	205	49 (24%)
Fagius,[5] 1983	91	67 (74%)
Konig et al,[6] 1984	70	10 (14%)
McLeod et al,[7] 1984	519	67 (13%)
Corvisier et al,[10] 1987	432	48 (11%)
Notermans et al,[11] 1993	500	75 (10%)
Wolfe et al,[2] 1999	402	93 (23%)
Jann et al,[12] 2001	222	48 (21%)

abnormal skin biopsy findings, found 50% to be idiopathic.[13] The authors' retrospective review looking at databases from 1 North American site and 2 South American sites (NASA) showed that CSPN represented approximately 25% of all referred PN patients (**Table 2**).[14,15] Likely reasons for the declining percentage include improvement in recognition of hereditary neuropathies and in the identification of immune-mediated neuropathies, as well as investigative plans becoming more sophisticated and the use of modern pattern-based diagnostic approaches.[10,11,16]

For a relatively common clinical problem, there are surprisingly few detailed reports of CSPN. The types of PN patients included differ between studies, making generalization somewhat difficult. Earlier studies did not provide detailed laboratory and electrophysiologic data. Nevertheless, the bulk of information available suggests that CSPN is predominantly sensory distal dying-back axonopathy that progresses little or slowly over time.

DIAGNOSTIC CRITERIA

CSPN is in essence a diagnosis of exclusion, established after a careful medical, family, and social history, neurologic examination, and directed laboratory testing. England and colleagues[17,18] recently reported the recommendations of the American Academy of Neurology (AAN) Practice Parameter Committee for the evaluation of distal symmetric polyneuropathy (DSP). Tests with the highest yield of abnormality in PN evaluation are blood glucose, serum vitamin B_{12} with metabolites (methylmalonic acid with or without homocysteine), and serum protein immunofixation electrophoresis. The level

Table 2 Total number of cases and diagnosis rate in 6 major categories		
Major Category	North America, n (%)	South America, n (%)
Total no. of cases	1090	1034
Immune mediated	215 (19.7)	191 (18)
Diabetic	148 (13.5)	236 (23)
Hereditary/degenerative	292 (26.7)	103 (10)
Infectious/inflammatory	53 (4.8)	141 (14)
Systemic/metabolic/toxic (nondiabetic)	71 (6.5)	124 (12)
Cryptogenic	311 (28.5)	239 (23)

of evidence in the literature allowed for the highest level of recommendation is class C. If routine testing of blood glucose is negative for diabetes mellitus, testing for impaired glucose tolerance may be considered. Nerve conduction studies (NCS) are indicated to define whether the neuropathy is axonal or demyelinating, focal or generalized, and hereditary or acquired. Skin biopsy also received a level C recommendation as having a role in the evaluation of DSP, particularly small-fiber sensory neuropathy. The purpose of such a clinical and laboratory evaluation is to rule out identifiable causes of neuropathy such as diabetes, chronic alcoholism, metabolic disturbances, endocrine abnormalities, connective tissue diseases, malignancy or amyloidosis, human immunodeficiency virus (HIV) or other infections, pertinent toxic or pharmacologic exposures, and hereditary factors. Genetic testing is recommended for the accurate diagnosis and classification of hereditary neuropathies and may be considered in patients with cryptogenic PN who exhibit a hereditary neuropathy phenotype by virtue of family history and long-standing high arches or hammer toes.[17,18] The literature is inconclusive about the utility of nerve biopsy in the evaluation of DSP.

CLINICAL FEATURES

The onset of idiopathic PNs occurs mainly in the sixth and seventh decades of life. The mean age of patients in published series ranges from 51 to 63 years old.[2,7,13,19–22] There appears to be no difference in the age of onset between sensorimotor and sensory groups. CSPN is usually diagnosed on the basis of pain, numbness, and/or tingling in the distal extremities, without symptoms of weakness. Sensory symptoms have to occur in a roughly symmetric pattern in the distal lower extremities or upper extremities or both, and evolve over weeks to months. On examination, patients have to demonstrate distal sensory deficits not confined to an individual peripheral nerve. Slight distal weakness, Medical Research Council (MRC) grade 4 or greater, in intrinsic muscles of the foot or hand is permitted as long as motor symptoms are not the presenting complaint. Series of patients with idiopathic sensorimotor neuropathies or mixed groups report a greater number of men than women, although it is unclear whether this truly reflects differences in disease prevalence or referral bias.[7,11,12,22,23] In series of patients with sensory-only or small-fiber neuropathy, there appear to be equal numbers of men and women represented, and in 1 study of small-fiber neuropathy, half of whom were idiopathic, there was a greater number of women than men.[2,13] Other studies of painful sensory neuropathy also failed to find a male predominance.[19,24]

In patients with sensorimotor idiopathic neuropathy, pain is reported in 27% to 42% of patients, sensory loss in 65%, paresthesias in 33% to 68%, weakness in 26% to 82%, and difficulty with balance in 33%.[7,11,12,21,22] In series of patients with sensory-only neuropathy or small-fiber neuropathy, the most common symptoms are pain in 54% to 100% of patients, sensory loss in 86%, and paresthesias in 86% to 100%.[2,11,20,21,23,24] In both groups, upper extremity symptoms are usually preceded by lower extremity involvement.[2,11] Worsening of sensory symptoms with heat exposure, activity, or fatigue is commonly reported in patients.[24] Approximately one-third to one-half of patients will have symptoms confined to their lower extremities.[11,24] The average time for symptoms to spread to the upper extremities appears to be about 5 years.[11] It is rare for patients to report symptoms restricted to the upper extremities.[23] Autonomic and cranial nerve findings are rare.[24]

On examination of CSPN patients, the most common findings are reduced or absent lower extremity light touch in 59% to 91%, pinprick in 53% to 95%, vibratory sense in 80% to 100%; proprioception is usually spared, being abnormal in 9% to 18%. Sensory abnormalities in the hands occur in 36% of patients. On motor examination, there is distal lower extremity weakness primarily affecting toe flexion and extension in 39% to 100% of patients, and intrinsic hand muscle weakness in 10%. Reduced or absent ankle-jerk reflexes are reported in 78% to 100% of patients.[2,7,11,12,22] Distal atrophy may be present and, as expected, foot deformities may develop after a decade from neuropathy onset.

DIAGNOSIS
Laboratory

The basic and highest-yield laboratory studies in DSP include blood glucose, vitamin B_{12} level with metabolites (methylmalonic acid and homocysteine), and serum protein immunofixation electrophoresis.[17] If those studies are normal, oral glucose tolerance testing should be completed, especially if the clinical presentation includes pain.[17,18] Other laboratory studies also recommended in routine laboratory testing include a basic metabolic panel, complete blood count, erythrocyte sedimentation rate, and antinuclear antigen. The following studies are rarely useful in CSPN cases but should also be considered in the appropriate clinical scenario: urine protein electrophoresis, antineutrophil cytoplasmic antigen antibodies, serologies for immunoglobulin G (IgG) and immunoglobulin A (IgA) antigliadin antibodies, IgA antitransglutaminase antibodies, HIV antibody, Lyme antibodies and Western blot, levels of heavy metals, and paraneoplastic and other antibody assays.

Testing for vitamin B_{12} deficiency is relatively high yield and should include testing levels of cobalamin metabolites, methylmalonic acid, and homocysteine. In 2 series of patients with PN, between 2.2% and 8% of patients had vitamin B_{12} deficiency,[25,26] and in 5% to 10% of patients with serum B_{12} levels in the low to normal range, methylmalonic acid and homocysteine levels were elevated.[27,28]

The incidence of monoclonal proteins in chronic idiopathic PN is as high as 10%, representing a monoclonal gammopathy of uncertain significance in most patients.[29–32] Patients with an immunoglobulin-M monoclonal gammopathy commonly have specific antibody binding against peripheral nerve antigens, implicating an auto-antibody pathogenesis of associated neuropathies.[33] However, PN patients with monoclonal gammopathy of uncertain significance are difficult to distinguish on clinical and electrophysiologic grounds from idiopathic PN patients without a paraprotein, raising questions about the pathogenic role of the immunoglobulin and whether the monoclonal gammopathy of uncertain significance, particularly IgG and IgA, is a coincidental discovery.[34,35] Incidental paraproteins are found in up to 3% of the general elderly population, the age group with the highest prevalence of PNs.[29]

Data on antisulfatide antibodies have produced conflicting results that render testing of limited value in CSPN. In earlier studies of idiopathic sensory–predominant PN, approximately one-quarter of patients selected from case records or a clinic population had antisulfatide antibodies.[36,37] However, other series have found antisulfatide antibodies in none or only a small percentage of patients with idiopathic PN.[2,11,19,20] Other antibodies including autoantibodies targeting voltage-gated potassium channel (VGKC) complexes have been associated with neuropathic pain. These patients have normal peripheral nervous system function but display neuronal hyperexcitability.[38] Antiganglionic acetylcholine receptor antibodies have been seen in some idiopathic autonomic neuropathy patients suggesting an immune mechanism.[39,40]

Lumbar Puncture

Cerebrospinal fluid (CSF) analysis is not essential to the diagnosis of CSPN. In earlier series, it is largely unremarkable. The mean CSF protein from 73 unclassified patients in a series was 43 mg/dL.[10] CSF was normal in 4 of 5 patients from another series.[2] In a 2001 series of 8 patients who had lumbar puncture for idiopathic neuropathy, none had elevated protein.[12] Although typically normal in idiopathic PNs, CSF analysis should be considered in patients with rapidly progressive symptoms, or if there is clinical suspicion of sensory chronic inflammatory demyelinating polyneuropathy (CIDP) as also suggested by NCS.

Genetic Testing

Genetic testing is not generally indicated in CSPN. Patients with unexplained family history of neuropathy (such as unrelated to diabetes), distal weakness as the presenting complaint, life-long foot deformities preceding the onset of numbness, or markedly demyelinating electrophysiology should be suspected to have a genetic origin for their neuropathy. In this small subgroup of CSPN, genetic testing may be appropriate. Otherwise it should be reserved for hereditary peripheral neuropathies, such as Charcot-Marie-Tooth disease, in which genetic mutations are detectable in 54% to 100% of individuals.[41–44] One recent study showed that 29% patients with idiopathic small fiber neuropathy have mutations in the SCN9A gene.[45] The role of genetic testing in CSPN patients without the classic phenotype is unknown.[17]

Electrophysiology

Nerve conduction studies

Besides assessing severity, NCS are indicated to define whether a neuropathy is axonal or demyelinating, and focal or generalized. CSPN is almost exclusively an axonal neuropathy, as none of the CSPN patients in the series of Wolfe and colleagues[2] had demyelinating features on NCS. NCS abnormalities should be expected in the vast majority (77%–97%) of CSPN patients.[2,7,11] Sural sensory nerve action potential testing has the greatest yield, being abnormal in 69% of CSPN patients and at least 83% in sensorimotor PN patients.[11] Sensory and motor NCS abnormalities typically consist of reduced amplitudes with normal or minimal changes in distal latency and conduction velocity. However, Gorson and Ropper[24] reported normal NCS in 45% of patients presenting with burning, painful paresthesias from presumed idiopathic distal small-fiber neuropathy.

Electromyography

A majority of patients demonstrate abnormalities on needle electromyography (EMG), even if there is no evidence of motor nerve involvement by history or examination.[2,24,46] In a large study, 70% of patients had an abnormal EMG.[2] Distal leg fibrillations potentials were present in 42% and neurogenic motor unit potentials in 63%. EMG abnormalities have also been found in smaller series of patients with pure sensory presentations.[24] Therefore, it is not uncommon for cryptogenic PN patients who only have sensory symptoms and signs to demonstrate subclinical motor involvement on electrophysiologic studies. Absence of the sural nerve sensory nerve action potential or the presence of spontaneous muscle fiber activity (ie, fibrillation potentials, positive sharp waves, or complex repetitive discharges) in the anterior tibial muscle were found in 72% of young and old CSPN patients.[47] In comparison, only 2% of the young and old control group (n = 49) had such an abnormality; one had absent sural nerve action potential and another mild positive sharp waves of the anterior tibial muscle.

Quantitative sensory testing

Quantitative sensory testing (QST) has been applied in several studies of idiopathic PNs. By measuring thermal thresholds, QST has a potential advantage over routine NCS in the assessment of small sensory fibers, the fiber population predominantly affected by many idiopathic PNs. QST commonly demonstrates abnormalities in patients with symptoms of neuropathy, and was slightly more sensitive than NCS in one large study.[2,20,48] However, no concordance was observed between QST and intraepidermal nerve-fiber density measurements in another study.[20] QST also requires subjective patient input and may reflect abnormalities outside of the peripheral nervous system.[49–51] Despite good test-retest and interobserver reliability following standardized training, QST results should not be the sole diagnostic criteria, because malingering and other nonorganic factors can influence the test results.[52,53]

Autonomic testing
Autonomic testing should be considered for patients with PN, particularly if there is clinical evidence for autonomic neuropathy or distal small-fiber sensory PN. Measurements of heart rate variability and quantitative sudomotor axon reflex testing have been shown to be sensitive and specific for PN, especially when used in combination.[18]

Pathology

Nerve biopsy generally confirms the axonal nature of idiopathic PNs. All 31 nerve specimens from a large series showed axonal degeneration.[11] There was no evidence of demyelination, inflammation, vasculitis, or amyloidosis. Of 14 sural nerve biopsies from another large series, 13 demonstrated typical features of axonal degeneration.[2] These studies suggest that sural nerve biopsy is rarely helpful in patients with idiopathic sensory neuropathies. Although biopsy findings typically demonstrate evidence of axonal damage, a recent series reported 8 patients with cryptogenic sensory neuropathy who had pathologic findings consistent with chronic myelinopathy.[54] Nerve biopsy should be considered, however, when there is clinical suspicion of certain types of neuropathies, including amyloid neuropathy, mononeuritis multiplex due to vasculitis, or atypical CIDP.[18]

Skin biopsy for the measurement of intraepidermal nerve fiber (IENF) density should be considered in the workup of distal sensory neuropathy, particularly in cases of small-fiber sensory neuropathy. The most commonly used technique involves a 3-mm punch biopsy of skin from the leg, which is sectioned and examined using immunostaining techniques for antiprotein gene product 9.5 (PGP 9.5) antibodies to count the IENF density.[18] Skin biopsy for IENF density has been shown to be reliable and valid in patients with distal sensory neuropathy, particularly those with small-fiber neuropathy, with a reported diagnostic efficiency of 88%.[55,56] It is more sensitive than QST or sudomotor autonomic testing, and one series demonstrated reduced IENF density in three-quarters of patients with painful sensory symptoms and normal NCS.[20] In another study, IENF on skin biopsy was abnormal in 39% of 158 patients with clinically suspected small-fiber neuropathy, of which 50% were of idiopathic origin.[13] High concordance has been reported between reduced IENF density and loss of pinprick on clinical examination.[57] Skin biopsy for IENF density has also been shown to be more sensitive than sural nerve biopsy for small-fiber sensory neuropathy, but is typically normal in demyelinating neuropathies.[58] Guidelines from both the AAN and the European Federation of Neurological Societies have recommended that skin biopsy for determination of IENF density is a valid and reliable method for the diagnosis of distal sensory neuropathy, particularly small-fiber sensory neuropathy.[18,59] IENF density in CSPN patients may not be significantly different from that in diabetic neuropathy patients.[60]

CLINICAL COURSE

Consistent with other prior reports,[8,11,19,35] fewer than 10% of CSPN patient in the series reported by Wolfe and colleagues[2] showed progression on follow-up. All remained ambulatory during the mean follow-up period of 8 months. Most patients with idiopathic sensory and sensorimotor PNs follow a stable to slowly progressive course over years.[2,7,8,11,12,19,21,24] A plateau phase of relative stability is particularly characteristic of pure sensory PNs.[11] Independent ambulation is maintained in nearly all patients, even after follow-up intervals stretching as long as 9 years.[23] However, walking canes and ankle bracing may be required over time in the sensorimotor population.[18] The need for assistive devices in patients with pure sensory presentations appears to be uncommon. In the series of Vrancken and colleagues,[47] 35 of 127 patients used walking aids such as a cane, adjusted shoes, ankle-foot orthoses, or a wheeled walker. These investigators also found that chronic idiopathic axonal PN seems to have a greater influence on the daily life of nonretired patients with onset before the age of 65 years.

YIELD OF REEVALUATIONS

There is controversy as to whether reevaluation of CSPN patients uncovers a cause in a sizable number of patients. Dyck and colleagues[16] found that intensive evaluation of referred unclassified neuropathies yielded an identifiable cause in 76%. Grahmann and colleagues[8] found that only 17.5% of outpatients remained unclassified after an initial evaluation. Reevaluation on an outpatient basis further classified 12 of 41 patients (29%) initially diagnosed as CSPN. McLeod and colleagues[7] reported a cause over time in 17 of 47 unclassified patients (36%). Notermans and colleagues[11] determined a cause in only 4 of 75 patients despite a follow-up period of more than 5 years. Repeating laboratory studies on a routine basis, including serum immunoelectrophoresis, was not informative. Differences in referral populations and in the breadth of the preliminary workup are the most obvious explanations for these contrasting yields on reevaluations. The authors, therefore, do not recommend repeat testing in CSPN. However, all patients with suspected CSPN should undergo a 2-hour glucose tolerance test even in the setting of a normal fasting blood glucose and normal hemoglobin A_{1c}, particularly those experiencing pain.

Hereditary neuropathies may account for a large number of undiagnosed PNs. The groups of McLeod, Notermans, and Dyck found evidence of a hereditary process in 42% of referred patients with idiopathic PN.[7,16,19,34] In approximately 30% of these cases inheritance was not revealed by review of family history and medical records, and was only identified after direct examination and electrophysiologic testing of relatives. In the Wolfe series[2] 29.9% were hereditary, and in the NASA series this represented 27% of North American cases.[15] Hereditary motor and sensory neuropathy (HMSN) type 2 should be considered when motor symptoms predominate and skeletal deformities are present.[61] Muscle cramping in the legs and feet and the absence of paresthesias may favor a hereditary neuropathy over other causes.[16] Onset late in life does not exclude HMSN, as it is estimated that 15% of patients with autosomal dominant HMSN type 2 present after the age of 50 years. Alcohol abuse may explain other cases.[7,19,34]

MANAGEMENT

Treatment of neuropathic pain is the primary focus of management for most CSPN patients. However, treatment of painful paresthesias and dysesthesias is rarely mentioned in prior series of CSPN. Most studies on the treatment of neuropathic pain have focused on painful diabetic and HIV-associated neuropathies, and postherpetic and trigeminal neuralgias. Medications studied for other forms of painful PN are borrowed and applied to the idiopathic group, with some success. The authors performed a retrospective chart review of 143 patients who were started on pregabalin or duloxetine for neuropathic pain.[62] No statistically significant difference was found in the proportion of patients who reported improvement in pain or adverse events with pregabalin (33% and 30%) and duloxetine (21% and 38%), respectively. Therefore, these limited data suggest that both pregabalin and duloxetine are probably effective for neuropathic pain, including that attributable to CSPN.

Several review articles have stratified medications for painful PN into first-line, second-line, and third-line therapies based on the evidence supporting their benefit and potential risks and side effects.[62–66] All agree that first-line therapies for peripheral neuropathic pain include tricyclic antidepressants and calcium channel $\alpha2\delta$ ligands (gabapentin and pregabalin). Topical lidocaine, available in patch and gel forms, is considered first-line or second-line therapy for localized peripheral neuropathic pain, with the greatest evidence for post-herpetic neuralgia. Antidepressants with dual serotonin and norepinephrine reuptake activity (duloxetine and venlafaxine) are first-line therapy in some reviews and second-line in others. Opioid medications and tramadol have been demonstrated to have good efficacy for neuropathic pain, particularly in combination with gabapentin, but most investigators consider these agents to be second-line or third-line therapies, based on concern for side effects and dependence.[67] Other medications that are typically classified as third-line or fourth-line therapies with inconsistent results for efficacy include other antidepressants (selective serotonin reuptake inhibitors), other antiepileptics (carbamazepine, oxcarbamazepine, lamotrigine, valproate, topiramate), topical capsaicin, cannabinoids, mexiletine, clonidine, and N-methyl-D-aspartate receptor antagonists (memantine, dextromethorphan). The AAN recently published evidence-based guidelines on the treatment of painful diabetic neuropathy.[68]

For further details, the reader is referred to the article by Trivedi and colleagues elsewhere in this issue on the treatment of painful peripheral neuropathy. There are limited data to support the empiric use of immunosuppressive agents in patients with predominantly sensory idiopathic PNs. Some studies have shown use of immunosuppressive agents in idiopathic axonal sensorimotor PN. Intravenous gammaglobulin produced nearly complete resolution of burning pain in 3 patients with small-fiber neuropathy who were refractory to other agents.[24] Two patients required repeat infusions to control their symptoms. Prednisone and methotrexate have been advocated to improve sensory and motor function in a preliminary report of 13 patients with idiopathic axonal neuropathy.[69] However, 9 of these patients had asymmetric sensory or motor deficits, 5 had elevated antinuclear antibody titers, and 7 had perivascular inflammation on muscle or nerve biopsy, all suggesting an immune-mediated process.[69] There have been individual reports of improvement of pain or motor function with intravenous immune globulin or other immunosuppressants, but evidence is limited and empirical treatment without a known cause is generally not recommended, particularly if the course is benign.[24,70] Arguments against the use of these agents include the potential for serious adverse events, the significant cost, the lack of concrete evidence for an autoimmune or inflammatory cause of the PN, and the relatively favorable long-term prognosis. Therefore, the authors do not recommend immunosuppressive therapy for CSPN.

As noted by Vrancken and colleagues,[47] up to 79% or 18% of CSPN patients complain of gait instability or loss of finger dexterity, respectively. Falls in this elderly group carries major risks related to long-bone and hip fractures. In a cross-sectional study of 82 subjects aged 50 to 85 years with clinical and electrodiagnostic evidence of PN, 48.8%, 34.1%, and 22.0% of subjects reported over the last 2 years a history of at least 1 fall, multiple falls, and injurious falls, respectively.[71] Hence, rehabilitative measures are an important consideration, including hand occupational therapy in some cases. Despite limited data, the authors also recommend gait-training physical therapy for patients with impaired balance and those experiencing falls or near falling. A recent literature review supports the safety and efficacy of strength and balance training in reducing falls and improving lower extremity strength and balance for individuals with peripheral neuropathy.[72]

Patient education plays an important role in the management of idiopathic PN. Patients are often anxious about their future, with many having been told by other physicians that their prognosis is bleak and that they will become physically incapacitated over time. The clinician can be a source of reassurance by referring to available literature stating that the vast majority of patients remain stable or progress slowly over time, suffer limited motor disability, and have a relatively favorable long-term prognosis. Simply relaying this natural history to patients can provide considerable emotional and even physical comfort.

Case study

A 68-year-old man developed numbness and tingling in his toes, progressing up to his ankles over 5 years. He described burning pain in his feet mainly at night and recently, started noticing symptoms of numbness and tingling in distal fingers. He denied any weakness.

Examination showed normal strength, with decreased pinprick and light touch sensations to the ankles and distal fingers. Timed vibration was 2 to 3 seconds and proprioception was normal, at the toes. Reflexes were normal in the arms and at the knees, whereas ankle reflexes were absent. Gait was normal.

The results of laboratory studies, including vitamin B_{12} level and a 2-hour glucose tolerance test, were normal, and serum monoclonal protein was absent. Nerve conduction studies showed decreased peroneal motor amplitude and the absence of sural sensory responses, indicating a mild to moderate axonal sensorimotor peripheral polyneuropathy.

He was started on gabapentin with the improvement of pain. Over the next 2 years, the numbness spread up to the wrists, but the strength remained normal.

REFERENCES

1. Beghi E, Monticelli ML. Chronic symmetric symptomatic polyneuropathy in the elderly: a field screening investigation in two Italian regions. I. Prevalence and general characteristics of the sample. Italian General Practitioner Study Group (IGPSG). Neurology 1995;45(10):1832–6.
2. Wolfe GI, Baker NS, Amato AA, et al. Chronic cryptogenic sensory polyneuropathy: clinical and laboratory characteristics. Arch Neurol 1999;56(5): 540–7.
3. Matthews WB. Cryptogenic polyneuritis. Proc R Soc Med 1952;45:667–9.
4. Rose FC. Peripheral neuropathy. Proc R Soc Med 1960;53:51–3.
5. Fagius J. Chronic cryptogenic polyneuropathy: the search for a cause. Acta Neurol Scand 1983;67:173–80.
6. König F, Neundörfer B, Kömpf D. Polyneuropathies in old age. Dtsch Med Wochenschr 1984;109(19):735–7.
7. McLeod JG, Tuck RR, Pollard JD, et al. Chronic polyneuropathy of undetermined cause. J Neurol Neurosurg Psychiatry 1984;47:530–5.
8. Grahmann F, Winterholler M, Neundörfer B. Cryptogenic polyneuropathies: an out-patient follow-up study. Acta Neurol Scand 1991;84:221–5.

9. Hopf HC, Althaus HH, Vogel P. An evaluation of the course of peripheral neuropathies based on clinical and neurographical re-examinations. Eur Neurol 1973;9: 90–104.
10. Corvisier N, Vallat JM, Hugon J, et al. Les neuropathies de cause indéterminée. Rev Neurol (Paris) 1987;143:279–83.
11. Notermans NC, Wokke JH, Franssen H, et al. Chronic idiopathic polyneuropathy presenting in middle or old age: a clinical and electrophysiological study of 75 patients. J Neurol Neurosurg Psychiatry 1993;56:1066–71.
12. Jann S, Beretta S, Bramerio M, et al. Prospective follow-up study of chronic polyneuropathy of undetermined cause. Muscle Nerve 2001;24(9):1197–201.
13. De Sousa EA, Hays AP, Chin RL, et al. Characteristics of patients with sensory neuropathy diagnosed with abnormal small nerve fibres on skin biopsy. J Neurol Neurosurg Psychiatry 2006;77(8):983–5.
14. Khan S, Wolfe G, Nascimento O, et al. North American and South America (NA-SA) Neuropathy project [abstract]. Neurology 2006;66:A84.
15. Pasnoor M, Nascimento O, Trivedi J. North America and South America (NA-SA) Neuropathy Project. Submitted to International Journal of Neuroscience 2013.
16. Dyck PJ, Oviatt KF, Lambert EH. Intensive evaluation of referred unclassified neuropathies yields improved diagnosis. Ann Neurol 1981;10(3):222–6.
17. England JD, Gronseth GS, Franklin G, et al. Practice parameter: evaluation of distal symmetric polyneuropathy: role of laboratory and genetic testing (an evidence-based review). Report of the American Academy of Neurology, American Association of Neuromuscular and Electrodiagnostic Medicine, and American Academy of Physical Medicine and Rehabilitation. Neurology 2009;72(2): 185–92.
18. England JD, Gronseth GS, Franklin G, et al. Practice parameter: evaluation of distal symmetric polyneuropathy: role of autonomic testing, nerve biopsy, and skin biopsy (an evidence-based review). Report of the American Academy of Neurology, American Association of Neuromuscular and Electrodiagnostic Medicine, and American Academy of Physical Medicine and Rehabilitation. Neurology 2009;72(2):177–84.
19. Notermans NC, Wokke JH, van der Graaf Y, et al. Chronic idiopathic axonal polyneuropathy: a five year follow up. J Neurol Neurosurg Psychiatry 1994;57(12): 1525–7.
20. Periquet MI, Novak V, Collins MP, et al. Painful sensory neuropathy: prospective evaluation using skin biopsy. Neurology 1999;53(8):1641–7.
21. Hughes RA, Umapathi T, Gray IA, et al. A controlled investigation of the cause of chronic idiopathic axonal polyneuropathy. Brain 2004;127(Pt 8):1723–30.
22. Lindh J, Tondel M, Osterberg A, et al. Cryptogenic polyneuropathy: clinical and neurophysiological findings. J Peripher Nerv Syst 2005;10(1):31–7.
23. Prineas J. Polyneuropathies of undetermined cause. Acta Neurol Scand Suppl 1970;44:3–72.
24. Gorson KC, Ropper AH. Idiopathic distal small fiber neuropathy. Acta Neurol Scand 1995;92(5):376–82.
25. Barohn RJ. Approach to peripheral neuropathy and neuronopathy. Semin Neurol 1998;18(1):7–18.
26. Saperstein DS, Wolfe GI, Gronseth GS, et al. Challenges in the identification of cobalamin-deficiency polyneuropathy. Arch Neurol 2003;60(9):1296–301.
27. Allen RH, Stabler SP, Savage DG, et al. Diagnosis of cobalamin deficiency I: usefulness of serum methylmalonic acid and total homocysteine concentrations. Am J Hematol 1990;34(2):90–8.

28. Savage DG, Lindenbaum J, Stabler SP, et al. Sensitivity of serum methylmalonic acid and total homocysteine determinations for diagnosing cobalamin and folate deficiencies. Am J Med 1994;96(3):239–46.
29. Kyle RA. 'Benign' monoclonal gammopathy. A misnomer. JAMA 1984;251(14):1849–54.
30. Bosch EP, Smith BE. Peripheral neuropathies associated with monoclonal proteins. Med Clin North Am 1993;77(1):125–39.
31. Kissel JT, Mendell JR. Neuropathies associated with monoclonal gammopathies. Neuromuscul Disord 1996;6(1):3–18.
32. Ropper AH, Gorson KC. Neuropathies associated with paraproteinemia. N Engl J Med 1998;338(22):1601–7.
33. Latov N. Pathogenesis and therapy of neuropathies associated with monoclonal gammopathies. Ann Neurol 1995;37(Suppl 1):S32–42.
34. Notermans NC, Wokke JH, Lokhorst HM, et al. Polyneuropathy associated with monoclonal gammopathy of undetermined significance. A prospective study of the prognostic value of clinical and laboratory abnormalities. Brain 1994;117(Pt 6):1385–93.
35. Notermans NC, Wokke JH, van den Berg LH, et al. Chronic idiopathic axonal polyneuropathy. Comparison of patients with and without monoclonal gammopathy. Brain 1996;119(Pt 2):421–7.
36. Pestronk A, Li F, Griffin J, et al. Polyneuropathy syndromes associated with serum antibodies to sulfatide and myelin-associated glycoprotein. Neurology 1991;41(3):357–62.
37. Nemni R, Fazio R, Quattrini A, et al. Antibodies to sulfatide and to chondroitin sulfate C in patients with chronic sensory neuropathy. J Neuroimmunol 1993;43(1–2):79–85.
38. Klein CJ, Lennon VA, Aston PA, et al. Chronic pain as a manifestation of potassium channel-complex autoimmunity. Neurology 2012;79(11):1136–44. http://dx.doi.org/10.1212/WNL.0b013e3182698cab. Epub 2012 Aug 15.
39. Sandroni P, Vernino S, Klein CM, et al. Idiopathic autonomic neuropathy: comparison of cases seropositive and seronegative for ganglionic acetylcholine receptor antibody. Arch Neurol 2004;61(1):44–8.
40. Koike H, Watanabe H, Sobue G. The spectrum of immune-mediated autonomic neuropathies: insights from the clinicopathological features. J Neurol Neurosurg Psychiatry 2013;84(1):98–106. http://dx.doi.org/10.1136/jnnp-2012-302833. Epub 2012 Aug 20.
41. Wise CA, Garcia CA, Davis SN, et al. Molecular analyses of unrelated Charcot-Marie-Tooth (CMT) disease patients suggest a high frequency of the CMTIA duplication. Am J Hum Genet 1993;53(4):853–63.
42. Nelis E, Van Broeckhoven C, De Jonghe P, et al. Estimation of the mutation frequencies in Charcot-Marie-Tooth disease type 1 and hereditary neuropathy with liability to pressure palsies: a European collaborative study. Eur J Hum Genet 1996;4(1):25–33.
43. Leonardis L, Zidar J, Ekici A, et al. Autosomal dominant Charcot-Marie-Tooth disease type 1A and hereditary neuropathy with liability to pressure palsies: detection of the recombination in Slovene patients and exclusion of the potentially recessive Thr118Met PMP22 point mutation. Int J Mol Med 1998;1(2):495–501.
44. Choi BO, Lee MS, Shin SH, et al. Mutational analysis of PMP22, MPZ, GJB1, EGR2 and NEFL in Korean Charcot-Marie-Tooth neuropathy patients. Hum Mutat 2004;24(2):185–6.

45. Faber CG, Hoeijmakers JG, Ahn HS, et al. Gain of function Na1.7 mutations in idiopathic small fiber neuropathy. Ann Neurol 2012;71(1):26–9. http://dx.doi.org/10.1002/ana.22485. Epub 2011 Jun 22.
46. Schecht HM, Olney RK. Clinically sensory distal axonal polyneuropathy: early motor involvement. Electroencephalogr Clin Neurophysiol 1996;98(3):26P.
47. Vrancken AF, Franssen H, Wokke JH, et al. Chronic idiopathic axonal polyneuropathy and successful aging of the peripheral nervous system in elderly people. Arch Neurol 2002;59(4):533–40.
48. Holland NR, Crawford TO, Hauer P, et al. Small-fiber sensory neuropathies: clinical course and neuropathology of idiopathic cases. Ann Neurol 1998;44(1):47–59.
49. Gruener G, Dyck PJ. Quantitative sensory testing: methodology, applications, and future directions. J Clin Neurophysiol 1994;11(6):568–83.
50. Finnerup NB, Johannesen IL, Fuglsang-Frederiksen A, et al. Sensory function in spinal cord injury patients with and without central pain. Brain 2003;126(Pt 1): 57–70.
51. Freeman R, Chase KP, Risk MR. Quantitative sensory testing cannot differentiate simulated sensory loss from sensory neuropathy. Neurology 2003;60(3): 465–70.
52. Geber C, Klein T, Azad S, et al. Test-retest and interobserver reliability of quantitative sensory testing according to the protocol of the German Research Network on Neuropathic Pain (DFNS): a multi-centre study. Pain 2011;152(3): 548–56.
53. Shy ME, Frohman EM, So YT, et al. Therapeutics and technology assessment subcommittee of the American academy of neurology. Quantitative sensory testing: report of the therapeutics and technology assessment subcommittee of the American academy of neurology. Neurology 2003;60(6):898–904.
54. Chin RL, Latov N, Sander HW, et al. Sensory CIDP presenting as cryptogenic sensory polyneuropathy. J Peripher Nerv Syst 2004;9(3):132–7.
55. McArthur JC, Stocks EA, Hauer P, et al. Epidermal nerve fiber density: normative reference range and diagnostic efficiency. Arch Neurol 1998;55(12): 1513–20.
56. Devigili G, Tugnoli V, Penza P, et al. The diagnostic criteria for small fibre neuropathy: from symptoms to neuropathology. Brain 2008;131(Pt 7):1912–25.
57. Walk D, Wendelschafer-Crabb G, Davey C, et al. Concordance between epidermal nerve fiber density and sensory examination in patients with symptoms of idiopathic small fiber neuropathy. J Neurol Sci 2007;255(1–2):23–6.
58. Herrmann DN, Griffin JW, Hauer P, et al. Epidermal nerve fiber density and sural nerve morphometry in peripheral neuropathies. Neurology 1999;53(8):1634–40.
59. Lauria G, Cornblath DR, Johansson O, et al. EFNS guidelines on the use of skin biopsy in the diagnosis of peripheral neuropathy. Eur J Neurol 2005;12(10): 747–58.
60. Pasnoor M, Herbelin L, Johnson M, et al. Clinical electrophysiologic and skin biopsy findings in cryptogenic sensorimotor polyneuropathy compared to diabetic polyneuropathy and normal controls [abstract]. Neurology 2009;72(Suppl 3): A217.
61. Teunissen LL, Notermans NC, Franssen H, et al. Differences between hereditary motor and sensory neuropathy type 2 and chronic idiopathic axonal neuropathy. A clinical and electrophysiological study. Brain 1997;120(Pt 6):955–62.
62. Mittal M, Pasnoor M, Mummaneni RB, et al. Retrospective chart review of duloxetine and pregabalin in the treatment of painful neuropathy. Int J Neurosci 2011; 121(9):521–7.

63. Attal N, Cruccu G, Haanpaa M, et al. EFNS guidelines on the pharmacological treatment of neuropathic pain. Eur J Neurol 2006;13(11):1153–69.
64. Dworkin RH, O'Connor AB, Backonja M, et al. Pharmacologic management of neuropathic pain: evidence-based recommendations. Pain 2007;132(3):237–51.
65. Moulin DE, Clark AJ, Gilron I, et al. Pharmacological management of chronic neuropathic pain—consensus statement and guidelines from the Canadian Pain Society. Pain Res Manag 2007;12(1):13–21.
66. O'Connor AB, Dworkin RH. Treatment of neuropathic pain: an overview of recent guidelines. Am J Med 2009;122(Suppl 10):S22–32.
67. Gilron I, Bailey JM, Tu D, et al. Morphine, gabapentin, or their combination for neuropathic pain. N Engl J Med 2005;352(13):1324–34.
68. Bril V, England J, Franklin GM, et al. Evidence-based guideline: treatment of painful diabetic peripheral neuropathy. Neurology 2011;76:1758–65.
69. Slogosky SL, Chavin JM, Heiman-Patterson T, et al. Idiopathic axonal neuropathy responsive to immunosuppression [abstract]. Ann Neurol 1995;38:336.
70. Donofrio PD, Berger A, Brannagan TH 3rd, et al. Consensus statement: the use of intravenous immunoglobulin in the treatment of neuromuscular conditions report of the AANEM ad hoc committee. Muscle Nerve 2009;40(5):890–900.
71. Richardson JK. Factors associated with falls in older patients with diffuse polyneuropathy. J Am Geriatr Soc 2002;50(11):1767–73.
72. Tofthagen C, Visovsky C, Berry DL. Strength and balance training for adults with peripheral neuropathy and high risk of fall: current evidence and implications for future research. Oncol Nurs Forum 2012;39(5):E416–24.

Nutritional Neuropathies

Nancy Hammond, MD*, Yunxia Wang, MD,
Mazen M. Dimachkie, MD, Richard J. Barohn, MD

KEYWORDS

- Neuropathy • Thiamine • Vitamin B12 • Copper • Vitamin B6 • Bariatric surgery

KEY POINTS

- Neuropathies due to nutritional problems can affect certain patient populations and have a varied presentation because of multiple coexistent nutritional deficiencies.
- Clinicians should consider nutritional neuropathies in patients presenting with neuropathies.
- Clinicians should be alert for signs and symptoms of neuropathy in patients who have had bariatric surgery.

INTRODUCTION

Malnutrition can affect all areas of the nervous system. Risk factors for malnutrition include alcohol abuse, eating disorders, older age, pregnancy, homelessness, and lower economic status. Any medical condition that affects the gastrointestinal tract can also impair absorption of essential vitamins. Nutritional deficiencies have been described in patients with inflammatory bowel disease, fat malabsorption, chronic liver disease, pancreatic disease, gastritis, and small bowel resections. Patients receiving total parental nutrition (TPN) are also at risk for vitamin deficiency, and TPN formulations should be carefully formulated to include supplemental vitamins and trace minerals. Neurologic complications following gastric bypass surgery are increasingly recognized.

Nutritional neuropathies manifest either acutely, subacutely, or chronically. They can be either demyelinating or axonal.

A unique class of peripheral neuropathy with coexistent myelopathy, also called myeloneuropathy, can also been seen with nutritional neuropathies. Myeloneuropathy has been described with deficiencies of vitamin B12 and copper.

Patients with myeloneuropathy present with both upper motor neuron and lower motor neuron signs. Peripheral neuropathy may mask the symptoms and signs of the myelopathy presenting a diagnostic challenge. Hyperreflexia may be difficult to

University of Kansas Medical Center, 3599 Rainbow Boulevard, Mail Stop 2012, Kansas City, KS 66160, USA
* Corresponding author.
E-mail address: nhammond@kumc.edu

Neurol Clin 31 (2013) 477–489
http://dx.doi.org/10.1016/j.ncl.2013.02.002   **neurologic.theclinics.com**

assess in the presence of severe peripheral neuropathy, and ankle jerks may be absent. Muscle weakness may impair the toe extensors, so Babinski sign may not be present. Besides spinal cord/cauda equina arteriovenous malformation, the clinician should suspect myeloneuropathy when the predominant complaint is gait impairment or bowel or bladder dysfunction in the setting of a peripheral neuropathy.

THIAMINE DEFICIENCY
Pathogenesis

Thiamine (vitamin B1) is a water-soluble vitamin present in most animal and plant tissues. Neuropathy due to thiamine deficiency, known as beriberi, was the first clinically described deficiency syndrome in humans. Beriberi may manifest with heart failure (wet beriberi) or without heart failure (dry beriberi). Thiamine deficiency is also responsible for Wernicke encephalopathy and Korsakoff syndrome. Thiamine is absorbed in the small intestine by both passive diffusion and active transport and rapidly converted to thiamine diphosphate (TDP). TDP serves as an essential cofactor in cellular respiration, ATP production, synthesis of glutamate and γ-aminobutyric acid[1] and myelin sheath maintenance. Only about 20 days of thiamine are stored in the body, and thiamine deficiency can start to manifest in as little as 3 weeks. The recommended daily allowance (RDA) for thiamine ranges from 1.0 mg per day for young healthy adults to 1.5 mg per day for breastfeeding women.[2] Athletes and patients with higher metabolic needs as seen during pregnancy, systemic infections, and certain cancers need a higher daily intake of thiamine. Thiamine deficiency is rare in industrialized countries and is most commonly seen in the setting of chronic alcohol abuse, recurrent vomiting, AIDS, long-term total parenteral nutrition, eating disorders, and weight reduction surgery.

Clinical Features

Symptoms usually develop gradually over weeks to months, but sometimes they may manifest rapidly over a few days mimicking Guillain Barré Syndrome.[3,4] Fatigue, irritability, and muscle cramps may appear within days to weeks of nutritional deficiency.[5] Clinical features of thiamine deficiency begin with distal sensory loss, burning pain, paraesthesias or muscle weakness in the toes and feet.[6] There is often associated aching and cramping in the lower legs. Left untreated, the neuropathy will cause ascending weakness in the legs and eventually evolve to a sensorimotor neuropathy in the hands. Beriberi may include involvement of the recurrent laryngeal nerve, producing hoarseness and cranial nerve involvement manifesting as tongue and facial weakness.[7] Oculomotor muscle weakness and nystagmus have been attributed to beriberi, but these manifestations are more likely because of coexistent Wernicke disease. Approximately 25% of patients with thiamine-deficient polyneuropathy may also have Wernicke encephalopathy, which manifests as ophthalmoplegia, ataxia, nystagmus, and encephalopathy.[6]

Diagnosis

Blood and urine assays for thiamine are not reliable for diagnosis of deficiency. Measurement of thiamine pyrophosphate by high-performance liquid chromatography[8] or erythrocyte transketolase activation may be preferred for assessment of thiamine status.[9] However, the precise sensitivity and specificity for those assays has not been established. Testing must be performed before thiamine supplementation is given. Electrodiagnostic testing shows an axonal sensorimotor polyneuropathy worse in the lower extremities, and nerve biopsies demonstrate axonal degeneration.[6]

Management

When a diagnosis of thiamine deficiency is made or suspected, thiamine replacement should be provided until proper nutrition is restored. Thiamine is usually given intravenously or intramuscularly at an initial dose of 100 mg followed by 100 mg per day. Cardiac manifestations may improve within hours to days, whereas neurologic improvement may take 3 to 6 months with motor manifestations responding better than sensory symptoms.[10] Some improvement is expected in most patients, but this typically occurs slowly, and in patients with severe neuropathy, there may be permanent deficits.[11]

VITAMIN B12
Pathogenesis

Vitamin B12 (cobalamin [Cbl]) is present in animal and dairy products and is synthesized by specific microorganisms. Humans depend on nutritional intake for their vitamin B12 supply. Vitamin B12 deficiency has been observed in 5% to 20% of older adults, and up to 40% of older adults have low serum vitamin B12 levels.[12] The RDA for vitamin B12 is 2.4 mcg daily.[2]

Vitamin B12 is an integral component of 2 biochemical reactions in human. The first is the formation of methionine by methylation of homocysteine (Hcy). A byproduct of this reaction is the formation of tetrahydrofolate, an important precursor of purine and pyrimidine synthesis. The second important reaction is the conversion of L-methylmalonyl coenzyme A into succinyl coenzyme A, which is essential for formation of the myelin sheath.

Vitamin B12 is liberated from food by stomach acid and pepsin. Liberated B12 then binds to R proteins secreted in the saliva and gastric secretions. Cbl is released from the R protein in the small intestine and binds to intrinsic factor. The vitamin B12–intrinsic factor complex is then absorbed in the terminal ileum.

Cases of vitamin B12 deficiency are because of malabsorption, pernicious anemia, gastrointestinal surgeries, and weight reduction surgery. As vitamin B12 is only found in animal products, strict vegan diets lack vitamin B12 and must be supplemented. Certain medications may contribute to vitamin B12 deficiency namely proton pump inhibitors[13] and metformin.[14] An underappreciated cause of Cbl deficiency is food-Cbl malabosrption. This difficulty typically occurs in older individuals and results from an inability to adequately absorb Cbl bound in food protein. These patients can absorb free Cbl without difficulty. Therefore, Schilling tests will be normal. No apparent cause of deficiency is identified in a significant number of patients with Cbl deficiency.

The most common cause of B12 deficiency is pernicious anemia. This autoimmune disorder is characterized by destruction of the gastric mucosa and the presence of parietal cell and intrinsic factor antibody leading to impaired B12 absorption. The disorder is more common in African Americans and in patients with Northern European background.

Chronic exposure to nitrous oxide has been associated with subacute combined degeneration.[15] The mechanism by which nitrous oxide induces vitamin B12 deficiency is by inactivation of methyl-Cbl, thereby inhibiting the conversion of Hcy to methionine and methyltetrahydrofolate and 5-methylene-tetrahydrofolate, which are required for myelin sheath protein and DNA synthesis.

Clinical Features

Vitamin B12 (Cbl) deficiency is associated with hematologic, neurologic, and psychiatric manifestations. Subacute combined degeneration, neuropsychiatric symptoms, peripheral neuropathy, and optic neuropathy are the classic neurologic consequences of B12 deficiency. Patients may present with neurologic symptoms regardless of a normal hematological picture. The neuropathy associated with B12 deficiency usually begins with sensory symptoms in the feet.

Differentiating vitamin B12 deficiency–related polyneuropathy from cryptogenic sensory polyneuropathy can be difficult on clinical grounds only. Clinical features useful to identify vitamin B12 deficiency–related peripheral neuropathy are the acuteness of symptoms onset and concomitant involvement of upper and lower extremities.[16] Sometimes the sensory symptoms and signs first appear in the upper extremities or the "numb hand syndrome."[17–19] When this occurs with other findings of a myeloneuropathy, immediately consider B12 as well as copper deficiency (see later discussion). The myeloneuropathy findings often consist of significant proprioception and vibration, increased tone, weakness in a corticospinal tract distribution, (eg, hip and knee flexors), brisk knee and arm reflexes, Hoffman signs in the fingers, and extensor plantar responses in the toes.

Histopathological studies have showed breakdown and vacuolization of central nervous system myelin under B12 deficiency states.[20] In contrast to the demyelinating features seen in the spinal cord, axonal neuropathy is seen on nerve biopsies and nerve conduction studies in vitamin B12 polyneuropathy.

Diagnosis

Diagnosis of B12 deficiency is usually made in the presence of typical neurologic symptoms, hematological abnormalities, and serum vitamin B12 levels less than 200 pg/mL, although a significant proportion of vitamin B12 deficiency patients may have serum levels that are within the low normal range up to 400 pg/mL. Measurement of the serum metabolites methylmalonic acid (MMA) and Hcy can improve the sensitivity significantly in patients with low normal range of B12 (300–400 pg/mL) when there is high clinical suspicion.[21] Although elevated MMA and Hcy suggest B12 deficiency, it is necessary to rule out other conditions associated with such abnormal levels, such as renal insufficiency and hypovolemia. Isolated Hcy elevation may also be seen in hypothyroidism, deficiency of folic acid and pyridoxine, cigarette smoking, and advanced age.

Historically, the Schilling test was used to diagnose pernicious anemia. Today, it is difficult to obtain a Schilling test because of the unavailability of the radioisotope. Anti-intrinsic factor and antiparietal cell antibodies are helpful in the diagnosis of pernicious anemia with high specificity and low sensitivity for the former and high sensitivity and low specificity for the latter.

In typical cases with myelopathic symptoms, increased T2 signal intensity is seen in the posterior column on magnetic resonance imaging (MRI) studies (see later discussion for imaging for copper deficiency, which is similar).

Treatment

Early diagnosis is critical because patients with advanced disease may be left with major residual disability.[17] Common treatment regimen includes administration of 1000 mcg intramuscularly (IM) daily for 5 to 7 days, followed by 1000 mcg IM monthly. Other approaches are a once-a-week injections for four weeks, and then monthly injections. Either is probably acceptable. B12 levels should be monitored occasionally to prevent inadequate treatment or noncompliance. Initial severity and duration of symptoms, and the initial hemoglobin measurements correlate with the residual neurologic damage after Cbl therapy. This inverse correlation between severity of anemia and neurologic damage is not understood. If a neurologic response occurs, it does so within the first six months of therapy, although further improvement may occur with time. On the other hand, sometimes treatment only prevents further neurologic impairment, and often patients are left with the neurologic deficits found before treatment.

Patients with food-Cbl malabsorption can absorb free Cbl and, therefore can be treated with oral cobalamin supplementation. Oral Cbl replacement therapy may also be an option for patients with pernicious anemia. The daily requirement for Cbl is 1 to 2 µg, and approximately 1% of orally administered Cbl can be absorbed by patients with pernicious anemia. Therefore, theoretically, an oral Cbl dose of 1000 mg per day should be sufficient. Although oral Cbl may seem preferable to IM injections, parenteral therapy is actually less expensive (if it is self-administered). Given the absence of convincing data regarding oral replacement in patients with neurologic deficits, the investigators' practice is to use IM Cbl therapy when the cause is pernicious anemia. However, a reasonable compromise may be to switch to oral therapy after several months and periodically monitor MMA or Hcy levels.

There is no clear evidence that folic acid therapy precipitates or exacerbates B12 deficiency–related neuropathy; however, pharmacologic doses of folic acid may reverse the hematological abnormalities of Cbl deficiency, masking early recognition of symptoms, therefore, resulting in the development or progression of neurologic symptoms.

VITAMIN E DEFICIENCY
Pathogenesis

Vitamin E is abundantly available in the diet and is present in animal fat, nuts, vegetable oils, and grains. Alpha-tocopherol is the biologically active form of vitamin E in humans. The RDA of vitamin E is 15 mg per day of alpha-tocopherol.[22] Dietary vitamin E is incorporated into chylomicrons and passively absorbed in the intestines. This process requires bile acids, fatty acids, and monoglycerides for absorption.[9] Vitamin E is delivered to tissues via the chylomicrons and then chylomicron remnants when vitamin E is transferred to very low-density lipoproteins via alpha-tocopherol transfer protein. Most vitamin E deficiencies occur in patients with malabsorption or transport deficiencies. Patients with cystic fibrosis who have malabsorption can develop vitamin E deficiency.

The pathogenesis of vitamin E deficiency is poorly understood. Vitamin E is an antioxidant and a free radical scavenger, and it is postulated that the neurologic manifestations of vitamin E deficiency are primarily related to the loss of this protective function. Fat malabsorption is the main cause of vitamin E deficiency. Isolated vitamin E deficiency is a rare autosomal recessive disorder caused by a mutation in the alpha-tocopherol transfer protein gene on chromosome 8q13.[23] Another hereditary disorder leading to vitamin E deficiency is abetalipoproteinemia, a rare autosomal dominant disorder resulting from mutations in the microsomal triglyceride transfer protein.[24] Patients with this disorder have fat malabsorption and deficiencies of many fat-soluble vitamins. If left untreated, patients with this disorder develop pigmented retinopathy, loss of vibration, and proprioception, loss of deep tendon reflexes, ataxia, and cerebellar degeneration as well as generalized muscle weakness.[25]

Clinical Features

Because alpha-tocopherol is stored in adipose tissues, symptoms of vitamin E deficiency may take 5 to 10 years to manifest. The onset of symptoms is usually slow and progressive. Clinical features of vitamin E deficiency mimic that of Friedrich ataxia and include ataxia, hyporeflexia, and loss of proprioception and vibration. Other findings on neurologic examination may include dysarthria, nystagmus, ophthalmoparesis, retinopathy, head titubation, decreased sensation, and proximal muscle weakness. Pes cavus and scoliosis may be present.

Nerve conduction studies in vitamin E deficiency show a sensory predominant axonal neuropathy. Nerve biopsy shows loss of large myelinated fibers with evidence of regeneration.[26] Electromyography is often normal, although mild signs of denervation may occur. Somatosensory evoked potential may show abnormalities consistent with posterior column involvement.[27] The principal pathologic features of vitamin E deficiency include swelling and degeneration of large myelinated axons in the posterior columns, peripheral nerves, and sensory roots.[9]

Diagnosis

Diagnosis is made by measuring alpha-tocopherol levels in the serum. Serum vitamin E levels may be normal even when deficiency is present. The ratio of total serum vitamin E to the total serum lipid concentration has been suggested as a superior assessment of vitamin E status.[28]

Management

Treatment of Vitamin E deficiency may reverse or halt the progression of the neurologic symptoms. Treatment begins with oral supplementation of Vitamin E 400 international units twice daily, with a gradual increase in the dose until normalization of serum vitamin E levels. Patients with abetalipoproteinemia may require very large doses of vitamin E to normalize serum vitamin E levels. Malabsorption syndromes may require treatment with water-miscible or intramuscular preparations of vitamin E.

VITAMIN B6
Pathogenesis

Vitamin B6, or pyridoxine, is unique in that either a deficiency or an excess can cause a neuropathy. Pyridoxine is readily available in the diet and dietary deficiency of B6 is rare. Humans are not able to synthesize B6, so dietary intake is essential. After absorption, pyridoxine is converted into pyridoxal phosphate, which is an important cofactor in numerous metabolic reactions. The RDA for pyridoxine is 1.3 mg daily with the upper limit of 100 mg daily.[2] Doses of 50 mg to 100 mg of vitamin B6 should mainly be used in certain conditions such as pyridoxine-deficient seizures and patients taking certain medications to avoid toxicity.

Vitamin B6 deficiency is most commonly seen in patients treated with the certain medications that are B6 antagonists, namely isoniazid, phenelzine,[29] hydralazine,[30] and penicillamine. B6 deficiency can also be seen in patients receiving chronic hemodialysis.[31] Vitamin B6 deficiency may also result from the malnutrition because of chronic alcoholism and in patients with high metabolic needs such as the pregnant or lactating woman. Risk factors for vitamin B6 toxicity are excessive intake of supplements.[32,33]

Clinical Features

In infants, pyridoxine deficiency is a cause of seizures. In adults, neuropathy due to B6 deficiency starts with numbness, paresthesias, or burning pain in the feet, which then ascends to affect the legs and eventually the hands. Neurologic examination reveals a length dependent polyneuropathy with decreased distal sensation, reduction of deep tendon reflexes, ataxia, and mild distal weakness.

Vitamin B6 toxicity produces a sensory ataxia, areflexia, and impaired cutaneous sensation. Patients often complain of burning or paresthesias. Electrodiagnostic testing usually shows a sensory neuronopathy, but with severe toxicity motor nerves can be affected as well.[33] Symptoms of toxicity are seen with doses as low as 100 mg per day.[34]

Diagnosis

Vitamin B6 deficiency can be detected by direct assay of blood or urine. Pyridoxal phosphate can also be measured in the blood. Nerve conduction studies reveal severely reduced sensory nerve action potentials with preserved compound muscle action potential. Sural nerve biopsy confirms axonal degeneration of small and large myelinated fibers.

Management

Vitamin B6 supplementation with 50 mg per day is suggested for patients being treated with isoniazid or hydralazine. Daily B6 doses of 10 mg to 50 mg are recommended for patients undergoing hemodialysis.[31]

The treatment of B6 toxicity is to stop the exogenous B6. Patients may continue to have symptom progression for 2 to 3 weeks following the discontinuation of vitamin B6 before a gradual improvement starts, a phenomenon known as coasting.

PELLAGRA (NIACIN DEFICIENCY)
Pathogenesis

Pellagra is the clinical manifestation of nicotinic acid (niacin or B3) deficiency. The classic clinical triad of pellagra is dermatitis, dementia, and diarrhea. Pellagra was once endemic in the United States and Europe and is still occasionally encountered. Most modern patients with pellagra have other risk factors for malnutrition such as homelessness,[35] anorexia,[36–38] certain cancers, or malabsorption.[39]

Niacin is absorbed in the intestine by simple diffusion. The RDA for niacin for adults is 14 mg to 16 mg per day.[2] Niacin and its derivatives are important in carbohydrate metabolism.

Clinical Features

Early neurologic symptoms are predominantly neuropsychiatric including apathy, inattention, irritability, and depression. Without treatment, symptoms can progress to stupor or coma. Isolated niacin is not known to be a cause of neuropathy and most patients deficient in niacin have other nutritional deficiencies because niacin alone will not improve neuropathy.[9]

Diagnosis

There is no reliable measure of serum niacin.

Management

Oral replacement of nicotinic acid of 50 mg 2 or 3 times a day is recommended for treatment, but dose may be limited because of flushing. Nicotinamide is used as a substitute in patients unable to tolerate nicotinic acid. Pellagra should be considered in any patient deficient in vitamin B12 or thiamine whose cognition does not improve with supplementation.

COPPER DEFICIENCY
Pathogenesis

Copper deficiency has long been recognized as a cause of hematologic abnormalities in humans, but neurologic abnormalities due to copper deficiency were not reported until 2001.[40] Since then copper deficiency has been reported to cause either myelopathy or a myeloneuropathy.[41] Copper deficiency has also been reported in association with peripheral neuropathy,[42,43] but it is not clear from these case reports if the neuropathy was isolated or in association with other neurologic manifestations. Copper sources are common in most western diets, and copper rich foods include seafood, nuts, wheat, and grains. The RDA for copper for adults is 900 mcg daily.[44]

Copper is essential in many oxidative reactions in the body. These reactions can generate free radicals, which are toxic to the cell and so both the absorption and excretion of copper are tightly regulated by cells.

Gastric acid is needed to solubilize dietary copper. Afterward, it is absorbed by both active and passive mechanisms in the intestines. The active transport mechanism predominates when dietary copper is low and augmented by passive diffusion when dietary copper is high. Gastric acid is needed to solubilize dietary copper. Once copper enters the serum, it is bound to plasma proteins and transported via the portal vein to the liver. Here copper is incorporated into ceruloplasmin for delivery to cells. If copper supplies are high, the liver excretes excess copper into the bile.

The most common cause of copper deficiency is prior gastric surgery. Exogenous zinc intake from either excessive intakes of zinc supplements[45] or use of older zinc-containing denture creams[46,47] has also been postulated as a cause of copper deficiency with neurologic manifestations. Both zinc and copper bind to metallothionein in the enterocytes. Excessive zinc intake leads to up-regulation of these complexes, and copper has a higher affinity for these receptors than zinc leading copper to displace zinc. The zinc is then absorbed into the bloodstream and the copper/metallothionein complex remains in the enterocyte and is excreted in the feces following normal sloughing of these cells. Copper deficiency can also be seen in association with excess iron consumption and malabsorption syndromes.

Clinical Features

Most patients present with gait difficulty and lower limb paresthesias. Neurologic examination reveals loss of proprioception and vibration because of dorsal column dysfunction and sensory ataxia. Upper motor neuron signs such as bladder dysfunction, brisk knee jerks, and extensor plantar reflexes can also be elicited.[41] A motor neuron disease–like presentation has also been reported.[48,49]

MRI studies of the spinal cord are reportedly abnormal in 47% of cases showing increased T2 signal in the posterior columns in both the cervical and thoracic spinal cord (**Fig. 1**).[50]

Neurophysiologic studies are abnormal in most patients with a copper myelopathy. Nerve conduction studies are compatible with mixed, motor, and sensory axonal polyneuropathy.[41]

Diagnosis

Hematologic abnormalities are common in patients with copper deficiency, particularly anemia or occasionally myelodysplastic syndrome. In copper deficiency serum copper, ceruloplasmin and urinary excretion of copper will be low and zinc often will

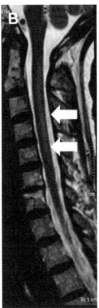
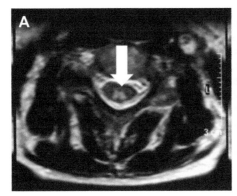

Fig. 1. Axial (*A*) and sagittal (*B*) T2-weighted MRI scans demonstrating posterior column hyperintensity (*arrows*).

be high. Ceruloplasmin is an acute phase reactant, so this may not be an adequate marker in certain patients.

Management

In patients with copper deficiency due to excessive zinc intake, it is important to discontinue the exogenous zinc. Replacement with 2 mg of elemental copper 3 times a day orally is the preferred method of copper replacement. The authors' clinic combines oral replacement with a 2 mg weekly intravenous infusion for 1 month. Copper salts (copper gluconate or copper chloride) may be given intravenously. Hematologic abnormalities due to copper deficiency often respond completely and promptly. While copper replacement will stop progression of neurologic abnormalities, patients are often left with residual symptoms.[41]

NEUROPATHY FOLLOWING BARIATRIC SURGERY

Obesity is an increasing medical challenge in both developed and developing counties. In 2010, more than 35% of Americans were obese, and 5% of Americans were morbidly obese. Bariatric surgery is an effective procedure for weight loss in morbidly obese patients refractory to a diet and exercise program. More than 200,000 bariatric surgeries were performed in 2008. The number expected to rise with the increase obesity population.

Neurologic complications have gained attention in association with bariatric surgery. Neurologic complications can involve the entire nervous system ranging from diffuse encephalopathy to peripheral neuropathy to myopathy. Among the neurologic complications seen after bariatric surgery, peripheral neuropathies were the most common and may affect up to 16% of operated patients.[51] There were

3 dominant peripheral neuropathy patterns seen after bariatric surgery: sensory-predominant polyneuropathy (acute, subacute, and chronic), mononeuropathy, and radiculoplexopathy, with the first 2 being more common than the radiculoplexopathy.[51] Onset of symptoms could be subacute to insidious; the time of onset varies from months to years, post-surgery.[52,53] Protracted vomiting and fast weight loss were risk factors to develop peripheral neuropathy after bariatric surgery.[51,54]

Malnutrition was not uncommon for morbidly obese patients before their bariatric surgery. As reported by Flancbaum, among 379 consecutive patients undergoing bariatric surgery 29% of patients were thiamine deficient.[55] The most common nutrient deficiencies following bariatric surgery are deficiencies of thiamine, vitamin B12, vitamin E, vitamin D, and copper.[56] Bariatric procedures cause or worsen malnutrition by restriction of intake or combined restriction of intake and impaired absorption. Peripheral neurologic complications after bariatric surgery are probably related to multiple nutritional deficiencies. Thiamine deficiency often was seen in painful polyneuropathy after bariatric surgery, which can present without central involvement (encephalopathy). B12 or copper deficiencies were the cause of myeloneuropathy, although data were not consistent.[51]

Thiamine, B12, and copper should be a part of baseline metabolic work-up for patient undergoing bariatric surgery, especially patients who were on a diet before surgery. Education regarding the importance of adherence to nutritional supplements after surgery is the key to prevent peripheral neuropathy developed after bariatric surgery.

Case study

A 46-year-old woman developed numbness and tingling in the fingers and toes simultaneously over several weeks. She then complained of an unsteady gait that progressed over several months, and she needed a walker to ambulate. On examination, motor strength was normal except for mildly weak hip flexors. Sensation showed decreased light touch and pin prick to the ankles and wrists; vibration and proprioception was absent at the toes and ankles. Reflexes were brisk with spread at the knees, absent at the ankles, and Hoffman signs were present in the fingers. The plantar responses were extensor. The gait was unsteady, and she could not perform tandem walking. Nerve conduction studies showed absent sural responses, low amplitude, and mild reduced peroneal (1 mv) and tibial (2 mv) motor potentials with mildly slow velocities, and needle electromyography showed occasional fibrillations in the gastrocnemius muscle and neurogenic motor units.

Blood tests showed a white blood cell (WBC) count of 1200 cells/μl, hemoglobin 7.7 g/dl, hematocrit 25%, mean corpuscular volume 108 fL, and B12 115 pg/ml. Bone marrow biopsy showed no malignancy. MRI showed increased signal in the cervical cord over several segments. She received B12 injections, 1000 units daily over 5 days, and then monthly injections. After several months, the B12 level was 1020 pg/ml, and the WBC count had increased to 3000. Neurologic symptoms and signs were unchanged. Further laboratory testing at this time revealed serum copper 14 ug (normal >80), zinc 176 ug/dl (normal 20–60), and ceruloplasmin 5 mg/dl (normal 17–54). Further questioning of the patient revealed that she used denture cream that contained zinc. Additional treatment consisted of stopping the use of the zinc-containing denture cream and beginning copper gluconate 2 mg orally 3 times a day. After a month, the copper normalized, but the WBC count was still 3000 cells/μl. She was then given weekly infusions of cupric sulfate 2 mg in 250 ml D5W over 1 hour for 2 months. Gait improved significantly so that she did not need a walker, and light touch and pin prick was now only in the finger tips and toes; other aspects on the exam were unchanged. After 2 months, the intravenous copper therapy was discontinued, and she continued to take daily oral copper and monthly B12 injections. The authors considered this a case of combined B12 and copper deficiency, with the copper deficiency most likely related to the zinc-containing denture cream. The exact cause of the B12 deficiency was unclear.

REFERENCES

1. Butterworth RF. Effects of thiamine deficiency on brain metabolism: implications for the pathogenesis of the Wernicke-Korsakoff syndrome. Alcohol Alcohol 1989;24(4):271–9.
2. Institute of Medicine (US) Standing Committee on the Scientific Evaluation of Dietary Reference Intakes and its Panel on Folate, Other B Vitamins, and Choline. Dietary Reference Intakes for Thiamin, Riboflavin, Niacin, Vitamin B6, Folate, Vitamin B12, Pantothenic Acid, Biotin, and Choline. Washington (DC): National Academies Press (US); 1998.
3. Koike H, Ito S, Morozumi S, et al. Rapidly developing weakness mimicking Guillain-Barre syndrome in beriberi neuropathy: two case reports. Nutrition 2008;24(7–8):776–80.
4. Murphy C, Bangash IH, Varma A. Dry beriberi mimicking the Guillain-Barre syndrome. Pract Neurol 2009;9(4):221–4.
5. Blass J. Vitamin and nutritional deficiencies. In: Siegel GJ, editor. Basic neurochemistry. 5th edition. New York: Raven Press; 1994. p. 749–60.
6. Koike H, Iijima M, Mori K, et al. Postgastrectomy polyneuropathy with thiamine deficiency is identical to beriberi neuropathy. Nutrition 2004;20(11–12):961–6.
7. Saperstein DB, Barohn RJ. Polyneuropathy caused by nutritional and vitamin deficiency. In: Dyck P, editor. Peripheral neuropathy. Philadelphia: Elsevier; 2005. p. 2051–62.
8. Floridi A, Pupita M, Palmerini CA, et al. Thiamine pyrophosphate determination in whole blood and erythrocytes by high performance liquid chromatography. Int J Vitam Nutr Res 1984;54(2–3):165–71.
9. Kumar N. Nutritional neuropathies. Neurol Clin 2007;25(1):209–55.
10. Koike H, Misu K, Hattori N, et al. Postgastrectomy polyneuropathy with thiamine deficiency. J Neurol Neurosurg Psychiatry 2001;71(3):357–62.
11. Hong CZ. Electrodiagnostic findings of persisting polyneuropathies due to previous nutritional deficiency in former prisoners of war. Electromyogr Clin Neurophysiol 1986;26(5–6):351–63.
12. Leishear K, Boudreau RM, Studenski SA, et al. Relationship between vitamin B12 and sensory and motor peripheral nerve function in older adults. J Am Geriatr Soc 2012;60(6):1057–63.
13. Yang YX, Metz DC. Safety of proton pump inhibitor exposure. Gastroenterology 2010;139(4):1115–27.
14. Reinstatler L, Qi YP, Williamson RS, et al. Association of biochemical B(1)(2) deficiency with metformin therapy and vitamin B(1)(2) supplements: the National Health and Nutrition Examination Survey, 1999-2006. Diabetes Care 2012; 35(2):327–33.
15. Kinsella LJ, Green R. Anesthesia paresthetica: nitrous oxide-induced cobalamin deficiency. Neurology 1995;45:1608–10.
16. Saperstein DS, Wolfe GI, Gronseth GS, et al. Challenges in the identification of cobalamin-deficiency polyneuropathy. Arch Neurol 2003;60(9):1296–301.
17. Saperstein DS, Barohn RJ. Peripheral neuropathy due to cobalamin deficiency. Curr Treat Options Neurol 2002;4:197–201.
18. Jackson CE, Barohn RJ. Lesion localization of numb hand syndrome in B12 deficiency. Muscle & Nerve 1993:1111.
19. Saperstein DS, Jackson CE, Nations SP, et al. Uncommon neurologic manifestations of pernicious anemia with cobalamin deficiency. Neurology 2001;56: A417.

20. Weir DG, Scott JM. The biochemical basis of the neuropathy in cobalamin deficiency. Baillieres Clin Haematol 1995;8(3):479–97.
21. Saperstein D, Barohn RJ. Neuropathy associated with nutritional and vitamin deficiencies. In: Dyck PJ, Thomas PK, editors. Peripheral neuropathy, vol. 2. Philadelphia: Elsevier Saunders; 2005. p. 2051–62.
22. Monsen ER. Dietary reference intakes for the antioxidant nutrients: vitamin C, vitamin E, selenium, and carotenoids. J Am Diet Assoc 2000;100(6):637–40.
23. Jackson CE, Amato AA, Barohn RJ. Isolated vitamin E deficiency. Muscle Nerve 1996;19(9):1161–5.
24. Chardon L. Identification of two novel mutations and long-term follow-up in abetalipoproteinemia: a report of four cases. Eur J Pediatr 2009;168(8):983–9.
25. Muller DP. Vitamin E and neurological function. Mol Nutr Food Res 2010;54(5):710–8.
26. Zouari M, Feki M, Ben Hamida C, et al. Electrophysiological and nerve biopsy: comparative study in Friedreich's ataxia and Friedreich's ataxia phenotype with vitamin E deficiency. Neuromuscul Disord 1998;8(6):416–25.
27. Puri V, Chaudhry N, Tatke M, et al. Isolated vitamin E deficiency with demyelinating neuropathy. Muscle Nerve 2005;32(2):230–5.
28. Sokol RJ, Heubi JE, Iannaccone ST, et al. Vitamin E deficiency with normal serum vitamin E concentrations in children with chronic cholestasis. N Engl J Med 1984; 310(19):1209–12.
29. Heller CA, Friedman PA. Pyridoxine deficiency and peripheral neuropathy associated with long-term phenelzine therapy. Am J Med 1983;75(5):887–8.
30. Raskin NH, Fishman RA. Pyridoxine-deficiency neuropathy due to hydralazine. N Engl J Med 1965;273(22):1182–5.
31. Corken M, Porter J. Is vitamin B(6) deficiency an under-recognized risk in patients receiving haemodialysis? A systematic review: 2000-2010. Nephrology (Carlton) 2011;16(7):619–25.
32. Silva CD, D'Cruz DP. Pyridoxine toxicity courtesy of your local health food store. Ann Rheum Dis 2006;65(12):1666–7.
33. Gdynia HJ, Müller T, Sperfeld AD, et al. Severe sensorimotor neuropathy after intake of highest dosages of vitamin B6. Neuromuscul Disord 2008;18(2):156–8.
34. So YT, Roger P. Deficiency diseases of the nervous system. In: Bradley WD, Fenichel G, Jankovic J, editors. Neurology in clinical practice. Boston: Butterworth-Heinemann; 2008. p. 1643–56.
35. Kertesz SG. Pellagra in 2 homeless men. Mayo Clin Proc 2001;76(3):315–8.
36. Jagielska G, Tomaszewicz-Libudzic EC, Brzozowska A. Pellagra: a rare complication of anorexia nervosa. Eur Child Adolesc Psychiatry 2007;16(7):417–20.
37. Prousky JE. Pellagra may be a rare secondary complication of anorexia nervosa: a systematic review of the literature. Altern Med Rev 2003;8(2):180–5.
38. Rapaport MJ. Pellagra in a patient with anorexia nervosa. Arch Dermatol 1985; 121(2):255–7.
39. Jarrett P, Duffill M, Oakley A, et al. Pellagra, azathioprine and inflammatory bowel disease. Clin Exp Dermatol 1997;22(1):44–5.
40. Schleper B, Stuerenburg HJ. Copper deficiency-associated myelopathy in a 46-year-old woman. J Neurol 2001;248(8):705–6.
41. Kumar N. Copper deficiency myelopathy (human swayback). Mayo Clin Proc 2006;81(10):1371–84.
42. Gregg XT, Reddy V, Prchal JT. Copper deficiency masquerading as myelodysplastic syndrome. Blood 2002;100(4):1493–5.

43. Willis MS, Monaghan SA, Miller ML, et al. Zinc-induced copper deficiency: a report of three cases initially recognized on bone marrow examination. Am J Clin Pathol 2005;123(1):125–31.
44. Trumbo P, Yates AA, Schlicker S, et al. Dietary reference intakes: vitamin A, vitamin K, arsenic, boron, chromium, copper, iodine, iron, manganese, molybdenum, nickel, silicon, vanadium, and zinc. J Am Diet Assoc 2001;101(3): 294–301.
45. Rowin J, Lewis SL. Copper deficiency myeloneuropathy and pancytopenia secondary to overuse of zinc supplementation. J Neurol Neurosurg Psychiatry 2005;76(5):750–1.
46. Nations SP, Boyer PJ, Love LA, et al. Denture cream: an unusual source of excess zinc, leading to hypocupremia and neurologic disease. Neurology 2008;71(9): 639–43.
47. Hedera P, Peltier A, Fink JK, et al. Myelopolyneuropathy and pancytopenia due to copper deficiency and high zinc levels of unknown origin II. The denture cream is a primary source of excessive zinc. Neurotoxicology 2009;30(6):996–9.
48. Weihl CC, Lopate G. Motor neuron disease associated with copper deficiency. Muscle Nerve 2006;34(6):789–93.
49. Estephan B, Barohn RJ, Dimachkie MM, et al. A young man with motor neuron-like syndrome. J Clin Neuromuscul Dis 2011;12(3):21.
50. Jaiser SR, Winston GP. Copper deficiency myelopathy. J Neurol 2010;257(6): 869–81.
51. Thaisetthawatkul P, Collazo-Clavell ML, Sarr MG, et al. A controlled study of peripheral neuropathy after bariatric surgery. Neurology 2004;63(8):1462–70.
52. Abarbanel JM, Berginer VM, Osimani A, et al. Neurologic complications after gastric restriction surgery for morbid obesity. Neurology 1987;37(2):196–200.
53. Juhasz-Pocsine K, Rudnicki SA, Archer RL, et al. Neurologic complications of gastric bypass surgery for morbid obesity. Neurology 2007;68(21):1843–50.
54. Halverson JD. Metabolic risk of obesity surgery and long-term follow-up. Am J Clin Nutr 1992;55(Suppl 2):602S–5S.
55. Flancbaum L, Belsley S, Drake V, et al. Preoperative nutritional status of patients undergoing Roux-en-Y Gastric bypass for morbid obesity. J Gastrointest Surg 2006;10(7):1033–7.
56. Becker DA, Balcer LJ, Galetta SL. The neurological complications of nutritional deficiency following bariatric surgery. J Obes 2012;2012:608534.

Guillain-Barré Syndrome and Variants

Mazen M. Dimachkie, MD*, Richard J. Barohn, MD

KEYWORDS

- Guillain-Barré syndrome • Acute inflammatory demyelinating polyneuropathy
- Acute motor axonal neuropathy • Acute motor and sensory axonal neuropathy
- Miller Fisher syndrome • Bickerstaff brainstem encephalitis • Diagnosis
- Nerve conduction testing

KEY POINTS

- Besides the classic presentation of ascending paralysis in demyelinating GBS, clinical variants are based on the types of nerve fibers involved (motor, sensory, sensory and motor, cranial, or autonomic); predominant mode of fiber injury (demyelinating vs axonal); and the presence of alteration in consciousness.
- All patients should be treated with either PE or IVIG, even if the disease is mild.
- Although therapy should be initiated within 2 weeks of onset, it is still appropriate to treat patients after 2 weeks, particularly if they are still progressing.
- PE and IVIG are equally effective in shortening the time to independent ambulation but the combination is no more effective.
- Newer prognostic tools are helpful in identifying in the first 2 weeks those at higher risk of poor recovery at 6 months.

HISTORICAL NOTE

Jean-Baptiste Octave Landry in 1859[1] first described a case of distal sensory "formications" and ascending weakness after a prodromal fever, malaise, and pain who progressed to paralysis over 3 weeks and died from respiratory failure, in addition to another four cases. Sixty years later, Georges Guillain, Jean-Alexandre Barré, and Andre Strohl[2] reported two cases with albuminocytologic dissociation on cerebrospinal fluid (CSF) testing and distinguished this syndrome from poliomyelitis-induced paralysis. Although occasionally referred to as Landry-Guillain-Barré-Strohl syndrome, it is commonly called Guillain-Barré-Strohl syndrome or, more often, Guillain-Barré syndrome (GBS), after the two French army neurologists.

Department of Neurology, University of Kansas Medical Center, 3599 Rainbow Boulevard, Mail Stop 2012, Kansas City, KS 66160, USA
* Corresponding author.
E-mail address: mdimachkie@kumc.edu

Neurol Clin 31 (2013) 491–510
http://dx.doi.org/10.1016/j.ncl.2013.01.005
0733-8619/13/$ – see front matter © 2013 Elsevier Inc. All rights reserved.

EPIDEMIOLOGY

GBS is an acute monophasic immune-mediated polyradiculoneuropathy with a mean age of onset of 40 years that affects slightly more males than females of all ages, races, and nationalities. The worldwide incidence of GBS ranges from 0.6 to 4 per 100,000 people.[3–7] A systematic literature review of the epidemiology of GBS found the overall incidence of GBS to be 1.1 to 1.8 per 100,000; however, it was lower in children at 0.34 to 1.34 per 100,000.[8] Compared with younger cases, the incidence of GBS increases after age 50 years from 1.7 to 3.3 per 100,000. Two-thirds of cases of GBS are associated with an antecedent infection. Most cases are sporadic, although summer epidemics in Northern China of the axonal variant with *Campylobacter jejuni* infection were reported. Although 5% of GBS in North America and Europe is caused by axonal GBS,[9] this variant is much more common in Northern China, Japan, and the rest of America.[10–13]

CLINICAL FEATURES

The most common initial symptom of GBS is acroparesthesia with little objective sensory loss.[14] Severe radicular back pain or neuropathic pain affects most cases. Within a few days, weakness ensues commonly in a symmetric "ascending pattern." Most patients present initially with leg weakness and arm weakness (32%) or selective proximal and distal leg weakness (56%) often spreading to the arm, whereas some have onset of weakness in the arms (12%). A descending presentation mimicking botulism, with onset in the face or arms, is less common. Besides prominent weakness, patients are hyporeflexic or areflexic within the first few days but this may be delayed by up to a week. Weakness can be somewhat asymmetric, and sensory loss can also be variable, rarely presenting with a pseudosensory level suggesting myelopathy. Facial nerve involvement occurs in up to 70% of cases; dysphagia in 40%; and rarely (5%) patients may develop ophthalmoplegia, ptosis, or both suggesting botulism or myasthenia gravis.[15] Hearing loss, papilledema, and vocal cord paralysis are less common. Axonal GBS occurs in up to one-third of cases and is more likely to be associated with antecedent *C jejuni* infection.

Nadir of weakness is reached within 2 weeks in 50% of cases, and in 90% by 4 weeks.[15] Symptom progression beyond 1 month suggests a subacute inflammatory demyelinating polyradiculoneuropathy, and if progression continues beyond 8 weeks chronic inflammatory demyelinating polyradiculoneuropathy (CIDP) is a consideration. Some patients progress rapidly to become ventilator dependent within hours or days, whereas others have very mild progression for several weeks and never lose ambulation. Occasional patients have a stuttering or step-wise progression. Weakness ranges from mild to severe flaccid quadriplegia and in up to 30% respiratory failure within a few days of onset. Dysautonomia affects most patients,[15] and consists most commonly of sinus tachycardia, but patients may experience bradycardia, labile blood pressure with hypertension and hypotension, orthostatic hypotension, cardiac arrhythmias, neurogenic pulmonary edema, and changes in sweat. Even more confusing and mimicking a spinal cord lesion are the 5% of cases that experience bladder (urinary retention) and gastrointestinal (constipation, ileus, gastric distention, diarrhea, fecal incontinence) dysfunction. The revised diagnostic criteria have been published (**Table 1**) several years ago and are well established. These include clinical, CSF, and electrophysiologic criteria (discussed later).

Moderate to severe neuropathic or radicular pain is commonly seen in the whole spectrum of GBS including Miller Fisher syndrome (MFS), mildly affected, and pure motor patients.[16] Persistent pain was reported in the 2 weeks preceding weakness

Table 1
Diagnostic criteria of Guillain-Barré syndrome

Required	Supportive	Exclusionary
Progressive symmetric weakness of >1 limb	Sensory symptoms or signs	Other causes excluded (toxins, botulism, porphyria, diphtheria)
Hyporeflexia or areflexia	Cranial nerve involvement especially bilateral VII	
Progression <4 wk	Autonomic dysfunction	
Symmetric weakness	CSF protein elevation CSF cell count <10/mm^3 Electrophysiologic features of demyelination Recovery	

Data from Barohn RJ. Approach to peripheral neuropathy and neuronopathy. Sem Neurol 1998;18:7–18.

in 36% of patients, whereas 66% reported pain in the acute phase and 38% reported pain after 1 year. The mean pain was most intense in patients with non-MFS GBS, those with sensory disturbances, and in severely affected patients.

GBS VARIANTS

Besides classic presentation of GBS, clinical variants are based on the types of nerve fibers involved (motor, sensory, sensory and motor, cranial, or autonomic); predominant mode of fiber injury (demyelinating vs axonal); and the presence of alteration in consciousness. The first GBS variant was MFS and consists of ophthalmoplegia, ataxia, and areflexia without any weakness.[17] Most of the patients with MFS present with at least two features and have in support an elevated CSF protein and characteristic autoantibody. Although MFS represents 5% to 10% of GBS cases in Western countries, it is more common in Eastern Asia, accounting for up to 25% of Japanese cases.[18] Some MFS cases may progress to otherwise classic GBS. In addition, 5% of typical GBS cases may have ophthalmoplegia. Bickerstaff brainstem encephalitis (BBE) is a variant of MFS characterized by alteration in consciousness, paradoxic hyperreflexia, ataxia, and ophthalmoparesis.[19] BBE cases represent a variant of MFS with antecedent infection (92%); elevated CSF protein (59%); and anti-GQ1b antibody (66%).[20,21] Brain magnetic resonance imaging (MRI) abnormalities are present in only 30% of BBE cases[21] and the frequency of BBE variant is 10% of that of MFS.[22] The pharyngeal-cervical-brachial motor variant manifests in up to 3% with ptosis, facial, pharyngeal, and neck flexor muscle weakness that spreads to the arms and spares leg strength, sensation, and reflexes thereby mimicking botulism. A less common paraparetic motor variant affects the legs selectively with areflexia mimicking an acute spinal cord lesion and is associated with back pain.[23] Other rare variants include ptosis without ophthalmoplegia, and facial diplegia or sixth nerve palsies with paresthesias.[23,24] Pure sensory ataxic and pandysautonomic variants are also less commonly reported without predominant weakness.

After the first detailed description of an axonal variant of GBS,[25] an axonal motor variant of GBS termed "acute motor axonal neuropathy" (AMAN) was reported in 1993 from Northern China, hence the name Chinese paralytic illness.[11] Soon after that, reports of an acute motor and sensory axonal neuropathy (AMSAN) were published.[26] Since then, these axonal variants have also been described from other countries. AMAN and AMSAN are associated with *C jejuni* infection, which is alone a poor prognostic factor.[27] As a group, patients with AMAN have a more rapid progression of weakness to an earlier nadir than in acute inflammatory demyelinating polyneuropathy (AIDP) resulting in prolonged paralysis and respiratory failure over a few days.[28] AMAN can present with transient conduction block without axonal loss, and this led to the term "acute motor conduction block neuropathy." In this AMAN variant, patients present with symmetric proximal and distal weakness without sensory abnormalities after *C jejuni* enteritis and may have normal or brisk tendon reflexes. The first two described cases had elevated titers of IgG antibody to GD1a and GM1 and serial nerve conduction studies (NCS) have shown transient partial conduction block in intermediate and distal nerve segments that dissipated within 2 to 5 weeks.[29]

PATHOGENESIS

Although GBS is presumed to be autoimmune, the precise molecular pathogenesis of GBS and its variants is uncertain. Data have implicated essentially every component of the cellular and humoral immune systems. GBS is a complex autoimmune disease of especially the proximal peripheral nerves and the nerve roots mediated in AIDP by lymphocytic mononuclear cell infiltration and intense macrophage-associated segmental demyelination. Much of the evidence for disease pathogenesis is derived from experimental allergic neuritis, which is the working animal model of GBS and is caused by a combination of T-cell–mediated autoimmunity to myelin proteins and antibodies to myelin glycolipids. Antibodies to peripheral nerve myelin were identified in the sera of patients with GBS with a decline in titers corresponding to clinical improvement. Antibodies to myelin glycolipids indicate humoral autoimmunity in GBS variants. An autopsy study supporting humoral autoimmunity demonstrated an antibody-mediated complement deposition on the Schwann cell abaxonal plasmalemma but not on the myelin sheath followed by vesicular paranodal myelin degeneration and retraction.[30] Macrophages are then recruited to strip off the myelin lamellae. Bystander axon loss may occur with severe inflammation.[15]

Unlike AIDP, AMAN is characterized by the paucity of lymphocytic infiltration and sparing of the dorsal nerve roots, dorsal root ganglia, and peripheral sensory nerves. The two early changes are the lengthening of the node of Ranvier followed by the recruitment of macrophages to the nodal region.[31] Nodal lengthening is reversible and results in impaired electrical impulse transmission caused by the absence of sodium channels, as in acute conduction block neuropathy. Subsequently, complement activation results in macrophage recruitment. Macrophages distort paranodal axons and myelin sheaths, separate myelin from the axolemma, and induce condensation of axoplasm in a reversible fashion. Alternatively, motor axons may undergo wallerian-like degeneration in severe cases, explaining the delayed recovery in some AMAN cases, which is still more readily accomplished given the involvement of distal motor nerve terminals. However, AMAN can be fatal and in seven such cases IgG and complement activation products were identified bound to the nodal axolemma of motor fibers. The suspected target autoantigen is likely GD1a because IgG antibodies to GD1a are detectable in 60% of AMAN cases and only 4% of AIDP.[32] Molecular mimicry is suggested because the pathogenetic mechanism of AMAN based on the strong association with *C jejuni* infection. The lipopolysaccharide capsule of the *C jejuni* shares epitopes with GM1 and GD1a resulting in cross-reacting antibodies. GM1 is found in high concentration at the nodes of Ranvier, where antibody binding might be particularly disruptive to nerve function. AMSAN shares many similarities with AMAN, although the attack in AMSAN is more severe or longer lasting resulting in more intense and ultimately diffuse wallerian-like degeneration of sensory and motor axons. In addition to AMAN and AMSAN, molecular mimicry is the most plausible mechanism in MFS where 90% of cases have antibodies to GQ1b. These autoantibodies have also been described in most BBE cases.[21]

ANTECEDENT EVENTS

An antecedent infection is noted 2 to 4 weeks before the onset in most GBS cases.[30] The most common are upper respiratory infections without any specific organism identified. Known viral precipitants, such as Epstein-Barr virus (mononucleosis or hepatitis) and cytomegalovirus (CMV), occur in only 6% of cases. CMV affects younger patients with cranial neuropathies, severe disease, and a higher likelihood of respiratory failure. In HIV, GBS occurs at the time of seroconversion or early in the disease. When suspected, it is important to obtain an HIV viral load measure through polymerase chain reaction, which is more sensitive than HIV antibodies. Bacterial infections, such as those caused by *Mycoplasma pneumonia* and Lyme disease, are rarely associated with GBS.

Campylobacter jejuni enteritis is the most common identifiable antecedent infection and precedes axonal GBS in up to 33% of patients. Because GBS develops about 9 days after the initial gastroenteritis, stool cultures for *C jejuni* are often negative but serologic evidence of recent infection remains. Although 2 million cases of *C jejuni* infection occur each year in the United States, only about 1 per 1000 of these patients have the genetic susceptibility to develops GBS[33] in association with specific HLA haplotypes.[34] Other anecdotal antecedent events that have been associated with GBS include surgery; epidural anesthesia; concurrent illnesses, such as Hodgkin's disease; and immunizations.

There was an increased incidence of GBS after the swine flu vaccine of 1976 in the United States with an excess risk of 10 cases per million vaccinations.[35] In the 1992 to 1993 and 1993 to 1994 seasons, the increased incidence of GBS within 6 weeks of the administration of influenza vaccine led to an estimated excess of one GBS case per million immunizations based on an adjusted relative risk of 1.7.[36] Besides influenza, the hepatitis vaccine has been associated with GBS but less frequently than the flu vaccine.[37] With the 2009 to 2010 H1N1 immunization campaign, Centers for Disease Control and Prevention surveillance data identified an excess GBS risk of 0.8 cases per million vaccinations,[38] which is similar to the risk conferred by seasonal influenza immunization. The 2009 H1N1 influenza virus has been associated with a hospitalization rate of 222 per million and a death rate of 9.7 per million inhabitants. Therefore, the risk of this illness outweighs the risk of the vaccines. A more complex question is whether patients who have experienced GBS within 6 weeks of influenza immunization should be allowed to be reimmunized with the flu vaccine a year later. In such cases, the established benefits of influenza vaccination might outweigh the risks for those who have a history of GBS and who also are at high risk for severe complications from influenza itself.[39] The limited available data suggest that if a patient's GBS episode was associated with the influenza vaccine, most will do well when rechallenged. There may be a small risk (3.5%) of a repeat episode but the frequency of serious GBS recurrence requiring admission is about 1.2%.[40]

ELECTROPHYSIOLOGIC FEATURES

When GBS is suspected, electrophysiologic studies are essential to confirm the diagnosis and exclude its mimics. The differential of pure motor syndrome includes other diseases associated with quadriparesis and paralysis, such as myasthenic crisis, acute presentation of the idiopathic inflammatory myopathies, and the unusual motor neuron disease patient presenting with acute respiratory failure. Associated clinical features are often helpful in distinguishing these from GBS. The finding of multifocal demyelination on early electrodiagnostic testing (or repeated a week later) is extremely helpful in confirming the diagnosis of AIDP with a high sensitivity and specificity. Needle electrode examination is nonspecific because it demonstrates reduced recruitment initially and fibrillations potentials 3 to 4 weeks after onset.

The earliest findings in AIDP are prolonged F-wave latencies or poor F-wave repeatability caused by demyelination of the nerve roots. This is followed by prolonged distal latencies (caused by distal demyelination) and temporal dispersion or conduction block. Slowing of nerve conduction velocities is less helpful because it tends to appear 2 to 3 weeks after the onset. However, the sensitivity of NCS based on reported criteria may be as low as 22% in early AIDP,[41] rising to 87% at 5 weeks into the illness.[42] There are several reasons for limited sensitivity of NCS in AIDP. First, the common sites of demyelination are at the level of the nerve roots, most distal nerve segments, and at entrapment sites. The nerve root is outside the reach of routine NCS, and entrapment sites are usually excluded when assessing the diagnosis of AIDP. However, slowing of nerve conduction velocities at multiple common entrapment sites is unusual in an otherwise normal young adult and may therefore support the clinical impression of GBS. Second, the number of motor nerves studied or those with an elicited response may be inadequate and finding prolongation of blink reflex latencies may be helpful. Finally, changes in the sensory NCS lag behind the motor abnormalities. However, a potential clue is the preservation of a normal sural nerve response when the median and ulnar sensory potentials are reduced in amplitude or absent.[42] A variety of motor NCS criteria have been published to optimize sensitivity while maintaining specificity (**Table 2**). A comparison of 10 published sets of criteria in 53 patients with AIDP, with amyotrophic lateral sclerosis and diabetic polyneuropathy control subjects, yielded a new set with 72% sensitivity and 100% specificity.[43] Clinicians should not expect each patient with ADIP to meet strict research criteria for demyelination, particularly early in the course. Because treatment is most effective when given earlier, patients with GBS should be treated based on clinical suspicion after the exclusion of potential mimics (**Box 1**).

In AMAN, Compound muscle action potential (CMAP) amplitudes are significantly reduced in the first few days and then in severe cases become absent.[25] It is difficult in AMAN to ascertain if the absence of CMAP is caused by axon loss, conduction block from sodium channel dysfunction distal to the most distal stimulation site, or an immune attack on the nodes of Ranvier. For this reason, fibrillation potentials may occur early on in the course of AMAN and needle electrode examination is helpful. In AMAN, nerve conduction testing may alternatively show transient partial conduction block in intermediate and distal nerve segments that disappears within 2 to 5 weeks.[29] In AMSAN the sensory potentials are reduced in amplitude and often absent.[26] Absence of H-reflexes may be the only abnormality in 75% of cases of MFS and BBE.[22]

LABORATORY FEATURES

Routine laboratory testing is unrevealing in GBS, such as a mild and nonspecific elevation of creatine kinase or transaminases. Hyponatremia should in the proper setting raise suspicion for porphyria or syndrome of inappropriate antidiuretic hormone. Marked vomiting, delayed hair loss, or Mees lines may support the need for heavy metal testing.

Table 2
GBS electrophysiologic criteria

	Amplitude	Percent Conduction Velocity Slowing			Percent Distal Latency Prolongation			Percent F-Wave Latency Prolongation			Amplitude Conduction Block		Abnormal Temporal Dispersion		Abnormal Parameters Required
		≥80% of LLN	<80% of LLN	No. of Nerves	≥80% of LLN	>80% of LLN	No. of Nerves	≥80% of LLN	<80% of LLN	No. of Nerves	%	No. of Nerves	%	No. of Nerves	
Albers,[42] 1985		>5	>15	2	>10	>20	2	>20	>20	2	>30	2	>30	1	1
Albers,[44] 1989		>10	>20	2	>15	>25	2	>25	>25	1	>30	1	>30	1	3
Asbury & Cornblath,[41] 1990		>20	>30	2	>25	>50	2	>20	>50	2	>20[a]	1	>15	1	3
Hadden,[9] 1998		>10[b]	>15	2	>10	>20[c]	2	>20	>20	2	>50[d]	2	—	—	1
Van denBergh,[43] 2004		>30	>30	2	>50	>50	2	>25	>50	2	>50[d]	2[e]	>30	2	1

Abbreviation: LLN, lower limit of normal.

a By area or amplitude.
b Distal amplitude >50% LLN.
c Distal amplitude less than LLN.
d Distal amplitude >20% of LLN.
e Alternatively one finding with another NCS abnormality.

Box 1
Mimics of GBS presenting as quadriparesis[a]

1. Anterior horn cell: poliomyelitis or West Nile virus infection (asymmetric weakness)
2. Peripheral nerve
   a. Critical illness neuropathy
   b. Lymphoma/leptomeningeal carcinomatous meningitis
   c. Toxic neuropathies: solvent or heavy metals
   d. Porphyria
   e. Lyme
   f. Diphtheria
   g. Vasculitic neuropathy
3. Neuromuscular junction
   a. Myasthenia gravis
   b. Botulism
   c. Tick paralysis (children)
4. Muscle
   a. Idiopathic inflammatory myopathies
   b. Periodic paralysis
   c. Critical illness myopathy
   d. Rhabdomyolysis
   e. Severe hypokalemia or hypophosphatemia
5. Acute spinal cord lesion

   [a] Psychogenic is an exclusion diagnosis.

CSF analysis is critically important in all GBS cases and reveals albuminocytologic dissociation, an elevated protein up to 1800 mg/dL[45] with 10 or less white cells in most cases. Half of GBS cases may have a normal CSF protein in the first week but that proportion declines to 10% if the test is repeated a week later.[15,46] Pleocytosis of 10 to 20 cells/mm^3 is seen in approximately 5% of cases and should not dissuade one from a diagnosis if the clinical and electrodiagnostic features are otherwise typical. If there are more than 50 cell/per mm^3 particularly 2 weeks after the onset of symptoms, one should consider early HIV infection, leptomeningeal carcinomatosis, CMV polyradiculitis, and sarcoidosis. Most MFS cases and half of BBE cases have albuminocytologic dissociation.[22]

Most cases of *C jejuni* enteritis are self-limited, resolving after several days, and require no specific treatment. Although antimicrobial therapy can hasten the clearance of *C jejuni* from the stool,[47] there is no evidence to suggest that such treatment has an effect on GBS after the onset of neuropathic symptoms. Therefore, stool cultures or antibody measurements of *C jejuni* do not change management of GBS cases but may indicate a less favorable prognosis for recovery.

Antibodies to GM1 gangliosides have been described more frequently in AMAN and some of the reports correlated coexistence of GM1 antibodies and AMAN with greater functional disability at 6 months.[48] *C jejuni* has GM1-like oligasacahrides on its surface that may cross-react with GM1, explaining why an antibody directed against the bacteria may also produce a neuropathy.[49] In another study, all three patients with GBS with poor recovery and inability to walk at 1 year had serologic evidence of recent *C jejuni* infection but no antibodies to GM1 or GD1b,[50] indicating that patients with GBS with antibodies to GM1 or GD1b may have excellent recovery. Antibodies to GM1 or GD1b do not necessarily mediate the extensive axonal damage seen in severely affected patients. However, IgG antibodies to GD1a are highly associated with AMAN, being detectable in 60% of AMAN cases and only 4% of AIDP.[32]

GT1a antibodies correlate with the presence of bulbar signs and symptoms and may be seen with BBE in addition to GQ1b antibodies. Although antibody testing in GBS is not recommended, MFS is a notable exception[51,52] because polyclonal GQ1b antibodies are highly sensitive and specific to MFS but can also be seen in typical GBS cases with prominent ophthalmoparesis. These may also be seen in GBS cases with marked ophthalmoparesis and in 66% of BBE cases.[18]

Gadolinium-enhanced MRI scan of the lumbosacral spine reveals cauda equina nerve root enhancement in most AIDP cases.[53,54] MRI can be especially useful in the paraparetic variant of GBS because it establishes the site of the lesion in the setting of typically unrevealing NCS.

TREATMENT
General Supportive Care

Observational studies and expert opinion consensus provide guidance to the general management of GBS.[55] Given that up to 30% of GBS cases progress to respiratory failure, good supportive care is the most important element of management. Patients with GBS are mostly admitted to the neurologic intensive care unit or an intermediary care telemetry unit to allow for close and frequent monitoring of respiratory, bulbar, and autonomic function. A rapid decline of the expiratory forced vital capacities to less than 15 mL/kg of ideal body weight (adjusted for age) or of the negative inspiratory force to less than 60 cm H_2O each indicate the need for urgent intubation and mechanical ventilation before hypoxemia supervenes.[15] This is associated with marked weakness of neck muscles and inability to count out loud till 20. Patients with severe dysphagia may require nasogastric or feeding tubes. Intubation should also be considered for patients who cannot handle their secretions or who have an ineffective cough. After 2 weeks of intubation, tracheostomy should be considered in those without improved pulmonary mechanics. In those intubated but with improved pulmonary parameters at 2 weeks, an additional week of intubation may be judicious to allow for successful weaning from the ventilator.[55] It is important when managing autonomic instability to be conservative and avoid aggressively treating blood pressure fluctuations because patients are sensitive to medications and use of long-acting antihypertensives is contraindicated. For those with marked radicular back pain or neuropathic pain refractory to acetaminophen or nonsteroidal anti-inflammatory drugs, treatment with pain-modulating drugs, such as antidepressants, gabapentin, pregabalin, carbamazepine, tramadol, and mexiletene, is indicated.[55] Bed-ridden patients should have deep venous thrombosis prophylaxis with compressive hose or anticoagulants in the form of subcutaneous heparin or enoxaprin. Bedside passive range of motion can help prevent muscle contractures in paralyzed patients but it is also important to be mindful that these patients are most often alert and cognitively intact. A means for communication must be established for patients who are on mechanical ventilation. Vigilance toward urinary and pulmonary infections is important because most severe cases develop one or the other. Treatment with plasmapheresis or intravenous immunoglobulin (IVIG) is indicated for patients with weakness impairing function or any respiratory involvement. Before initiating any of these therapies, patients and their families should be educated that it takes on average 2 to 3 months for patients to walk without aids no matter what therapy is used.

Plasma Exchange

Plasma exchange (PE) directly removes humoral factors, such as autoantibodies, immune complexes, complement, cytokines, and other nonspecific inflammatory mediators, and was the first treatment shown in randomized controlled trials to be effective in GBS (**Table 3**).[56,57] In both studies, PE performed within 2 weeks from symptom onset consistently demonstrated a statistically significant reduction in the time to weaning from the ventilator by 13 to 14 days and time to walk unaided by 32 to 41 days. In addition, the French Cooperative Group showed a reduction in the proportion of patients who required assisted ventilation, a decrease in the time to onset of motor recovery, and a reduction in time to walk with assistance.[56] The Guillain-Barré Syndrome Study Group identified similar benefits with more PE recipients improved at 4 weeks, and the one-grade improvement occurring 3 weeks earlier.[56,57] The volume of PE is well-defined at 50 mL/kg administered five times, daily or every other day for 5 to 10 days, totaling 250 mL/kg. PE beyond the standard amount does not offer additional benefits.[58] The French Cooperative Group on Plasma Exchange in Guillain-Barré Syndrome showed that patients with mild GBS on admission (could walk with or without aid but not run, or those who could stand up unaided) would benefit from two PEs.[58] For those who could not stand up unaided (moderate group), four PEs were more beneficial than two for time to walk with assistance (median, 20 vs 24 days) and for 1-year full

Table 3 Guillain-Barré syndrome: North American and French plasmapheresis trials	Plasma Exchange[a]	Control[a]
North American (1985)		
Number of patients	122	123
Time to improve one grade	19 d	40 d
Time to walk unaided, all patients	53 d	85 d
Time to walk unaided, respirator	97 d	169 d
Time on ventilator	9 d	23 d
% Improved one grade at 1 mo	59%	39%
% Improved at 6 mo	97%	87%
French (1987)		
Number of patients	109	111
Time to weaning	18 d	31 d
Time to walk unaided	70 d	111 d
Time in hospital	28 d	45 d
% Patients to ventilator after entry	21%	42%

[a] All differences in both columns are statistically significant.

Data from Guillain-Barré Syndrome Study Group. Plasmapheresis and acute Guillain-Barré syndrome. Neurology 1985;35:1096–104; and French Cooperative Group on Plasma Exchange in Guillain-Barré Syndrome: role of replacement fluids. Ann Neurol 1987;22:753–61.

muscle-strength recovery rate (64% vs 46%). Six exchanges were no more beneficial than four in the severe mechanically ventilated GBS cases.

PE is performed at specialized centers and involves removing 3 to 6 L of plasma over several hours and replacing it with preferably albumin or in some cases fresh frozen plasma. Limitations include intravenous access because it requires large double-lumen catheter through subclavian, internal jugular, or femoral venous access. Potential complications include pneumothorax, hypotension, sepsis, pulmonary embolism, hemorrhage from vein puncture, low platelets, prolonged clotting parameters, hypocalcemia, citrate toxicity, and anemia. For a 70-kg adult, the total exchange volume is approximately 15,000 mL. During PE, it is important to monitor blood pressure, pulse, and amount of fluid intake and output. We obtain daily complete blood count, platelets, calcium, prothrombin time, partial thromboplastin time, and international normalized ratio and hold apheresis 1 to 2 days if coagulation parameters become abnormal.

Although the PE-treated groups in the North American and French studies did better than control subjects, the time to walk and to discharge and the time spent on a ventilator were still fairly long, even in PE-treated patients. Therefore, physicians, patients, and family members need to have realistic expectations about the extent of the effect of PE and IVIG (discussed next). Dramatic improvement within days of beginning treatment is not the rule and if this occurs, it may have happened regardless of treatment.

Intravenous Immunoglobulin

The postulated mechanisms of action of IVIG in neuromuscular disorders include interference with costimulatory molecules involved in antigen presentation and modulation of autoantibodies, cyotokines and adhesion molecules production, and macrophage Fc receptor. It also disrupts complement activation and membrane attack complex formation.[59] Sialylated IgG Fc fragments are important for the in vivo activity of IVIG[60] because they initiate an anti-inflammatory cascade through the lectin receptor SIGN-R1 or DC-SIGN. This leads to upregulated surface expression of the inhibitory Fc receptor, Fc gamma receptor IIb, on inflammatory cells, thereby attenuating autoantibody-initiated inflammation.

The first large study to demonstrate a favorable response to IVIG in GBS was by the Dutch Guillain-Barré Study Group two decades ago.[61] They compared the efficacy of IVIG with PE in 147 patients and there was no control group. Their results showed not only that IVIG was effective but that it was possibly more effective than PE (**Table 4**).

Table 4
Guillain-Barré syndrome: Dutch IVIG versus plasmapheresis study[65] compared with the North American plasmaphersis study

	Dutch		North American	
	IVIG	PE	PE	Control
Total patients	74	73	108	120
Improved one grade (4 wk)	53%	34%	59%	39%
Days to improve one grade (median)	27	41	19	40
Days to grade 2	55	69	19	40
Number of multiple complications	5	6	—	—
Ventilator dependent by Week 2	27%	42%	—	—

Data from Guillain-Barré Syndrome Study Group. Plasmapheresis and acute Guillain-Barré syndrome. Neurology 1985;35:1096–104; and French Cooperative Group on Plasma Exchange in Guillain-Barré syndrome: role of replacement fluids. Ann Neurol 1987;22:753–61.

However, there may have been a group imbalance to account for the later because PE efficacy in the Dutch trial did not match up with that of the North American study, such as in the rate of one-grade improvement at 4 weeks. A subsequent larger study by the Plasma Exchange and Sandoglobulin Guillain-Barré Syndrome Trial Group[62] has conclusively shown that there is no difference between the outcomes with IVIG or PE.

The total dose of IVIG is 2 g/kg administered over 2 to 5 days. Because most patients with GBS are in the hospital for longer than 2 days, there is probably no advantage to giving it in less than 5 days for this disorder. Although the side effects are usually mild, the infusions are generally better tolerated if given over 5 days We closely monitor patients with the first infusion, starting at a very slow rate of 25 to 50 mL/h for 30 minutes and increasing it progressively by 50 mL/h every 15 to 20 minutes up to 150 to 200 mL/h. Mild reactions (headache, nausea, chills, myalgia, chest discomfort, back pain) occur in 10% and are improved with slowing the infusion rate and are preventable with premedication with acetaminophen, Benadryl, and if need be intravenous methylprednisolone. Moderate rare reactions include chemical meningitis neutropenia and delayed red, macular skin reaction of the palms, soles, and trunk with desquamation. Acute renal failure is uncommon and related to patient dehydration and the prior use of sucrose or maltose diluents. Other severe and rare reactions are anaphylaxis, stroke, myocardial infarction, or pulmonary emboli caused by hyperviscocity syndrome. The latter is more likely to occur in old age, immobility, diabetes, thrombocytemia, hypercholesterolemia, hypergammaglobunemia, and cryoglobunemia. We avoid using IVIG in patients with several of these risk factors and place IVIG recipients on 81-mg daily aspirin prophylactically. Total IgA deficiency is extremely rare but such patients may experience anaphylaxis when given IVIG. However, obtaining quantitative IgA levels is not practical in this urgent scenario. Manufacturers take steps to eliminate the possibility of hepatitis virus transmission (heat pasteurization and solvent or detergent inactivation), so this potential issue has been eliminated. There has never been a reported case of HIV infection transmitted by IVIG. Nanofiltration and caprylate treatment reduce the risk of prion disease transmission.

Two reports raised the issue of relapses after treatment with IVIG,[63,64] also referred to as "treatment-related fluctuations," causing confusion for doctors attempting to make a rational treatment decision for a patient with GBS. However, relapses had also been reported with PE.[57] In the French study, the PE group had a relapse rate of 5.5% compared with 1% for the control group.[58] Physicians have to accept that rarely some patients with GBS may have minor relapses. Although the relapse rate may be slightly higher with either IVIG or PE compared with no treatment, the weight of all available clinical and research evidence indicates it is better to treat patients with GBS than not to treat. PE and IVIG are equally effective, but in the hemodynamically unstable patient, PE is contraindicated and furthermore IVIG is more often readily available in most hospitals.

PE Followed by IVIG

The management of the patient with severe GBS who does not improve 10 to 14 days after PE or IVIG is problematic. The Plasma Exchange Sandoglobulin Guillain-Barré study group conducted a multicenter trial comparing PE monotherapy, IVIG monotherapy, and PE followed by IVIG.[65] Combined treatment produced no significant difference in patient outcomes compared with either therapy given alone (**Table 5**). This study also showed that PE and IVIG treatments were equally effective in GBS and found no significant difference in the incidence of side effects, thus further settling

Table 5 Guillain-Barré syndrome: PE monotherapy, IVIG monotherapy, versus PE followed by IVIG			
	PE	IVIG	PE Followed by IVIG
Total patients	121	130	128
Days to walk unaided	49	51	40
Median days to hospital discharge	63	53	51
% Unable to walk unaided after 48 wk	16.7	16.5	13.7
Median days to stop artificial ventilation	29	26	18
Deaths	4.1%	4.6%	6.3%

From The Dutch Guillain-Barré Study Group. Treatment of Guillain-Barré syndrome with high-dose immune globulins combined with methylprednisolone: a pilot study. Ann Neurol 1994;35(6):749–52; with permission.

the lingering question from the Dutch IVIG study. Based on that, there is no added benefit in treating PE recipients subsequently with IVIG.[65]

Corticosteroids

Corticosteroids (CS) are of no benefit in the treatment of GBS. In one of the early studies, patients treated with oral CS did worse than the control subjects.[66] Intravenous methylprednisolone was evaluated in GBS in three studies. In the large randomized British study, 124 patients received methylprednisolone, 500 mg daily, for 5 days within 15 days of onset and 118 patients received placebo[67] and about half the patients in both groups received PE. There was no difference between the two groups in the degree of improvement at 4 weeks or in secondary outcome measures. The researchers concluded that "a short course of high-dose methylprednisolone given early in GBS is ineffective." In the second study, a smaller Dutch open-label pilot study[68] suggested that 25 patients receiving intravenous methylprednisolone and IVIG did better than 74 patients from the earlier Dutch study who received IVIG alone. This led to a randomized controlled study by the Dutch group in patients unable to walk independently and who had been treated within 14 days after onset of weakness with IVIG to receive either intravenous methylprednisolone (500 mg/day; n = 116) or placebo (n = 117) for 5 days within 48 hours of administration of first dose of IVIG.[69] There was no statistically significant difference between the groups in the prespecified primary outcome measure of improvement from baseline in GBS disability score of one or more grades at 4 weeks after randomization (68% in the methylprednisolone group vs 56% in the control subjects; $P = .06$). Thus, intravenous CS is not recommended therapy for GBS.

American Academy of Neurology Practice Parameters

The American Academy of Neurology[70] recommends PE for nonambulant adult patients with GBS who seek treatment within 4 weeks of the onset of symptoms (level A). PE should also be considered for ambulant patients examined within 2 weeks of the onset of symptoms (level B). IVIG is recommended for nonambulant adult patients with GBS within 2 (level A) or possibly 4 weeks (level B) of the onset of neuropathic symptoms. It also indicates that sequential treatment with PE followed by IVIG, or immunoabsorption followed by IVIG, is not recommended for patients with GBS. CSs are not recommended for the management of GBS. In children with severe GBS, PE and IVIG are treatment options.

PROGNOSIS

Most patients with GBS begin to recover at 28 days with mean time to complete recovery being 200 days in 80% of cases. However, many (65%) have minor residual signs or symptoms often making recovery less than complete.[15,46] Besides that, major residual neurologic deficits affect 10% to 15% of patients. In a study of 79 cases a year after the onset of GBS, 8% had died (all older than 60); 4% remained bedbound or ventilator dependent; 9% were unable to walk unaided; 17% were unable to run; and 62% had made a complete or almost complete recovery.[71]

In most GBS cases with complete to almost complete recovery, functionally significant residual deficits are commonly detectable on careful evaluation. Forty patients with GBS were compared at a mean of 7 years after the acute attack with 40 healthy control subjects showing residual neuropathy affecting large- and medium-sized myelinated motor and sensory fibers in approximately half of all patients.[72] There was also a trend toward impaired self-reported physical health status, and other long-term studies have demonstrated similar functionally relevant neurologic deficits up to 7 years after the acute GBS attack. These deficits were predominantly in the lower extremities and in some cases there was evidence of persistent dysautonomia.[73,74]

Five percent of GBS cases succumb to their illness because of complications of critical illness (infections, adult respiratory distress syndrome, pulmonary embolism), and rarely dysautonomia. The relapse rate is 5% and it usually occurs within the first 8 weeks. The alternative diagnosis of relapsing-remitting CIDP should be considered in relapsing cases.[75] When the first relapse is delayed by more than 2 months after an acute attack or the number of relapses exceeds two instances, either should raise suspicion for relapsing-remitting (CIDP).[76] Further clues favoring CIDP in relapsing cases include maintaining the ability to ambulate independently at nadir, absence of cranial nerve dysfunction, and the presence of marked demyelinating slowing on NCS.

Slowed recovery and a reduced likelihood of walking unaided at 6 months may be attributable to a suboptimal increase in IgG levels at 2 weeks after infusion.[75] After a standard dose of IVIG treatment, patients with GBS show a large variation in its pharmacokinetics, which is thought to be related to clinical outcome. In a retrospective analysis of 174 patients with GBS enrolled previously in a randomized controlled clinical trial, patients with a minor increase of serum IgG level 2 weeks after standard single IVIG dose recovered significantly slower.[75] Additionally, fewer of these patients reached the ability to walk unaided at 6 months after correction for known clinical prognostic factors. This may indicate that patients with a small increase in serum IgG level at 2 weeks could benefit from a higher dosage or second course of IVIG, but this hypothesis is yet to be tested in a prospectively designed study.

McKhann and colleagues[77] identified four factors that indicated a poor prognosis in the North American GBS study (regardless of whether patients received plasmapheresis): (1) older age (>50–60); (2) rapid onset before presentation within 7 days; (3) the need for mechanical ventilation; and (4) severely reduced distal motor amplitudes (to 20% or less of the lower limit of normal). A preceding diarrheal illness with *C jejuni* can be added to this list but not GM1 autoantibodies. A preceding infection with CMV may also result in a delayed recovery (see **Table 5**).[78]

Recently, the Erasmus GBS outcome score was derived from data of 388 patients enrolled in two randomized controlled trials and one pilot study.[79] This 1 to 7 score consists of three items: (1) age (0 = up to 40 years, 0.5 = 41–60 years, or 1 = for age >60); (2) preceding diarrhea (0 or 1); and (3) modified GBS disability score at 2 weeks after entry (1–5). This score obtained at 2 weeks was validated in another GBS sample as a predictor of the probability of independent ambulation at 6 months.

Predictions corresponding to these prognostic scores ranged from 1% to 83% for the inability to walk independently at 6 months with a very good discriminative ability (area under the curve, 0·85) in both data sets (**Box 2**). Of patients with an Erasmus GBS outcome score of 5 at 2 weeks, 27% are unable to walk independently at 6 months, whereas a score of 5.5 to 7 markedly raises that proportion to 52%. More recently, an earlier clinical model in the first week of disease accurately predicted the outcome of GBS in 397 patients at 6 months.[80] High age (>60), preceding diarrhea, and low Medical Research Council sumscore (<31; range, 0–60 scale) at hospital admission and at 1 week were independently associated with being unable to walk at 4 weeks, 3 months, and 6 months.

Most patients with AMAN have more delayed recovery than AIDP,[81] whereas some cases recover quicker.[82] Motor nerve terminal degeneration provides a potential mechanism for rapid recovery in AMAN after *Campylobacter* infection. In the later report, Ho and colleagues demonstrated on motor-point biopsy denervation of the neuromuscular junction and reduction in the intramuscular nerve fiber count. Because GM1 antibodies can bind at nodes of Ranvier, they suggested that these might induce failure of electrical conduction. Quicker recovery may therefore be caused by reversible changes of the sodium channels at nodes of Ranvier as acute motor conduction block variant of AMAN or by degeneration followed by regeneration of motor nerve terminals and intramuscular axons.

Most patients with MFS recover by 6 months.[83] In that study, all 28 untreated MFS cases returned to normal activities with a respective median period of 32 days between onset and disappearance of ataxia and 88 days for ophthalmoplegia. In a follow-up study, Mori and colleagues[83] analyzed the clinical recovery of 92 patients with MFS who had been treated with IVIG (n = 28), plasmapheresis (n = 23), and no immune treatment (n = 41). Although IVIG slightly hastened the amelioration of ophthalmoplegia and ataxia, 96% of cases were free of all symptoms and signs 1 year after the onset of neurologic symptoms, whether or not they received immunotherapy. In a large case series, most of the 62 patients with BBE with and without limb weakness were given immunotherapy including steroids, plasmapheresis, and IVIG.[21] Six months after BBE onset, 37 (66%) of 56 for whom outcome data were available showed complete remission with no residual symptoms. A Cochrane review indicates that there are no randomized controlled trials of immunomodulatory therapy in MFS or related disorders on which to base practice.[18]

Box 2
Poor prognostic factors in GBS

1. Older age (>50–60)

2. Rapid onset before presentation (<7 days)

3. Ventilator dependency

4. Severely reduced distal CMAP amplitudes (<20% lower limit of normal)

5. Preceding infection with CMV

6. Preceding diarrheal illness or *C jejuni*

7. Erasmus GBS outcome score at 2 weeks ≥ 5[79]

   a. Ventilator dependence, or

   b. Bedbound or chairbound and elderly (>60), or

   c. Bedbound or chairbound and preceding diarrheal illness

Case report

A 25 year-old woman developed numbness and tingling of the feet and hands followed by progressive leg more than arm muscle weakness over the last week. She experienced a diarrheal illness 3 weeks ago that had resolved within 10 days.

Examination showed marked bifacial weakness and absent muscle stretch reflexes. She had with normal pinprick, light touch and proprioception but vibration was reduced at the toes. Leg strength is 2 to 3/5 and arm strength is 3 to 4/5, with proximal and distal weakness. She could not stand up or walk with assistance. Forced vital capacity was 2.0 liters.

Laboratory studies including vitamin B12 level and 2 hour glucose tolerance test were normal and there was no serum monoclonal protein. Cerebrospinal fluid evaluation showed no white cells but protein was 82 mg/dl. Nerve conduction studies showed 50% delay in tibial and median F wave latencies. Sensory conductions showed normal sural and absent median potentials.

She was started on intravenous gammaglobulin for the diagnosis of GBS. She started improving in strength 2 weeks later. She could ambulate with a walker at 2 months and independently at 6 months.

REFERENCES

1. Landry O. Nore sur la paralysie ascendante aigue. Gaz Hebd Med Paris 1859;6: 472–4.
2. Guillain G, Barré JA, Strohl A. Sur un syndrome de radilculonévrite avec hyperalbuminose du liquid céphalo-rachidien sans reaction cellulaire. Remarques sur les catactères cliniques et graphiques de reflexes tendineux. Bull Mem Soc Med Hop Paris 1916;40:1462–70.
3. Alter M. The epidemiology of Guillain-Barré syndrome. Ann Neurol 1990;27:S7–12.
4. Hughes RA, Cornblath DR. Guillain-Barré syndrome. Lancet 2005;366(9497): 1653–66.
5. Hughes RA, Rees JH. Clinical and epidemiologic features of Guillain-Barré syndrome. J Infect Dis 1997;176(Suppl 2):S92–8.
6. Van Koningsveld R, Van Doorn PA, Schmitz PI, et al. Mild forms of Guillain-Barré syndrome in an epidemiologic survey in The Netherlands. Neurology 2000;54(3): 620–5.
7. Govoni V, Granieri E. Epidemiology of the Guillain-Barré syndrome. Curr Opin Neurol 2001;14(5):605–13.
8. McGrogan A, Madle GC, Seaman HE, et al. The epidemiology of Guillain-Barré syndrome worldwide. A systematic literature review. Neuroepidemiology 2009; 32(2):150–63.
9. Hadden RD, Cornblath DR, Hughes RA, et al. Electrophysiological classification of Guillain-Barré syndrome: clinical associations and outcome. Plasma Exchange/Sandoglobulin Guillain-Barré Syndrome Trial Group. Ann Neurol 1998;44(5):780–8.
10. McKhann GM, Cornblath DR, Ho T, et al. Clinical and electrophysiological aspects of acute paralytic disease of children and young adults in northern China. Lancet 1991;338(8767):593–7.
11. McKhann GM, Cornblath DR, Griffin JW, et al. Acute motor axonal neuropathy: a frequent cause of acute flaccid paralysis in China. Ann Neurol 1993;33(4):333–42.
12. Ogawara K, Kuwabara S, Mori M, et al. Axonal Guillain-Barré syndrome: relation to anti-ganglioside antibodies and *Campylobacter jejuni* infection in Japan. Ann Neurol 2000;48(4):624–31.

13. Paradiso G, Tripoli J, Galicchio S, et al. Epidemiological, clinical, and electrodiagnostic findings in childhood Guillain-Barré syndrome: a reappraisal. Ann Neurol 1999;46(5):701–7.

14. Barohn RJ, Saperstein DS. Guillain-Barré syndrome and chronic inflammatory demyelinating polyneuropathy. Semin Neurol 1998;18(1):49–61.

15. Ropper AH, Wijdicks EF, Truax BT. Guillain-barré syndrome, contemporary neurology series 34. Clinical features of the typical syndrome. Philadelphia: FA Davis; 1991.

16. Ruts L, Drenthen J, Jongen JL, et al. Pain in Guillain-Barre syndrome: a long-term follow-up study. Neurology 2010;75(16):1439–47.

17. Fisher CM. An unusual variant of acute idiopathic polyneuritis (syndrome of ophthalmoplegia, ataxia and areflexia). N Engl J Med 1956;255:57–65.

18. Overell JR, Hsieh ST, Odaka M, et al. Treatment for Fisher syndrome, Bickerstaff's brainstem encephalitis and related disorders. Cochrane Database Syst Rev 2007;(1):CD004761.

19. Bickerstaff E, Cloake P. Mesencephalitis and rhombencephalitis. Br Med J 1951; 2:77–81.

20. Yuki N, Sato S, Tsuji S, et al. An immunologic abnormality common to Bickerstaff's brain stem encephalitis and Fisher's syndrome. J Neurol Sci 1993;118(1):83–7.

21. Odaka M, Yuki N, Yamada M, et al. Bickerstaff's brainstem encephalitis: clinical features of 62 cases and a subgroup associated with Guillain Barre syndrome. Brain 2003;126:2279–90.

22. Ito M, Kuwabara S, Odaka M, et al. Bickerstaff's brainstem encephalitis and Fisher syndrome form a continuous spectrum: clinical analysis of 581 cases. J Neurol 2008;255(5):674–82.

23. Ropper AH. Unusual clinical variants and signs in Guillain-Barré syndrome. Arch Neurol 1986;43(11):1150–2.

24. Ropper AH. Further regional variants of acute immune polyneuropathy. Bifacial weakness or sixth nerve paresis with paresthesias lumbar polyradiculopathy and ataxia with pharyngeal-cervical-brachial weakness. Arch Neurol 1994; 51(7):671–5.

25. Feasby TE, Gilbert JJ, Brown WF, et al. An acute axonal form of Guillain-Barré polyneuropathy. Brain 1986;109(Pt 6):1115–26.

26. Griffin JW, Li CY, Ho TW, et al. Pathology of the motor-sensory axonal Guillain-Barré syndrome. Ann Neurol 1996;39(1):17–28.

27. Ho TW, Mishu B, Cy Li, et al. Guillain-Barré syndrome in northern China. Relationship to Campylobacter jejuni infection and anti-glycolipid antibodies. Brain 1995; 118:597–605.

28. Hiraga A, Mori M, Ogawara K, et al. Differences in patterns of progression in demyelinating and axonal Guillain-Barre syndromes. Neurology 2003;61(4): 471–4.

29. Capasso M, Caporale CM, Pomilio F, et al. Acute motor conduction block neuropathy: another Guillain-Barre syndrome variant. Neurology 2003;61:617–22.

30. Hafer-Macko C, Sheikh KA, Li CY, et al. Immune attack on the Schwann cell surface in acute inflammatory demyelinating polyneuropathy. Ann Neurol 1996; 39:625–35.

31. Griffin JW, Li CY, Macko C, et al. Early nodal changes in the acute motor axonal neuropathy pattern of the Guillain-Barré syndrome. J Neurocytol 1996;25:33–51.

32. Ho TW, Willison HJ, Nachamkin I, et al. Anti-GD1a antibody is associated with axonal but not demyelinating forms of Guillain-Barré syndrome. Ann Neurol 1999;45:168–73.

33. Allos BM. Association between *Campylobacter* infection and Guillain-Barré syndrome. J Infect Dis 1997;176(Suppl 2):S25–127.
34. Magira EE, Papaioakim M, Nachamkin I, et al. Differential distribution of HLA-DQ beta/DR beta epitopes in the two forms of Guillain-Barré syndrome, acute motor axonal neuropathy and acute inflammatory demyelinating polyneuropathy (AIDP): identification of DQ beta epitopes associated with susceptibility to and protection from AIDP. J Immunol 2003;170(60):3074–4080.
35. Schonberger LB, Bregman DJ, Sullivan-Bolyai JZ, et al. Guillain-Barré syndrome following vaccination in the National Influenza Immunization Program, United States, 1976–1977. Am J Epidemiol 1979;110:105–23.
36. Lasky T, Terracciano GJ, Magder L, et al. The Guillain-Barré syndrome and the 1992-1993 and 1993-1994 influenza vaccines. N Engl J Med 1998;339(25):1797–802.
37. Souayah N, Nasar A, Suri MF, et al. Guillain-Barre syndrome after vaccination in United States a report from the CDC/FDA Vaccine Adverse Event Reporting System. Vaccine 2007;25(29):5253–5.
38. Centers for Disease Control and Prevention. Preliminary results: surveillance for Guillain-Barré syndrome after receipt of influenza A (H1N1) 2009 monovalent vaccine—United States, 2009–2010. MMWR Morb Mortal Wkly Rep 2010;59(Early Release):1–5. Available at: http://www.cdc.gov/mmwr/preview/mmwrhtml/mm59e0602a1. htm?s_cid=mm59e0602a1_e. Accessed February 3, 2011.
39. Fiore AE, Uyeki TM, Broder K, et al, Centers for Disease Control and Prevention (CDC). Prevention and control of influenza with vaccines: recommendations of the Advisory Committee on Immunization Practices (ACIP), 2010. MMWR Recomm Rep 2010;59(RR-8):1–62.
40. Pritchard J, Mukherjee R, Hughes RA. Risk of relapse of Guillain-Barré syndrome or chronic inflammatory demyelinating polyradiculoneuropathy following immunisation. J Neurol Neurosurg Psychiatry 2002;73(3):348–9.
41. Asbury AK, Cornblath DR. Assessment of current diagnostic criteria for Guillain-Barré syndrome. Ann Neurol 1990;27(Suppl):S21–4.
42. Albers JW, Donofrio PD, McGonagle TK. Sequential electrodiagnostic abnormalities in acute inflammatory demyelinating polyradiculoneuropathy. Muscle Nerve 1985;8(6):528–39.
43. Van den Bergh PY, Piéret F. Electrodiagnostic criteria for acute and chronic inflammatory demyelinating polyradiculoneuropathy. Muscle Nerve 2004;29(4):565–74.
44. Albers JW, Kelly JJ Jr. Acquired inflammatory demyelinating polyneuropathies: clinical and electrodiagnostic features. Muscle Nerve 1989;12(6):435–51.
45. Wiederholt WC, Mulder DW, Lambert EH. The Landry-Guillain-Barré-Srohl syndrome or polyradiculoneuropathy. Historical review, report on 97 cases and present concepts. Mayo Clin Proc 1964;39:427–51.
46. Ropper AH. The Guillain-Barré syndrome. N Engl J Med 1992;326(17):1130–6.
47. Anders BJ, Lauer BA, Paisley JW, et al. Double-blind placebo controlled trial of erythromycin for treatment of *Campylobacter enteritis*. Lancet 1982;1(8264):131–2.
48. Kuwabara S, Yuki N, Koga M, et al. IgG anti-GM1 antibody is associated with reversible conduction failure and axonal degeneration in Guillain-Barré syndrome. Ann Neurol 1998;44(2):202–8.
49. Oomes PG, Jacobs BC, Hazenberg MP, et al. Anti-GM1 IgG antibodies and *Campylobacter* bacteria in Guillain-Barré syndrome: evidence of molecular mimicry. Ann Neurol 1995;38(2):170–5.

50. Vriesendorp FJ, Mishu B, Blaser MJ, et al. Serum antibodies to GM1, GD1b, peripheral nerve myelin, and *Campylobacter jejuni* in patients with Guillain-Barré syndrome and controls: correlation and prognosis. Ann Neurol 1993;34(2): 130–5.

51. Willison HJ, Veitch J, Paterson G, et al. Miller Fisher syndrome is associated with serum antibodies to GQ1b ganglioside. J Neurol Neurosurg Psychiatry 1993; 56(2):204–6.

52. Yuki N, Sato S, Tsuji S, et al. Frequent presence of anti-GQ1b antibody in Fisher's syndrome. Neurology 1993;43(2):414–7.

53. Morgan GW, Barohn RJ, Bazan C, et al. Nerve root enhancement with MRI in inflammatory demyelinating polyradiculoneuropathy. Neurology 1993;43(3 Pt 1):618–20.

54. Gorson KC, Ropper AH, Muriello MA, et al. Prospective evaluation of MRI lumbosacral nerve root enhancement in acute Guillain-Barré syndrome. Neurology 1996;47(3):813–7.

55. Hughes RA, Wijdicks EF, Benson E, et al, Multidisciplinary Consensus Group. Supportive care for patients with Guillain-Barré syndrome. Arch Neurol 2005; 62(8):1194–8.

56. French Cooperative Group on Plasma Exchange in Guillain-Barré Syndrome. Efficiency of plasma exchange in Guillain-Barré syndrome: role of replacement fluids. Ann Neurol 1987;22:753–61.

57. The Guillain-Barré syndrome Study Group. Plasmapheresis and acute Guillain-Barré syndrome. Neurology 1985;35(8):1096–104.

58. French Cooperative Group on Plasma Exchange in Guillain-Barré Syndrome. Appropriate number of plasma exchanges in Guillain-Barré syndrome. Ann Neurol 1997;41:298–306.

59. Dalakas MC. Intravenous immunoglobulin in autoimmune neuromuscular diseases. JAMA 2004;291(19):2367–75.

60. Anthony RM, Ravetch JV. A novel role for the IgG Fc glycan: the anti-inflammatory activity of sialylated IgG Fcs. J Clin Immunol 2010;30(Suppl 1):S9–14.

61. van der Meché FG, Schmitz PI. The Dutch Guillain-Barré Study Group. A randomized trial comparing intravenous immune globulin and plasma exchange in Guillain-Barré syndrome. N Engl J Med 1992;326:1123–9.

62. Plasma Exchange and Sandoglobulin Guillain-Barré; Syndrome Trial Group. Randomized trial of plasma exchange, intravenous immunoglobulin and combined treatments in Guillain-Barré syndrome. Lancet 1997;349:225–30.

63. Irani DN, Cornblath DR, Chaudhry V, et al. Relapse in Guillain-Barré syndrome after treatment with human immune globulin. Neurology 1993;43(5):872–5.

64. Castro LH, Ropper AH. Human immune globulin infusion in Guillain-Barré syndrome: worsening during and after treatment. Neurology 1993;43(5):1034–6.

65. Hughes RA. Plasma exchange versus intravenous immunoglobulin for Guillain-Barré syndrome. Ther Apher 1997;1:129–30.

66. Hughes RA, Newsom-Davis JM, Perkin GD, et al. Controlled trial prednisolone in acute polyneuropathy. Lancet 1978;2(8093):750–3.

67. Guillain-Barré Syndrome Steroid Trial Group. Double-blind trial of intravenous methylprednisolone in Guillain-Barré syndrome. Lancet 1993;341(8845):586–90.

68. The Dutch Guillain-Barré Study Group. Treatment of Guillain-Barré syndrome with high-dose immune globulins combined with methylprednisolone: a pilot study. Ann Neurol 1994;35(6):749–52.

69. van Koningsveld R, Schmitz PI, Meché FG, et al. Effect of methylprednisolone when added to standard treatment with intravenous immunoglobulin for Guillain-Barré syndrome: randomised trial. Lancet 2004;363(9404):192–6.

70. Hughes RA, Wijdicks EF, Barohn R, et al. Quality Standards Subcommittee of the American Academy of Neurology. Practice parameter: immunotherapy for Guillain-Barré syndrome: report of the Quality Standards Subcommittee of the American Academy of Neurology. Neurology 2003;61(6):736–40.
71. Rees JH, Thompson RD, Smeeton NC, et al. Epidemiological study of Guillain-Barré syndrome in south east England. J Neurol Neurosurg Psychiatry 1998;64(1):74–7.
72. Dornonville de la Cour C, Jakobsen J. Residual neuropathy in long-term population-based follow-up of Guillain-Barre syndrome. Neurology 2005;64(2):246–53.
73. Vedeler CA, Wik E, Nyland H. The long-term prognosis of Guillain-Barre syndrome. Evaluation of prognostic factors including plasma exchange. Acta Neurol Scand 1997;95:298–302.
74. Koeppen S, Kraywinkel K, Wessendorf TE, et al. Long-term outcome of Guillain-Barre syndrome. Neurocrit Care 2006;5:235–42.
75. Ruts L, Drenthen J, Jacobs BC, et al, Dutch GBS Study Group. Distinguishing acute-onset CIDP from fluctuating Guillain-Barre syndrome: a prospective study. Neurology 2010;74(21):1680–6.
76. Kuitwaard K, de Gelder J, Tio-Gillen AP, et al. Pharmacokinetics of intravenous immunoglobulin and outcome in Guillain-Barré syndrome. Ann Neurol 2009; 66(5):597–603.
77. McKhann GM, Griffin JW, Cornblath DR, et al. Plasmapheresis and Guillain-Barré syndrome: analysis of prognostic factors and the effect of plasmapheresis. Ann Neurol 1988;23(4):347–53.
78. Visser LH, Schmitz PI, Meulstee J, et al. Dutch Guillain-Barré Study Group. Prognostic factors of Guillain-Barré syndrome after intravenous immunoglobulin or plasma exchange. Neurology 1999;53(3):598–604.
79. van Koningsveld R, Steyerberg EW, Hughes RA, et al. A clinical prognostic scoring system for Guillain-Barré syndrome. Lancet 2007;6(7):589–94.
80. Walgaard C, Lingsma HF, Ruts L, et al. Early recognition of poor prognosis in Gullain-Barre syndrome. Neurology 2011;76(11):968–75.
81. Ho TW, Li CY, Cornblath DR, et al. Patterns of recovery in the Guillain-Barre syndromes. Neurology 1997;48(3):695–700.
82. Ho TW, Hsieh ST, Nachamkin I, et al. Motor nerve terminal degernation provides a potential mechanism for rapid recovery in acute motor axonal neuropathy after *Campylobacter* infection. Neurology 1997;48:717–24.
83. Mori M, Kuwabara S, Fukutake T, et al. Intravenous immunoglobulin therapy for Miller Fisher syndrome. Neurology 2007;68(14):1144–6.

Chronic Inflammatory Demyelinating Polyneuropathy

Kenneth C. Gorson, MD[a],*, Jonathan Katz, MD[b]

KEYWORDS

- CIDP • Immune neuropathy • Demyelination • Monoclonal gammopathy • IVIg
- Corticosteroids • Plasma exchange

KEY POINTS

- Chronic inflammatory demyelinating polyradiculoneuropathy (CIDP) is a condition characterized by "classic" clinical features of progressive proximal limb weakness, areflexia, and large fiber sensory loss, but a large number of variant presentations have been described and should be recognized because they also respond to treatment in most cases.
- There are numerous published diagnostic criteria for CIDP but most have not been validated scientifically, and therefore the Koski criteria or European Federation of Neurologic Societies criteria are recommended to establish the diagnosis.
- There are proven effective therapies (corticosteroids, intravenous immunoglobulin, and plasma exchange) in CIDP, and these published treatment regimens should be used rather than alternative treatment approaches with often arbitrary dosing and duration intervals. Alternative immunomodulating agents should not be considered unless proven therapies have failed.
- The prognosis for CIDP is generally favorable, and for those patients who do not improve with any of the proven first-line treatments, the diagnosis of CIDP should be reconsidered.

INTRODUCTION

The term chronic inflammatory demyelinating polyradiculoneuropathy (CIDP) applies to the "classic presentation" among a spectrum of acquired immune-mediated demyelinating neuropathies. These conditions differ mainly in their time course and in the pattern of clinical involvement. As the name implies, CIDP is a chronic, acquired, immune-mediated condition affecting the peripheral nervous system. The pathogenesis is incompletely understood, but includes several humoral and cell-mediated

Disclosures: Dr Gorson has received compensation from Grifols Pharmaceuticals for speaking engagements and serves on an independent data safety monitoring board and as a consultant for CSL Behring. Dr Katz: None.
[a] Neuromuscular Service, Tufts University School of Medicine, St. Elizabeth's Medical Center, 736 Cambridge Street, Boston, MA 02135, USA; [b] Neuromuscular Service, California Pacific Medical Center, University of California, 2324 Sacramento Street, Suite 111, San Francisco, CA 94115, USA
* Corresponding author.
E-mail address: kengorson@comcast.net

Neurol Clin 31 (2013) 511–532
http://dx.doi.org/10.1016/j.ncl.2013.01.006
0733-8619/13/$ – see front matter © 2013 Elsevier Inc. All rights reserved.

mechanisms.[1–4] Pathologic studies have shown endoneurial inflammation and nerve demyelination mediated by complement pathways and antibodies directed against antigenic components of the myelin sheath.[1–8]

The classic description of CIDP includes (1) progressive limb weakness involving proximal and distal muscles, sensory loss, and areflexia, and a relapsing or progressive course; (2) electrophysiological features of segmental demyelination, including prolonged distal motor and F-wave latencies, reduced conduction velocities, conduction block, and temporal dispersion; (3) albumino-cytologic dissociation in the cerebrospinal fluid (CSF); and (4) inflammation, demyelination, and remyelination on nerve biopsy.[9,10] In most cases, the diagnosis can be confidently established by clinical and electromyography (EMG) criteria, and nerve biopsy is not needed. Response to immunomodulating therapy can be a supportive diagnostic feature. Many prospective, randomized, placebo-controlled trials have established the short-term and longer-term efficacy of immune therapy for CIDP, including corticosteroids, plasma exchange (PE), and intravenous immunoglobulin (IVIg).[11–20]

CLINICAL FEATURES

Acute inflammatory demyelinating neuropathy (AIDP, Guillain-Barré syndrome [GBS]) and CIDP have similar clinical findings, but as the terms imply, the time course is defined by a peak deficit within 4 weeks in AIDP, and after at least 8 weeks in CIDP. For an illness that reaches its nadir between 4 and 8 weeks, the term subacute demyelinating neuropathy has also been used.[21]

CIDP most commonly occurs in adults between the ages of 40 and 60, but can affect the elderly and children.[1–4,22] There is a slight predilection for men. The prevalence ranges from about 5 to 9 cases per 100,000 individuals.[23,24] Two-thirds of cases are progressive and the remainder relapsing. The term "relapse" often reflects the outcome from treatment withdrawal, but relapses may be triggered by infections or other systemic illnesses, and sometimes may occur spontaneously.

In its classic form, the initial features of CIDP are progressive, symmetric limb weakness and sensory loss that usually begin in the legs (**Box 1**). Patients report difficulty walking, climbing stairs, rising from a chair, and falls. Upper limb involvement may cause trouble using utensils, tying shoe laces, and gripping objects. A core clinical feature is proximal limb weakness, which distinguishes CIDP from the large group of far more commonly encountered distal polyneuropathies. Sensory involvement causes loss of feeling, distal paresthesias, poor balance, and impaired proprioception. Neuropathic pain occurs in a minority of cases.[1–4,9,10,25] A useful clinical finding is the discrepancy between the degree of weakness and the absence of atrophy in affected muscles. This finding strongly suggests nerve demyelination, as opposed to axonal loss in which atrophy may be prominent. Facial, oropharyngeal, and ocular involvement occurs in fewer than 15% of patients. Autonomic dysfunction and ventilatory failure develop in fewer than 10% of cases, in contrast to GBS.[3,26]

Box 1
Classic clinical features of CIDP

- Relapsing or progressive course >8 weeks
- Generalized symmetric weakness with a predilection for proximal and distal muscles
- Generalized hypoflexia or areflexia
- Large-fiber sensory loss in the distal limbs (light touch, vibration, and joint position sense)

CLINICAL VARIANTS

Several reports have highlighted a variety of clinical patterns that are considered variants of CIDP. These are also grouped within the category of chronic acquired demyelinating polyneuropathy, primarily because they share electrophysiological and CSF features.[27–45] Variants include pure motor, pure sensory, and ataxic patterns, as well as multifocal patterns in which weakness and sensory loss develop in the distributions of individual nerve territories (**Box 2**). The motor variant is a generalized, pure motor demyelinating neuropathy, which can be distinguished from multifocal motor neuropathy by the presence of widespread proximal and distal limb weakness, relative symmetry, no sensory involvement, and response to corticosteroids.[27,34]

The pure sensory syndrome causes a clinical pattern of distal predominant sensory loss, which can be identified because of the prominent demyelinating motor abnormalities on EMG studies. Another variant presentation may simulate a sensory ganglionopathy, with absent sensory potentials and normal motor studies, and nerve biopsy may be required to establish the diagnosis.[27–33] A third rare but striking sensory variant is a large fiber ataxic form, manifest by inflammation and demyelination isolated to the sensory roots. In this condition, routine electrodiagnostic studies are usually normal, whereas somatosensory evoked potentials demonstrate slowing at the level of the lumbar and cervical roots. The CSF protein level is elevated, and lumbar rootlet biopsy demonstrates characteristic pathologic features of CIDP. This pattern has been termed chronic inflammatory sensory polyradiculopathy (CISP).[33]

In contrast, "regional" variants are recognized, including a sensorimotor multifocal form that clinically simulates axonal mononeuritis multiplex, termed Lewis-Sumner syndrome or multifocal acquired demyelinating sensory and motor neuropathy.[35–38]

Box 2
Clinical variants of CIDP

Functional Variants

- Pure motor CIDP

- Pure sensory CIDP

- Ataxic CIDP

- CISP

Regional Variants

- Focal or multifocal CIDP (LSS, MADSAM)

- Upper limb pattern

- Paraparetic pattern

- Distal CIDP (DADS)

- Isolated cranial neuropathies

Temporal Course

- Subacute inflammatory demyelinating polyneuropathy (SIDP)

- Relapsing Guillain-Barré syndrome pattern

Abbreviations: CIDP, chronic inflammatory demyelinating polyneuropathy; CISP, chronic inflammatory sensory polyradiculopathy; DADS, distal acquired demyelinating symmetric neuropathy; LSS, Lewis-Sumner syndrome; MADSAM, multifocal acquired demyelinating sensory and motor neuropathy.

These conditions tend to involve distal muscles and affect the upper limbs more than the legs. At the extreme, there are descriptions of a purely upper limb demyelinating neuropathy that may be strikingly focal.[39] A paraparetic form of CIDP is associated with regional leg weakness, sensory loss, striking nerve root hypertrophy, and gadolinium enhancement of the lumbosacral nerve roots on magnetic resonance imaging (MRI) studies. This condition causes a phenotype emulating a progressive cauda equina syndrome.[40] A few patients have only prominent and isolated cranial nerve palsies.[3,27,41]

Finally, some experts have stressed a distal, symmetric, predominantly sensory, demyelinating polyneuropathy as a variant of CIDP. This has been termed distal acquired demyelinating symmetric [DADS] neuropathy.[42] This variant simulates a distal sensorimotor neuropathy clinically, and can be missed without careful electrodiagnostic evaluation. This pattern also can be difficult to separate from axonal neuropathies that have mild demyelinating features, and should be diagnosed only when nerve conduction studies and spinal fluid evaluation show unequivocal findings consistent with CIDP. These functional and regional variants seem to respond to the conventional therapies for CIDP with about the same frequency but have never been subjected carefully to controlled study.

Other similar illnesses have been distinguished from typical CIDP based on the temporal course. For example, investigators have identified patients with a time course between AIDP and CIDP, as previously noted.[26,43] Occasionally, the initial manifestations of CIDP may mimic a clinical pattern of acute relapsing GBS; such cases can be reclassified as CIDP only after 3 or more relapses or progression of symptoms and signs beyond 9 weeks.[44,45]

CIDP AND ASSOCIATED ILLNESSES

A number of medical conditions may occur contemporaneously with CIDP and have been implicated in its pathogenesis (**Box 3**). For example, most large series of patients with CIDP have found that approximately 15% to 20% have a monoclonal gammopathy detected by serum immunofixation.[1–4,25,27,46–48] A small number of these patients have a malignant plasma cell dyscrasia and an immunoglobulin G (IgG) (or less commonly IgA) paraprotein that causes the POEMS syndrome (polyneuropathy, organomegaly, endocrinopathy, M-spike, skin changes). Others may have lymphoma or Waldenström macroglobulinemia. However, most have a monoclonal gammopathy of undetermined significance (MGUS). Most patients with CIDP-MGUS and an IgG or IgA monoclonal protein have a disorder that is indistinguishable from idiopathic CIDP, including improvement with immune therapies.[1–3,46–48]

In contrast, demyelinating neuropathies with an IgM paraprotein usually need to be considered as a distinct syndrome. These cases typically present with a length-dependent sensorimotor phenotype marked by distal sensory loss, tremor, and relatively severe demyelination in distal compared with proximal nerve segments. In these cases, anti–myelin-associated glycoprotein antibodies or other pathogenic antineuronal antibodies may be detected in the serum in about half the cases. These patients are less responsive to the standard treatments for CIDP and likely constitute a different disease.[47–50]

A small number of patients with CIDP have an associated systemic medical disorder, although the precise relationship to the neuropathy may vary. **Box 3** lists disorders that have been linked to CIDP. A particularly vexing problem for the clinician is the relationship between diabetes mellitus and CIDP. Some investigators believe the risk of developing CIDP is increased in patients with diabetes, but this has not been proven. In fact, a recent well-conducted epidemiologic study indicated

---

Box 3
CIDP-associated illnesses

Paraprotein-associated disorders

Monoclonal gammopathy of undetermined significance (MGUS)

Osteosclerotic myeloma (POEMS syndrome)

Multiple myeloma

Waldenström macroglobulinemia

Amyloidosis

Castleman disease

Chronic Infections

HIV infection

Human T lymphotropic virus type I

Lyme disease

Hepatitis C

Cat scratch disease

Epstein-Barr infection

Connective tissue and autoimmune disorders

Systemic lupus erythematosus

Sjögren syndrome

Rheumatoid disease

Giant cell arteritis

Sarcoidosis

Inflammatory bowel disease

Myasthenia gravis

Chronic active hepatitis

Multiple sclerosis

Systemic medical disorders

Diabetes mellitus

Thyrotoxicosis

Chronic renal failure requiring dialysis

Membranous glomerulonephropathy

Malignancy

Hepatocellular carcinoma

Melanoma

Pancreatic carcinoma

Colon adenocarcinoma

Lymphoma

Paraneoplastic demyelinating neuropathy

Medications

Interferon alpha

Procainamide

Tacrolimus

Tumor necrosis factor antagonists

Other Possible Associations

Vaccinations

Solid organ transplantation

Hereditary neuropathy (CIDP and CMT)

Abbreviations: CMT, Charcot-Marie-Tooth disease; POEMS, polyneuropathy, organomegaly, endocrinopathy, M-spike, skin changes.

diabetes mellitus was not a predisposing risk factor for CIDP compared with the general population.[24] Clinical confusion arises when some patients with diabetes mellitus develop a severe, progressive, symmetric neuropathy that is out of proportion to the severity or duration of the diabetes. Occasionally, patients with diabetes mellitus have some demyelinating features on EMG studies, and the spinal fluid protein concentration can be raised in some diabetics. In such cases, it can be difficult to know whether these cases should be classified as CIDP in a diabetic patient and treated with standard immune therapies, or a neuropathy as a complication of diabetes. Until clinical trials can study this specific group of patients, it is difficult to draw firm conclusions.

LABORATORY EVALUATION

The laboratory studies indicated for patients suspected of CIDP are provided in **Box 4**. The detection of a monoclonal protein warrants investigation to exclude a plasma cell dyscrasia before concluding the monoclonal protein represents MGUS. When an M-protein has been detected, other useful tests include serum cryoglobulins, β-2 microglobulin, and viscosity (for IgM cases) when more than 3.0 g/dL of monoclonal protein is detected. Referral to a hematologist, bone scan, and bone marrow biopsy are generally indicated in patients who have more than 3.0 g/L of monoclonal protein or have systemic features suggesting myeloma (eg, fatigue, bone pain, weight loss, anemia, hypercalcemia, renal failure). A skeletal bone survey also is required to exclude bone lesions associated with osteosclerotic myeloma and the POEMS syndrome, especially if there is an IgG, IgA, or lambda light chain monoclonal protein. Suspicious sclerotic bone lesions should be biopsied. Chest and abdominal computed tomography scanning can be useful in selected cases when lymphoma or the POEMS syndrome associated with Castleman disease is considered.

A lumbar puncture is indicated in most patients suspected of having CIDP. An elevated CSF protein level (>45 mg/dL) is detected in at least 80% of patients.[1–4,25,27] The diagnosis of CIDP cannot be excluded based on a normal CSF protein concentration only. The cell count is usually normal, although as many 10% of patients have greater than 5 lymphocytes/mm³. The American Academy of Neurology (AAN) criteria has suggested that there should be fewer than 10 white blood cells in the spinal fluid, and fewer than 50 cells in patients with HIV infection.[9] Accordingly, the presence of a CSF pleocytosis should prompt an evaluation for HIV infection, as well as Lyme disease, lymphomatous meningitis, and sarcoidosis. In addition, an MRI of the lumbar spine with gadolinium sometimes can demonstrate nerve root enhancement in patients suspected of CIDP, as demonstrated in **Fig. 1**.[33]

Box 4
Diagnostic evaluation of patients suspected of CIDP

Complete blood count

Routine chemistries

Renal and liver function tests

Thyroid function studies

Fasting glucose and hemoglobin A1c

HIV titer

Antinuclear antibodies

Serum and urine immunofixation

Lumbar puncture for protein level and cells

Nerve conduction studies and electromyography

Additional laboratory studies in selected cases:

Serum cryoglobulins

Lyme titer

Hepatitis B and C titers

Serum anti-neutrophil cytoplasmic antibodies

Anti–Sjögren syndrome (SS) A and SSB antibodies

Genetic testing to exclude inherited demyelinating neuropathies (CMT 1A, 1B, CMT-X, hereditary liability to pressure palsies [HNPP])

Paraneoplastic antibody screening

Gadolinium-enhanced magnetic resonance imaging of the lumbar spine

Nerve biopsy

ELECTRODIAGNOSTIC CRITERIA

Nerve conduction studies establish the diagnosis of CIDP with confidence in the vast majority of cases. Many electrodiagnostic criteria have been proposed, all requiring some combination of (1) reduced conduction velocities (eg, <80% of the lower limit of normal [LLN] if the distal motor amplitude is normal, and <70% of LLN if the amplitude is substantially reduced); (2) prolonged distal motor latencies, (3) prolonged F-wave latencies (eg, >125% of the upper limit of normal [ULN] if the distal motor amplitude is normal, and >150% of ULN if the amplitude is reduced for distal latencies and F-waves); and, (4) conduction block/temporal dispersion (eg, conduction block is >50% reduction of proximal/distal [p/d] amplitude and abnormal temporal dispersion is >130% increase of p/d duration). According to the AAN criteria (**Box 5**), the presence of 3 of the 4 criteria in 2 or more nerves establishes the electrophysiological diagnosis of CIDP for research purposes.[9] For the practicing clinician, these criteria should be taken in context, as only 50% to 60% of patients with typical clinical features of CIDP fulfill strict AAN electrodiagnostic criteria.

Accordingly, over the past 20 years, at least 16 alternative EMG criteria have been proposed,[51] with varying degrees of sensitivity and specificity. As with any receiver operator characteristic, the greater the requirement to define "demyelination," the lower the sensitivity and the greater the specificity. Only one criterion has been

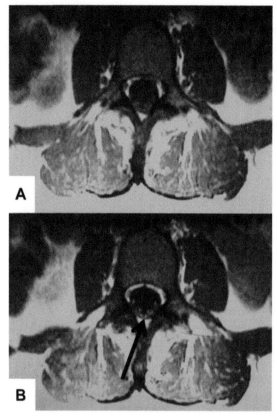

Fig. 1. Axial T1 MRI of the lumbar nerve roots, nonenhanced image (*A*) and gadolinium-enhanced image (*B*) showing nerve root enhancement (*arrow*).

validated in a rigorous manner (**Box 6**),[52] thus contributing to further controversy and confusion. As a general rule, because demyelination in CIDP is frequently a multifocal process, study of multiple motor nerves (at least 4 and probably more) is necessary. Similarly, proximal nerve and root stimulation may be required in some patients to confirm cases in which the involvement is predominantly in proximal segments. Indeed, exhaustive bilateral upper limb studies, including proximal stimulation across the Erb point, or 4-limb forearm and foreleg studies have been shown to increase the likelihood of detecting demyelination and satisfy EMG criteria for CIDP.[53] Computer simulation techniques have demonstrated that up to a 50% amplitude reduction between proximal and distal points of stimulation may occur in normal motor nerves, a phenomenon termed "pseudo-conduction block," which has been attributed to interphase cancellation of motor potential waveforms. Therefore, the criterion for definite conduction block has been increased from 20% (initial AAN criteria) to 50% amplitude reduction following proximal nerve stimulation, especially with studies of very proximal nerve or root segments.[54]

We recommend the use of the Koski criteria for electrodiagnostic confirmation of CIDP (see **Box 6**) because (1) the parameters have been derived in a statistically validated fashion; (2) the electrodiagnostic criteria can be satisfied by studying fewer nerves as long as an odd number of nerves are assessed; (3) those motor nerves with a high likelihood of being absent (eg, patients with severe foot atrophy) need

---

Box 5
AAN ad hoc subcommittee electrodiagnostic research criteria for CIDP

3 of 4 criteria must be fulfilled in 2 or more nerves:

1. Reduction in conduction velocity in 2 or motor nerves:

    a. <80% of lower limit of normal (LLN) if amplitude >80% of LLN

    b. <70% of LLN if amplitude is <80% of LLN

2. Partial conduction block in 1 or more motor nerves defined as <15% change in duration between proximal and distal sites and >20% drop in negative peak (−p) and/or peak-to-peak (p–p) area or peak-to-peak (p–p) amplitude between proximal and distal sites.

3. Prolonged distal motor latencies in 2 or more nerves:

    a. >125% of upper limit or normal (ULN) if amplitude is >80% of LLN

    b. >150% of ULN if amplitude is <80% of LLN

4. Absent F-waves or prolonged minimum F-wave latencies in 2 or more motor nerves:

    a. >120% of ULN if amplitude >80% of LLN

    b. >150% of ULN if amplitude <80% of LLN

Data from Cornblath DR, Asbury AK, Albers JW, et al. Report from an Ad Hoc Subcommittee of the American Academy of Neurology AIDS Task Force. Research criteria for the diagnosis of chronic inflammatory demyelinating polyneuropathy (CIDP). Neurology 1991;41:617–8.

---

not be studied, leading to diagnostic efficiency; and (4) it is easy to apply (see **Box 6**).[52] An alternative preferred criteria is from the European Federation of Neurologic Societies; most recent treatment trials have used these criteria for patient selection.[10]

PATHOLOGY

The classic pathologic features of CIDP include demyelination, remyelination (onion bulbs), endoneurial edema, and inflammatory cell infiltrates in the epineurium and endoneurium (**Fig. 2**), usually with preferential involvement of the nerve roots.[1–5,25] Chronically demyelinated and remyelinated nerve fibers form onion bulbs, identical to but less numerous than in hereditary demyelinating polyneuropathy (eg, Charcot-Marie-Tooth disease type I). Routine semithin plastic sections typically show an

---

Box 6
Electrodiagnostic criteria for the diagnosis of CIDP (Koski criteria)

There must be evidence of a chronic polyneuropathy for at least 2 months without a documented genetic abnormality or serum paraprotein, and:

At least 75% of motor nerves tested had a detected response, and 1 or more of the following conditions were satisfied:

Using AAN criteria for demyelination:

a. More than 50% of the motor nerves assessed had an abnormal distal latency, or

b. More than 50% of the motor nerves assessed had an abnormal conduction velocity, or

c. More than 50% of the motor nerves assessed had an abnormal F-latency

Data from Koski CL, Baumgarten M, Magder LS, et al. Derivation and validation of diagnostic criteria for chronic inflammatory demyelinating polyneuropathy. J Neurol Sci 2009;277:1–8.

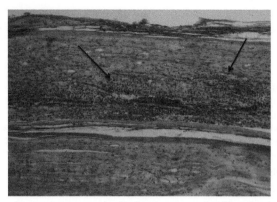

Fig. 2. Sural nerve demonstrating marked inflammatory cell infiltration (*arrows*) (hematoxylin-eosin stain [H&E], original magnification ×10).

excess of large, thinly myelinated nerve fibers usually associated with varying degrees of acute axonal degeneration and reduced axonal density (**Fig. 3**). Because CIDP is a multifocal process, nerve biopsy often does not yield a confirmatory diagnosis and recent large series have demonstrated inflammatory changes are found in only 10% to 50% of specimens,[1–3,55–58] features of only axonal degeneration in only 20% to 40%, and normal biopsies in approximately 20% of cases.[4,27] The inflammatory infiltrates are composed primarily of CD8+ and CD4+ lymphocytes and macrophages within the endoneurium. Analysis of teased fibers is probably the most sensitive method of demonstrating demyelinating changes, which are found in 50% to 80% of nerve biopsy specimens.[55,59] However, the procedure is cumbersome and time-consuming and is performed primarily at specialized centers. The utility of nerve biopsy in CIDP continues to engender controversy; many experts endorse the value of routine nerve biopsy, and especially teased fiber studies, in patients with suspected CIDP,[55,59] whereas others have shown that the procedure adds little to the diagnosis if other clinical and electrodiagnostic features support the diagnosis,[25,57,58] particularly if one considers that a normal biopsy is not likely to influence the decision to start therapy. Nerve biopsy can be especially helpful when CIDP is considered, but clinical and electrophysiological features are atypical or do not fulfill accepted

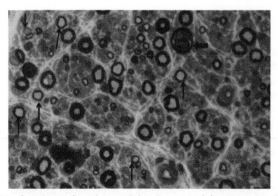

Fig. 3. Cross section showing reduced axonal density, axonal degeneration (*thick arrow*), and an excess of thinly myelinated nerve fibers (*thin arrows*) (H&E, original magnification ×25).

diagnostic criteria or when the differential diagnosis requires excluding the possibility of amyloid or nerve vasculitis.[60]

TREATMENT

The primary goal of treatment is to reduce symptoms (weakness, sensory loss, imbalance, and pain), improve functional status (reduce disability and handicap), and, if possible, maintain long-term remission in patients with CIDP. Conventional therapy for CIDP has included corticosteroids, PE, and IVIg (**Box 7**). Improvement can be expected in 40% to 80% of patients with one of these standard treatments.[1–4,11–20] Each of these therapies has been demonstrated to be effective in randomized, double-blind studies. Furthermore, randomized, prospective clinical trials have shown that PE versus IVIg, and IVIg versus prednisolone have similar short-term efficacy.[61,62] In another study, although IVIg was shown to be superior to IV pulse methylprednisolone after 6 months, the relapse rate was higher in IVIg-treated patients, and no patient who responded to IV methylprednisolone relapsed with 6-month follow-up off treatment.[13] The practical issues associated with all of these agents are the lack of a durable response in many patients, and the difficulties of using these therapies, which are ideally suited for short-term administration, over longer periods. IVIg is expensive and time-consuming, and may have limited availability in some circumstances. PE can be invasive for those who require central venous catheters and requires well-trained personnel at specialized centers. Corticosteroids have a large number of side effects and often are poorly tolerated. One reasonable algorithm for the treatment of CIDP is provided in **Fig. 4**.

Prednisone

In a 3-month, randomized, placebo-controlled trial of alternate-day, high-dose prednisone (120 mg) in 28 patients, corticosteroids were demonstrated to be more effective than placebo.[11] The effect was similar between patients with a progressive and relapsing course. The average time to induce a response with prednisone (60 mg/d) is approximately 2 months with maximal improvement not observed until after 6 months.[4] In some patients the addition of azathioprine, or other so-called "steroid-sparing" agents, may sustain a remission and reduce or eliminate the requirement for high-dose prednisone, but this benefit was not confirmed by randomized controlled trial.[63] However, it should be noted that this study was limited in trial design because of the short duration of exposure to azathioprine, as the benefits of the drug typically require up to 12 to 18 months of therapy. Because of concerns regarding long-term daily prednisone exposure, several alternative corticosteroid treatment regimens have been proposed. In a double-blind, placebo-controlled randomized trial, high-dose oral dexamethasone (40 mg) was administered daily for 4 days sequentially, every month for 6 months, and was shown to be as effective as 60 mg of daily oral prednisolone for 4 weeks followed by a tapering schedule over 6 months, with a 40% response rate for both drugs.[12] However, adverse effects were similar between the 2 groups[12,87]; In another comparative double-blind trial, 48% of patients improved with IV methylprednisolone administered as 500 mg/d for 4 days sequentially every month for 6 months, and none relapsed after an additional 6 months without further treatment.[13] Other retrospective case series have suggested benefit with weekly IV or oral high-dose prednisolone.[72,73]

PE

Two short-term randomized, placebo-controlled trials have demonstrated that PE is superior to placebo, with response rates ranging from 33% to 80%.[15,16] The

Box 7
Therapy for CIDP

Proven therapies from randomized controlled trials

Intravenous immunoglobulin (IVIg)

    2 g/kg loading dose, then 1 g/kg every 3 weeks for 6 months, or 0.5 g/kg daily for 4 days, monthly for 6 months[13,20]

Prednisone

    Daily for 3 months with a tapering regimen

    Prednisolone 60 mg for 4 weeks with tapering regimen over 22 weeks[12]

Plasma exchange

    Twice weekly for 3 weeks or 10 exchanges over 4 weeks[15,16]

Pulse oral dexamethasone

    40 mg daily for 4 days, monthly for 6 months[12]

Pulse IV methylprednisolone

    500 mg IV, daily for 4 days, monthly for 6 months[13]

Therapies probably ineffective based on randomized controlled trials. These studies had methodological issues with trial design:

Azathioprine[63]

Interferon B1a[64]

Methotrexate[65]

Alternative treatments of unproven benefit based on uncontrolled case series or clinical experience

Azathioprine[66,67]

Mycophenolate mofetil[68,69]

Subcutaneous immunoglobulin[70,71]

Pulse weekly IV methylprednisolone[72]

Pulse weekly oral prednisolone[73]

Cyclosporine A[74,75]

Cyclophosphamide[76,77]

Rituximab[78]

Interferon alpha 2a[79]

Etanercept[80]

Tacrolimus[81]

Alemtuzumab[82]

Hematopoietic stem cell transplantation[83–86]

beneficial effects of PE were subsequently supported by a Cochrane review.[88] Improvements were observed in the mean Neurologic Disability Score, grip strength, clinical disability grade, and summated mean motor potential amplitudes and conduction velocities. Patients improved within 4 weeks of initiating therapy, and those with a chronic progressive course responded as well as others with relapsing

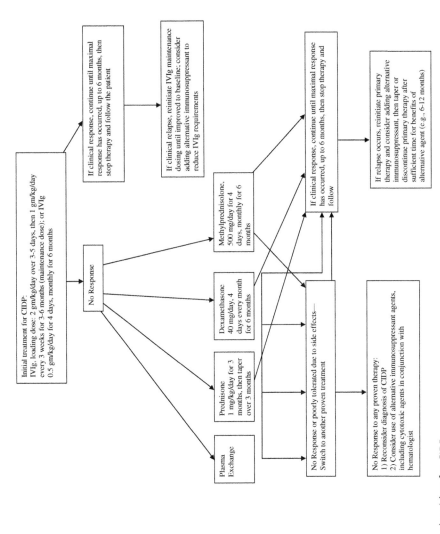

Fig. 4. Treatment algorithm for CIDP.

disease. Although the short-term efficacy of PE has been convincingly demonstrated, up to 50% to 67% of patients may deteriorate within weeks to months after treatment. Many require repeated exchanges or an alternative therapy to maintain improvement.[16,27] Long-term outpatient plasma exchange can be used successfully in selected patients if peripheral access can be maintained.[89] Although no specific guidelines have been established for the frequency or schedule of treatment beyond 4 weeks, the frequency of PE can be guided by the duration and degree of the clinical response and exchanges may be repeated periodically as necessary to maintain improvement.

IVIg

IVIg has been used as the primary therapy for CIDP over the past 2 decades. Multiple well-controlled studies have demonstrated that approximately 45% to 70% of patients respond to IVIg.[17–20] Improvement usually begins within a few weeks and occasionally may be dramatic. The IVIg in CIDP Efficacy (ICE) trial was the largest and longest randomized, double-blind, placebo-controlled trial in this disease. It demonstrated sustained efficacy using a loading dose of 2 g/kg administered over 2 to 5 days, followed by repeated infusions of 1 g/kg administered every 3 weeks for 6 months.[20] There were 117 subjects diagnosed with CIDP by the Inflammatory Neuropathy Cause and Treatment (INCAT) criteria enrolled in the trial. Patients were randomized to IVIg or placebo and treated for 6 months, followed by re-randomization to an open phase of treatment with IVIg or placebo for an additional 6 months of follow-up. This study showed 54% of treated patients in the blinded phase improved in measures of strength, functional disability, and quality of life compared with placebo-treated patients.[20] In the open phase, approximately half of those receiving placebo remained in remission after 6 months off treatment. These data suggest that many IVIg responders have a sustained remission off therapy, and therefore we now recognize that many patients on long-term (eg, more than 6 months) IVIg therapy may be inappropriately overtreated and are likely to remain in remission after IVIg is discontinued. In the ICE trial, IVIg responders were defined as having a 2-point or more improvement in the INCAT disability score, and most such patients could be identified after 3 cycles of treatment.[90] Therefore, it seems reasonable to offer patients with CIDP 3 cycles of IVIg every 3 weeks, and if there is no meaningful clinical response, consider an alternative first-line treatment regimen (corticosteroids or plasma exchange).

Because of the results of the ICE trial, the standard IVIg dosage is a loading dose of 2.0 g/kg administered IV over 2 to 5 days, followed by 1 g/kg over 1 day every 3 weeks. Those who initially respond and then relapse when therapy is discontinued will most likely require long-term IVIg, or an alternative oral immunosuppressant may be added (see later in this article) to decrease the frequency of IVIg administration. In IVIg responders, once the patient has stabilized, some tolerate IVIg dosage reduction or an increase of the treatment interval and still maintain clinical stability. The presence of axon loss as manifest by prominent muscle atrophy or by low or absent motor amplitudes on nerve-conduction studies is the major prognostic factor for lack of response to IVIg therapy.[91] Several reports have indicated an alternative approach to the administration of immunoglobulin by way of subcutaneous injection (SCIg). Data are limited to open-label case reports but suggest this is a viable option to administer the drug with similar efficacy to IVIg and allow greater patient autonomy with self-administered home infusion therapy.[70,71] A randomized, placebo-controlled trial to assess the efficacy of SCIg is currently under way.

ALTERNATIVE IMMUNOSUPPRESSIVE REGIMENS

The indications for considering alternative immunosuppressive agents for patients with CIDP are as follows: (1) the patient has not improved with sequential or combined trials of the previously outlined proven therapies from randomized controlled trials (see caveat at the end of this paragraph); (2) the patient has responded to these treatments but experiences frequent relapses, or (3) the proven therapies may be effective but have caused intolerable adverse effects. All of the alternative agents listed in **Box 7** have been reported to be effective in some patients with CIDP in single case reports, open-label case series, or retrospective reviews, but none have been submitted to rigorous trials to establish efficacy. Some of these agents (eg, azathioprine, methotrexate, interferon B1a) have been carefully studied in larger controlled trials and were proven ineffective, but these studies also had methodological shortcomings that make it difficult to be certain they have no benefit. In those individuals in whom there is a reasonable expectation that additional therapies are needed to stabilize the condition and halt further progression, a trial of an alternative immunosuppressive agent may be appropriate. In our experience, many of these treatments can be helpful to reduce the dependence on IVIg, allow for successful tapering of corticosteroids, or reduce the frequency of plasma exchange. We would advise using the least toxic agents first before pursuing therapies with potentially greater risk for serious adverse events. For example, interventions such as stem-cell transplantation for treatment-refractory CIDP should be undertaken only under the auspices of an institutional review board–approved experimental trial. *Before pursuing treatment trials with potentially toxic alternative immunosuppressant agents in so-called "treatment-refractory" patients, an important caveat is that if there is no response to any of the proven therapies for CIDP, this should prompt clinicians to reconsider the diagnosis,* as subsequent trials of sequential alternative therapies will have an even lower chance of benefit.

SUPPORTIVE THERAPIES

Patients certainly may benefit from canes, walking sticks, walkers, braces, ankle-foot orthotics, and other rehabilitation strategies to assist walking and other activities of daily living. Physical and occupational therapy may be helpful to maintain range of motion, prevent joint contractures in paretic limbs, and assist in gait retraining. A tolerable exercise regimen may help reduce physical fatigue and increase endurance. Symptomatic medications are available to offer relief of neuropathic and mechanical pain, fatigue, and alleviate depression and anxiety, but none have been studied in a rigorous fashion in CIDP.

PROGNOSIS

The available data on long-term outcome in CIDP are surprisingly limited. More than two-thirds of patients remain independent and able to work,[1–4,92–94] and recent experience suggests that approximately one-third of patients eventually have a complete remission with a normal neurologic examination and no functional disability (**Box 8**).[95] Older age of onset (>30 years), 4-limb weakness at onset, a progressive course, central nervous system involvement, and prominent axonal loss on EMG studies appear to be poor prognostic factors.[92–94]

We performed an analysis of 106 definite cases of CIDP evaluated at academic treatment centers to examine the reproducibility of a grading system for characterizing long-term outcomes, termed the CIDP Disease Activity Status (CDAS, **Box 8**).[52,95] By

---

Box 8
CIDP Disease Activity Status of patients with a consensus diagnosis of idiopathic CIDP

	Patients (n = 106), n (%)	
The CIDP Disease Activity Status is based on clinical assessment by the treating physician:		
1. Cure: ≥ 5 years off treatment		11% Cure
A. Normal examination	6 (6)	
B. Abnormal examination, stable/improving	5 (5)	
2. Remission: <5 years off treatment		20% Remission
A. Normal examination	12 (11)	
B. Abnormal examination, stable/improving	10 (9)	
3. Stable active disease: ≥ 1 year, on treatment		44% Stable disease
A. Normal examination	18 (17)	
B. Abnormal examination, stable/improving	29 (27)	
4. Improvement: ≥ 3 months <1 year, on treatment		7% Improving
A. Normal examination	0 (0)	
B. Abnormal examination, stable/improving	8 (7)	
5. Unstable active disease: abnormal examination with progressive or relapsing course[a]		18% Active disease
A. Treatment naïve or <3 months	6 (6)	
B. Off treatment	7 (7)	
C. On treatment	5 (5)	

[a] 5B and 5C refer to patients who were treatment refractory from prior therapy or worsening despite ongoing therapy.
Data from Gorson KC, Van Schaik IN, Merkies IS, et al. Chronic inflammatory demyelinating polyneuropathy disease activity status (CDAS): recommendations for clinical research standards and use in clinical practice. J Peripher Nerv Syst 2010;15:326–33.

---

applying the CDAS scale to patients with CIDP with a median of 5 years of follow-up, we found that 11% of the patients could be classified as cured, 20% as in remission, 44% as stable active disease on therapy, and 7% as improving on therapy. For those classified as cured, mean follow-up was 7.4 years (median, 8 years; range 5–12 years). Overall, 75% of treated patients had *long-term stability* off treatment, or they were stable or improving on treatment. In contrast, only 18% were either untreated at the time of classification or refractory to previously administered immune therapies (see **Box 8**).[95] Prospective 5-year follow-up data from the dexamethasone trial has also confirmed that roughly a third of patients were considered cured or in remission off therapy, another third were in remission but still required treatment, and 5% were improving with less than 5-year follow-up. Only 10% of patients were treatment refractory, and 18% were found to have an alternative diagnosis.[96] The results from the retrospective and prospective data sets were quite similar and indicate that most patients with CIDP have a favorable prognosis following treatment.[95,96]

Case study

A 43-year-old woman developed progressive limb weakness over 3 months. She noted difficulty getting out of a chair and climbing stairs. She had trouble combing her hair, putting on earrings, and using utensils. She complained of tingling in her hands and feet and poor balance. Her general health was excellent and there was no relevant family history.

Examination showed generalized, symmetric limb weakness affecting the arms and legs and she was not able to squat without assistance. She was areflexic. There was reduced touch and pinprick sensation in the fingers and feet, absent vibration sensation at the great toes, and a Romberg sign.

Routine laboratory studies were normal and there was no monoclonal protein in serum or urine. Spinal fluid showed a protein concentration of 126 mg/dL with no cells. Electrodiagnostic testing, including the assessment of 5 motor nerves in the arms and legs, found borderline low distal motor amplitudes. However, there was definite conduction block in 3 nerves, absent F-responses in 4, and slowed conduction velocity in the demyelinating range in 3, consistent with a generalized, acquired demyelinating polyneuropathy. These findings fulfilled criteria for the diagnosis of chronic inflammatory demyelinating polyradiculoneuropathy (CIDP).

The patient was treated with intravenous immune globulin (IVIg) with a loading dose of 1 g/kg/d for 2 days and then 1 g/kg/d every 3 weeks. She noted improvement within a week of completing the loading dose. After 3 cycles of therapy, there was clear improvement in strength and balance. Strength returned to normal after 6 months of therapy. IVIg was discontinued, and she has remained in clinical remission off therapy after 1 year of follow-up.

REFERENCES

1. Dalakas MC. Advances in the diagnosis, pathogenesis and treatment of CIDP. Nat Rev Neurol 2011;7:507–17.
2. Köller H, Kieseier BC, Jander S, et al. Chronic inflammatory demyelinating polyneuropathy. N Engl J Med 2005;352:1343–56.
3. Dyck PJ, Lais AC, Ohta M, et al. Chronic inflammatory polyradiculoneuropathy. Mayo Clin Proc 1975;50:621–37.
4. Barohn RJ, Kissel JT, Warmolts JR, et al. Chronic inflammatory demyelinating polyneuropathy. Clinical characteristics, course, and recommendations for diagnostic criteria. Arch Neurol 1989;46:878–84.
5. Hartung HP, Willison H, Jung S, et al. Auto-immune responses in peripheral nerve. Springer Semin Immunopathol 1996;18:97–123.
6. Rezania K, Gundogdu B, Soliven B. Pathogenesis of chronic inflammatory demyelinating polyradiculoneuropathy. Front Biosci 2004;9:939–45.
7. Yan WX, Taylor J, Andrias-Kauba S, et al. Passive transfer of demyelination by serum or IgG from chronic inflammatory demyelinating polyneuropathy patients. Ann Neurol 2000;47:765–75.
8. Yan WX, Archelos JJ, Hartung HP, et al. P0 protein is a target antigen in chronic inflammatory demyelinating polyradiculoneuropathy. Ann Neurol 2001;50:286–92.
9. Cornblath DR, Asbury AK, Albers JW, et al. Report from an Ad Hoc Subcommittee of the American Academy of Neurology AIDS Task Force. Research criteria for the diagnosis of chronic inflammatory demyelinating polyneuropathy (CIDP). Neurology 1991;41:617–8.
10. Joint Task Force of the EFNS and PNS. European Federation of Neurological Societies/Peripheral Nerve Society Guideline on the management of chronic inflammatory demyelinating polyradiculopathy: report of a joint task force of the European Federation of Neurological Societies and First Revision. J Peripher Nerv Syst 2010;15:1–9.
11. Dyck PJ, O'Brien PC, Oviatt KF, et al. Prednisone improves chronic inflammatory demyelinating polyradiculoneuropathy more than no treatment. Ann Neurol 1982;11:136–41.
12. van Schaik IN, Eftimov F, van Doorn PA, et al. Pulsed high-dose dexamethasone versus standard prednisolone treatment for chronic inflammatory demyelinating

polyradiculoneuropathy (PREDICT study): a double-blind, randomised, controlled trial. Lancet Neurol 2010;9:245–53.

13. Nobile-Orazio E, Cocito D, Jann S, et al. Intravenous immunoglobulin versus intravenous methylprednisolone for chronic inflammatory demyelinating polyradiculoneuropathy: a randomised controlled trial. Lancet Neurol 2012;11:493–502.

14. Mehndiratta MM, Hughes RA. Corticosteroids for chronic inflammatory demyelinating polyradiculoneuropathy [Cochrane Review]. Cochrane Database Syst Rev 2002;(1):CD002062.

15. Dyck PJ, Daube J, O'Brien P, et al. Plasma exchange in chronic inflammatory demyelinating polyneuropathy. N Engl J Med 1986;314:461–5.

16. Hahn AF, Bolton CF, Pillay N, et al. Plasma exchange therapy in chronic inflammatory demyelinating polyneuropathy. A double-blind sham-controlled, cross-over study. Brain 1996;119:1055–66.

17. Hahn AF, Bolton CF, Zochodne D, et al. Intravenous immunoglobulin treatment in chronic inflammatory demyelinating polyneuropathy. A double-blind, placebo-controlled cross-over study. Brain 1996;119:1067–77.

18. Mendell JR, Barohn RJ, Freimer ML, et al. Randomized controlled trial of IVIg in untreated chronic inflammatory demyelinating polyradiculopathy. Neurology 2001;56:445–9.

19. Van Schaik IN, Winer JB, de Haan R, et al. Intravenous immunoglobulin for chronic inflammatory demyelinating polyradiculoneuropathy. Cochrane Database Syst Rev 2002;(2):CD001797.

20. Hughes RA, Donofrio P, Bril V, et al, ICE Study Group. Intravenous immune globulin (10% caprylate-chromatography purified) for the treatment of chronic inflammatory demyelinating polyradiculoneuropathy (ICE study): a randomised placebo-controlled trial. Lancet Neurol 2008;7:136–44.

21. Oh SJ, Kurokawa K, de Almeida DF, et al. Subacute inflammatory demyelinating polyneuropathy. Neurology 2003;61:1507–12.

22. Simmons Z, Wald JJ, Albers JW. Chronic inflammatory demyelinating polyradiculoneuropathy in children: I. Presentation, electrodiagnostic studies, and initial clinical course, with comparison to adults. Muscle Nerve 1997;20:1008–15.

23. Rajabally YA, Simpson BS, Beri S, et al. Epidemiologic variability of chronic inflammatory demyelinating polyneuropathy with different diagnostic criteria: study of a UK population. Muscle Nerve 2009;39:432–8.

24. Laughlin RS, Dyck PJ, Melton LJ, et al. Incidence and prevalence of CIDP and the association of diabetes mellitus. Neurology 2009;73:39–45.

25. Saperstein DS, Katz JS, Amato AA, et al. Clinical spectrum of chronic acquired demyelinating polyneuropathies. Muscle Nerve 2001;24:311–24.

26. Henderson RD, Sandroni P, Wijdicks EF. Chronic inflammatory demyelinating polyneuropathy and respiratory failure. J Neurol 2005;252:1235–7.

27. Gorson KC, Allam G, Ropper AH. Chronic inflammatory demyelinating polyneuropathy: clinical features and response to treatment in 67 consecutive patients with and without monoclonal gammopathy. Neurology 1997;48:321–8.

28. Simmons Z, Tivakaran S. Acquired demyelinating polyneuropathy presenting as a pure clinical sensory syndrome. Muscle Nerve 1996;19:1174–6.

29. Oh SJ, Joy JL, Kuruoglu R. "Chronic sensory demyelinating neuropathy": chronic inflammatory demyelinating polyneuropathy presenting as a pure sensory neuropathy. J Neurol Neurosurg Psychiatry 1992;55:677–80.

30. Ohkoshi N, Harada K, Nagata H, et al. Ataxic form of chronic demyelinating polyradiculoneuropathy: clinical features and pathological study of the sural nerves. Eur Neurol 2001;45:241–8.

31. Yato M, Ohkoshi N, Sato A, et al. Ataxic form of chronic inflammatory demyelinating polyradiculoneuropathy. Eur J Neurol 2000;7:227–30.
32. Rotta FT, Sussman AT, Bradley WG, et al. The spectrum of chronic inflammatory demyelinating polyneuropathy. J Neurol Sci 2000;173:129–39.
33. Sinnreich M, Klein CJ, Daube JR, et al. Chronic immune sensory polyradiculopathy: a possibly treatable sensory ataxia. Neurology 2004;63:1662–9.
34. Sabatelli M, Madia F, Mignogna T, et al. Pure motor chronic inflammatory demyelinating polyneuropathy. J Neurol 2001;248:772–7.
35. Lewis RA, Sumner AJ, Brown MJ, et al. Multifocal demyelinating neuropathy with persistent conduction block. Neurology 1982;32:958–64.
36. Saperstein DS, Amato AA, Wolfe GI, et al. Multifocal acquired demyelinating sensory and motor neuropathy: the Lewis-Sumner syndrome. Muscle Nerve 1999;22:560–6.
37. Gorson KC, Ropper AH, Weinberg DH. Upper limb predominant, multifocal chronic inflammatory demyelinating polyneuropathy. Muscle Nerve 1999;22:758–65.
38. Oh SJ, LaGanke C, Powers R, et al. Multifocal motor sensory demyelinating neuropathy: inflammatory demyelinating polyradiculoneuropathy. Neurology 2005;65:1639–42.
39. Thomas PK, Claus D, Jaspert A. Focal upper limb demyelinating neuropathy. Brain 1996;119:765–74.
40. Goldstein JM, Parks BJ, Mayer PL, et al. Nerve root hypertrophy as a cause of lumbar stenosis in chronic inflammatory demyelinating polyradiculoneuropathy. Muscle Nerve 1996;19:892–6.
41. Guibord N, Chalk C, Win F, et al. Trigeminal nerve hypertrophy in chronic inflammatory demyelinating polyradiculoneuropathy. Neurology 1998;51:1459–62.
42. Katz JS, Saperstein DS, Gronseth G, et al. Distal acquired demyelinating symmetric neuropathy. Neurology 2000;54:615–20.
43. Hughes R, Sanders E, Hall S, et al. Subacute idiopathic demyelinating polyneuropathy. Arch Neurol 1992;49:612–6.
44. Mori K, Hattori N, Sugiura M, et al. Chronic inflammatory demyelinating polyneuropathy presenting with features of GBS. Neurology 2002;58:979–82.
45. Ruts L, van Koningsveld R, van Doorn PA. Distinguishing acute-onset CIDP from Guillain-Barre syndrome with treatment related fluctuations. Neurology 2005;65:138–40.
46. Simmons Z, Albers JW, Bromberg MB, et al. Presentation and initial clinical course in patients with chronic inflammatory demyelinating polyneuropathy: comparison of patients without and with monoclonal gammopathy. Neurology 1993;43:2202–9.
47. Gorson KC. The clinical features, evaluation and treatment of patients with polyneuropathy associated with monoclonal gammopathy of undetermined significance. J Clin Apheresis 1999;14:149–53.
48. Ropper AH, Gorson KC. Neuropathies associated with paraproteinemia. N Engl J Med 1998;338:1601–7.
49. Suarez GA, Kelly JJ Jr. Polyneuropathy associated with monoclonal gammopathy of undetermined significance: further evidence that IgM- MGUS neuropathies are different than IgG-MGUS. Neurology 1993;43:1304–8.
50. Gorson KC, Ropper AH, Weinberg DH, et al. Treatment experience in patients with anti-myelin-associated glycoprotein neuropathy. Muscle Nerve 2001;24:778–86.
51. Bromberg M. Review of the evolution of electrodiagnostic criteria for chronic inflammatory demyelinating polyradiculopathy. Muscle Nerve 2011;43:780–94.

52. Koski CL, Baumgarten M, Magder LS, et al. Derivation and validation of diagnostic criteria for chronic inflammatory demyelinating polyneuropathy. J Neurol Sci 2009;277:1–8.

53. Rajabally YA, Jacob S, Hbahbih M. Optimizing the use of electrophysiology in the diagnosis of chronic inflammatory demyelinating polyneuropathy: a study of 20 cases. J Peripher Nerv Syst 2005;10:282–92.

54. Olney RK. Consensus criteria for the diagnosis of partial conduction block. Muscle Nerve 1999;22(Suppl 8):225–9.

55. Vital C, Vital A, Lagueny A, et al. Chronic inflammatory demyelinating polyneuropathy: immunopathological and ultrastructural study of peripheral nerve biopsy in 42 cases. Ultrastruct Pathol 2000;24:363–9.

56. Krendel DA, Parks HP, Anthony DA, et al. Sural nerve biopsy in chronic inflammatory demyelinating polyradiculoneuropathy. Muscle Nerve 1989;12:257–64.

57. Bosboom WM, van den Berg LH, Franssen H, et al. Diagnostic value of sural nerve demyelination in chronic inflammatory demyelinating polyneuropathy. Brain 2001;124:2427–38.

58. Molenaar DS, Vermeulen M, de Haan R. Diagnostic value of sural nerve biopsy in chronic inflammatory demyelinating polyneuropathy. J Neurol Neurosurg Psychiatry 1998;64:84–9.

59. Nagamatsu M, Terao S, Misu K, et al. Axonal and perikaryal involvement in chronic inflammatory demyelinating polyneuropathy. J Neurol Neurosurg Psychiatry 1999;66:727–33.

60. Vallat JM, Tabaraud F, Magy L, et al. Diagnostic value of nerve biopsy for atypical chronic inflammatory demyelinating polyneuropathy: evaluation of eight cases. Muscle Nerve 2003;27:478–85.

61. Dyck PJ, Litchy WJ, Kratz KM, et al. A plasma exchange versus immune globulin infusion trial in chronic inflammatory demyelinating polyradiculoneuropathy. Ann Neurol 1994;36:838–45.

62. Hughes R, Bensa S, Willison H, et al. Randomized controlled trial of intravenous immunoglobulin versus oral prednisolone in chronic inflammatory demyelinating polyradiculoneuropathy. Ann Neurol 2002;50:195–201.

63. Dyck PJ, O'Brien P, Swanson C, et al. Combined azathioprine and prednisone in chronic inflammatory demyelinating polyneuropathy. Neurology 1985;35: 1173–6.

64. Hughes RA, Gorson KC, Cros D, et al. Intramuscular interferon beta 1a in chronic inflammatory demyelinating polyradiculoneuropathy. Neurology 2010;74:651–7.

65. RMC Trial Group. Randomised controlled trial of methotrexate for chronic inflammatory demyelinating polyradiculoneuropathy (RMC trial): a pilot, multicentre study. Lancet Neurol 2009;8:158–64.

66. Palmer KN. Polyradiculoneuropathy treated with cytotoxic drugs. Lancet 1966;1: 265.

67. Pentland B. Azathioprine in chronic relapsing idiopathic polyneuropathy. Postgrad Med J 1980;56:734–5.

68. Gorson KC, Amato AA, Ropper AH. Efficacy of mycophenolate mofetil in patients with chronic immune demyelinating polyneuropathy. Neurology 2004;63:715–7.

69. Bedi G, Brown A, Tong T, et al. Chronic inflammatory demyelinating polyneuropathy responsive to mycophenolate mofetil. J Neurol Neurosurg Psychiatry 2010; 81:634–6.

70. Magy L, Ghorab K, Calvo J, et al. Subcutaneous immunoglobulin as maintenance therapy in intravenous immunoglobulin-responsive CIDP patients. Long term response in 16 patients. J Peripher Nerv Syst 2009;14(Suppl 2):94.

71. Cocito D, Serra G, Falcone Y, et al. The efficacy of subcutaneous immunoglobulin administration in chronic inflammatory demyelinating polyneuropathy responders to intravenous immunoglobulin. J Peripher Nerv Syst 2011;16:150–2.
72. Lopate G, Pestronk A, Al-Lozi M. Treatment of chronic inflammatory demyelinating polyneuropathy with high-dose intermittent intravenous methylprednisolone. Arch Neurol 2005;62:249–54.
73. Muley SA, Kelkar P, Parry GJ. Treatment of chronic inflammatory demyelinating polyneuropathy with pulsed oral steroids. Arch Neurol 2008;65:1460–4.
74. Mahattanakul W, Crawford TO, Griffin JW, et al. Treatment of chronic inflammatory demyelinating polyneuropathy with cyclosporine-A. J Neurol Neurosurg Psychiatry 1996;60:185–7.
75. Odaka M, Tatsumoto M, Susuki K, et al. Intractable chronic inflammatory demyelinating polyneuropathy treated successfully with ciclosporin. J Neurol Neurosurg Psychiatry 2005;76:1115–20.
76. Good JL, Chehrenama M, Mayer RF, et al. Pulse cyclophosphamide therapy in chronic inflammatory demyelinating polyneuropathy. Neurology 1998;51:1735–8.
77. Brannagan TH, Pradhan A, Heiman-Patterson T, et al. High-dose cyclophosphamide without stem-cell rescue for refractory CIDP. Neurology 2002;58:1856–8.
78. Benedetti L, Briani C, Franciotta D, et al. Rituximab in patients with chronic inflammatory demyelinating polyradiculoneuropathy: a report of 13 cases and review of the literature. J Neurol Neurosurg Psychiatry 2011;82:306–8.
79. Gorson KC, Allam G, Simovic D, et al. Improvement following interferon-alpha 2A in chronic inflammatory demyelinating polyneuropathy. Neurology 1997;48:777–80.
80. Chin RL, Sherman WH, Sander HW, et al. Etanercept (Enbrel) therapy for chronic inflammatory demyelinating polyneuropathy. J Neurol Sci 2003;210:19–21.
81. Ahlmen J, Andersen G, Hallgren, et al. Positive effects of tacrolimus in a case of CIDP. Transplant Proc 1998;30:4194.
82. Marsh EA, Hirst CL, Llewelyn JG, et al. Alemtuzumab in the treatment of IVIG-dependent chronic inflammatory demyelinating polyneuropathy. J Neurol 2010;257:913–9.
83. Oyama Y, Sufit R, Loh Y, et al. Nonmyeloablative autologous hematopoietic stem cell transplantation for refractory CIDP. Neurology 2007;69:1802–3.
84. Remenyi P, Masszi T, Borbenyi Z, et al. CIDP cured by allogeneic hematopoietic stem cell transplantation. Eur J Neurol 2007;14:e1–2.
85. Axelson HW, Oberg G, Askmark H. Successful repeated treatment with high dose cyclophosphamide and autologous blood stem cell transplantation in CIDP. J Neurol Neurosurg Psychiatry 2008;79:612–4.
86. Mahdi-Rogers M, Kazmi M, Ferner R, et al. Autologous peripheral blood stem cell transplantation for chronic inflammatory demyelinating neuropathy. J Peripher Nerv Syst 2009;14:118–24.
87. Gorson KC. A new trick for an old dog: pulsed dexamethasone treatment for chronic inflammatory demyelinating polyneuropathy. Lancet Neurol 2010;9:228–9.
88. Mehndiratta MM, Hughes RA, Agarwal P. Plasma exchange for chronic inflammatory demyelinating polyradiculoneuropathy. Cochrane Database Syst Rev 2004;(3):CD003906.
89. Isose S, Mori M, Misawa S, et al. Long-term regular plasmapheresis as maintenance treatment for chronic inflammatory demyelinating polyneuropathy. J Peripher Nerv Syst 2010;15:147–9.
90. Latov N, Deng C, Dalakas MC, et al. Timing and course of clinical response to intravenous immunoglobulin in chronic inflammatory demyelinating polyradiculoneuropathy. Arch Neurol 2010;67:802–7.

91. Iijima M, Yamamoto M, Hirayama M, et al. Clinical and electrophysiologic corre-lates of IVIg responsiveness in CIDP. Neurology 2005;64:1471–5.
92. Simmons Z, Albers JW, Bromberg MB, et al. Long-term followup of patients with chronic inflammatory demyelinating polyradiculoneuropathy, with and without monoclonal gammopathy. Brain 1995;118:359–68.
93. Bouchard C, Lacroix C, Plante V, et al. Clinicopathologic findings and prognosis of chronic inflammatory demyelinating polyneuropathy. Neurology 1999;52: 498–503.
94. Sghirlanzoni A, Solari A, Ciano, et al. Chronic inflammatory demyelinating polyra-diculoneuropathy: long-term course and treatment of 60 patients. Neurol Sci 2000;21:31–7.
95. Gorson KC, Van Schaik IN, Merkies IS, et al. Chronic inflammatory demyelinating polyneuropathy disease activity status (CDAS): recommendations for clinical research standards and use in clinical practice. J Peripher Nerv Syst 2010;15: 326–33.
96. Eftimov F, Vermeulen M, van Doorn PA, et al. Long-term remission of CIDP after pulsed dexamethasone or short-term prednisolone treatment. Neurology 2012; 78:1079–84.

Multifocal Motor Neuropathy, Multifocal Acquired Demyelinating Sensory and Motor Neuropathy, and Other Chronic Acquired Demyelinating Polyneuropathy Variants

Mazen M. Dimachkie, MD[a],*, Richard J. Barohn, MD[a], Jonathan Katz, MD[b]

KEYWORDS

- Multifocal motor neuropathy
- Multifocal acquired demyelinating sensory and motor neuropathy
- Distal acquired demyelinating symmetric • CANOMAD
- Chronic inflammatory sensory polyradiculoneuropathy • Diagnosis
- Nerve conduction testing • Treatment

KEY POINTS

- Chronic acquired demyelinating neuropathies (CADP) constitute a heterogeneous group of immune-mediated neuromuscular disorders affecting myelin that includes multifocal motor neuropathy (MMN), multifocal acquired demyelinating sensory and motor neuropathy (MADSAM), distal acquired demyelinating symmetric (DADS) neuropathy, and other less common variants.
- MMN presents with asymmetric weakness affecting the arms are more commonly than the legs.
- Although sensory loss is limited at the onset to toe vibratory impairment, MMN patients may over several years of progression develop sensory loss in the territory of affected motor nerves.
- Markedly elevated GM1 antibody titers are detectable in the blood in up to 50% of MMN patients. Whereas MMN is refractory to corticosteroids, most patients respond to intravenous immunoglobulin G (IVIg).
- MADSAM patients have weakness and sensory loss at the onset, and an elevated cerebrospinal fluid protein.
- It is important to recognize MADSAM, because corticosteroids are also effective in addition to IVIg. DADS-M patients are refractory to corticosteroids, IVIg, and rituximab.

[a] Department of Neurology, University of Kansas Medical Center, 3599 Rainbow Boulevard, Mail Stop 2012, Kansas City, KS 66160, USA; [b] Neuromuscular Service, California Pacific Medical Center, University of California, 2324 Sacramento Street, Suite 111, San Francisco, CA 94115, USA
* Corresponding author.
E-mail address: mdimachkie@kumc.edu

Neurol Clin 31 (2013) 533–555
http://dx.doi.org/10.1016/j.ncl.2013.01.001
0733-8619/13/$ – see front matter © 2013 Elsevier Inc. All rights reserved.

neurologic.theclinics.com

HISTORICAL NOTE

The first case of recurrent neuritis was published by Eichhorst[1] in 1890. In 1958, Austin described the steroid responsiveness of this recurrent polyneuropathy.[2] The frequent occurrence of elevated cerebrospinal fluid (CSF) protein levels was subsequently observed. Dyck and colleagues[3] described the first large series of 54 patients with what they termed chronic inflammatory polyradiculoneuropathy. In addition to inflammatory pathology and demyelinating electrophysiology, these patients showed clinically a variety of neurologic deficit patterns including monophasic progression over 6 months, recurrent weakness, steady deterioration, or stepwise progression. A decade later, Dyck and Arnason[4] underscored the demyelinating nature of this disorder and coined the term chronic inflammatory demyelinating polyradiculoneuropathy (CIDP).[4–7]

In addition to classic CIDP, other phenotypes sharing some clinical and pathologic features, laboratory findings, and in most cases a response to immunomodulatory therapies has been described in the rubric of chronic acquired demyelinating polyneuropathies (CADP) (**Table 1**).[8,9] The 4 categories of CADP are largely based on the phenotypic differences. Symmetric proximal and distal weakness with or without sensory loss is highly suggestive of CIDP (see the article by Gorson and Katz on CIDP and symmetric variants elsewhere in this issue). The pattern of symmetric distal weakness and sensory loss should raise suspicion of distal acquired demyelinating symmetric (DADS) neuropathy.[10] When weakness is asymmetric, further classification hinges around the presence or absence of sensory signs. Asymmetric distal weakness without sensory loss indicates multifocal motor neuropathy (MMN), whereas sensory loss would suggest multifocal acquired demyelinating sensory and motor (MADSAM) neuropathy (Lewis-Sumner syndrome).[11–14] About half of the MMN patients also have serum GM-1 antibodies, and most DADS patients have an immunoglobulin M (IgM) monoclonal protein in the serum, often accompanied by antibodies to myelin-associated glycoprotein (MAG). In a report of 25 patients with the MADSAM phenotype, ganglioside antibodies were detected about half of the patients,[14] although in the authors' earlier series and in 2 other series these antibodies were not detected in any MADSAM patients.[12,13,15] The benefit of placing the CADP into various phenotypes is that it helps clinicians identify potentially treatable neuropathies in choosing the most appropriate therapy, and in determining the prognosis.

MULTIFOCAL MOTOR NEUROPATHY
Clinical Presentation

In 1988, Parry and Clarke[16] demonstrated the presence of multifocal conduction block in 5 patients with purely motor neuropathies, cramps, and fasciculations as well as relatively preserved reflexes suspicious for motor neuron disease, and pointed out that this electrodiagnostic finding distinguished these cases from those with motor neuron disease. Around that same time reports of similar patients emerged, often associated with the presence of anti-GM1 serum antibodies, and this entity became known as MMN with conduction block.[17–21] However, the authors' group as well as others subsequently reported that neither the presence of anti-GM1 antibodies nor conduction block are necessary to diagnose MMN.[22–25]

MMN is an immune-mediated demyelinating neuropathy that presents with chronic asymmetric distal-limb weakness atrophy and fasciculations affecting the distal arm more frequently than the leg, usually in the distribution of individual peripheral nerves with limited or no sensory symptoms.[16–22,26–31] There is a male-to-female ratio of approximately 3:1 with most cases beginning in the fifth decade of life, although the

Table 1
Comparison of the chronic acquired immune-mediated demyelinating polyneuropathies

	CIDP	DADS Neuropathy	MADSAM Neuropathy	MMN
Clinical Features				
Weakness	Symmetric; proximal + distal	Symmetric; distal only Mild or no weakness	Asymmetric; distal > proximal Upper limbs > lower limbs	Asymmetric; distal > proximal Upper limbs > lower limbs
Sensory deficits	Yes; symmetric	Yes; symmetric	Yes; multifocal (distribution of individual nerves)	No
Reflexes	Reduced or absent symmetrically	Reduced or absent symmetrically	Reduced or absent (multifocal or diffuse)	Reduced or absent (multifocal or diffuse)
Electrophysiology				
Abnormal CMAPs:				
Demyelinating features	Usually symmetric	Usually symmetric Prolonged distal latencies	Asymmetric (multifocal)	Asymmetric (multifocal)
Conduction block	Frequent	Uncommon	Frequent	Frequent
Abnormal SNAPs	Usually symmetric	Usually symmetric	Asymmetric (multifocal)	SNAPs are normal
Laboratory Findings				
CSF protein	Usually elevated	Usually elevated	Usually elevated	Usually normal
Monoclonal protein	Occasionally present Usually IgG or IgA	IgM-κ present in the majority 50%–70% are MAG positive	Rarely present	Rarely present
Anti-GM1 antibodies	Rarely present	Not present	Rarely present	Frequently present (50%)
Sensory nerve biopsy:				
Demyelination/ remyelination	Frequent	Frequent	Frequent Sometimes asymmetric	Occasional Minimal findings
Treatment Response				
Prednisone	Yes	Poor[a]	Yes	No
Plasma exchange	Yes	Poor[a]	Possible (more study needed)	No
IVIg	Yes	Poor[a]	Yes	Yes
Cyclophosphamide	Yes	Poor[a]	Possible (more study needed)	Yes

Treatment responses in DADS neuropathy patients without a monoclonal gammopathy of undetermined significance (MGUS) are more similar to those with CIDP.

Abbreviations: CIDP, chronic inflammatory demyelinating polyneuropathy; CMAPs, compound motor action potentials; CSF, cerebrospinal fluid; DADS, distal acquired demyelinating symmetric; IVIg, intravenous immunoglobulin; MADSAM, multifocal acquired demyelinating sensory and motor; MAG, myelin-associated glycoprotein; MMN, multifocal motor neuropathy; SNAPs, sensory nerve action potentials.

[a] When associated with an IgM-MGUS.

age of symptom onset ranges from childhood to the eighth decade of life. Most patients present with insidious intrinsic hand weakness, wrist drop, or foot drop, which progresses over the course of several years to involve other limbs, and weakness will rarely affect cranial innervated muscles. The lack of atrophy in muscles weakened by conduction block should heighten suspicion of MMN. However, patients with MMN may develop secondary axon loss with resultant denervation atrophy, leading to a misdiagnosis of amyotrophic lateral sclerosis (ALS). However, weakness in the latter is in a myotomal pattern, whereas in MMN it follows a peripheral nerve distribution. Deep tendon reflexes may be diminished but are often normal in unaffected nerves, although they occasionally can be brisk. Clonus, spasticity, and extensor plantar responses are not observed. In the authors' experience the incidence of MMN is much less than that of ALS.

More recently, sensory loss to a variable degree has been described in patients with otherwise typical MMN.[32,33] Five of 11 patients fulfilling American Association of Neuromuscular and Electrodiagnostic Medicine (AANEM) diagnostic criteria for MMN at the onset of disease developed sensory loss associated with electrophysiologic sensory abnormalities while being treated with intravenous immunoglobulin (IVIg).[32] The mean time to appearance of objective sensory signs was 7.2 years, being preceded by intermittent paresthesias in the same nerve territories as the motor involvement in three-fifths of cases. Anti-GM1 IgM antibodies were positive in 4 patients. Although these 5 cases overlap with MADSAM, they were closer to MMN on clinical and therapeutic grounds. Therefore, the Joint Task Force of the European Federation of Neurological Societies/Peripheral Nerve Society 2010 revised guideline on MMN[34] requires that there would not be any objective sensory abnormality except for minor vibration sense abnormalities in the lower limbs, but allows for sensory signs and symptoms that may develop over the course of MMN.

Laboratory Testing

As in **Table 1** and in contrast to CIDP, the CSF protein level in most cases of MMN is normal, and a significantly elevated CSF protein level should suggest an alternate diagnosis such as MADSAM or CIDP.[35] Although most patients do not have a serum M protein, polyclonal IgM GM1 antibodies are detected in the sera of 40% to 80% of MMN patients, and the relationship of these antibodies to pathogenesis is unclear.[20,36–41] Very high titers of IgM anti-GM1 antibodies appear to be specific for MMN,[42] but the sensitivity of standard anti-GM1 antibody testing is at best 50%.[22,43,44] Low titers of anti-GM1 antibodies are not specific to MMN, as they can be found in other neuropathies such as Guillain-Barré syndrome and CIDP.[40,45] Reports of very high sensitivity and specificity using a specialized enzyme-linked immunoassay (ELISA) technique[46] could not be reproduced by other investigators.[47] In a patient presenting with the MMN phenotype, the presence of anti-GM1 antibodies is supportive of, but not essential to, the diagnosis, and these antibodies do not predict response to treatment.

Pestronk and colleagues[48] recently identified serum IgM binding, using covalent antigen linkage to ELISA plates, to a disulfated heparin disaccharide (NS6S) in 43% of 75 patients with motor neuropathy with mostly distal predominant asymmetric arm weakness and objective sensory loss, mostly of the distal legs, in 28 patients. Motor conduction block was present in 42 patients; other features of demyelination were apparent in 3 while 30 had motor axon loss without evidence of demyelination, and without a detailed description of weakness pattern. High titers (≥7000) of serum NS6S or GM1 antibody in motor neuropathy increased sensitivity from 43%, based on GM1 antibody positivity alone, to 64% when either antibody was detected. Whereas none of the ALS or CIDP patients had an abnormal titer, 21% of 56 patients with sensory neuropathy had highly elevated NS6S antibody titers. Additional review of the 2113 sera revealed 27 patients with IgM GM1 positivity, of whom 2 had mild cryptogenic sensory neuropathy and high titers of IgM binding to NS6S, thereby suggesting 93% specificity. Given the retrospective approach, the presence of thoracic paraspinous denervation in 11 of the 25 patients tested, sensory neuropathy in 21% of patients, and the lack of detailed clinical data on 30 cases of motor axon loss, the value of NS6S IgM antibody in clinical practice is yet to be determined.

Electrophysiologic Findings

Although motor conduction block has been considered the electrophysiologic hallmark of MMN,[49] some otherwise typical MMN cases have no detectable conduction block. This situation may be due to proximal location of the conduction block, making it difficult to confirm electrophysiologically, or to the activity dependence of these blocks.[50] In addition, the authors and others have described prolonged distal latencies, temporal dispersion, slow conduction velocity, and delayed or absent F-waves on motor nerve conduction studies (NCS) in MMN.[22,25,29,51,52] Conduction block is not essential to the diagnosis of MMN if other features of demyelination are detected.[22,25] In the authors' series of MMN patients,[22] only 31% had conduction block; 44% had temporal dispersion, and 94% had other electrodiagnostic features of demyelination with superimposed axonal degeneration (**Table 2**). The authors and others found that response to treatment was no different between patients with or without conduction block.[22–24]

Vucic and colleagues[53] described needle cervical root stimulation (CRS) findings in 13 MMN patients meeting the American Academy of Electrodiagnostic Medicine (AAEM) criteria of either possible (n = 7) or definite (n = 6) MMN. The sensitivity of the established neurophysiologic criteria for definite MMN was 46.1% with conventional NCS and after CRS all patients showed either conduction block, prolonged onset latency of compound motor action potentials, or both, thereby establishing the diagnosis of MMN.

The AANEM consensus criteria for definite or probable MMN[49] include patients without objective sensory loss, with normal sensory nerve conduction velocity across the same segments with demonstrated motor conduction block and normal sensory NCS on all tested nerves, with a minimum of 3 nerves tested. Therefore, sensory

Table 2								
Nerve conduction study values needed to be considered "demyelinating"								
	NCV (m/s)			**DL (ms)**			**F-Waves (ms)**		
	LLN	<80%[a]	<70%[b]	ULN	>125%[a]	>150%[b]	ULN	>120%[a]	>150%[b]
Median	49	39.2	34.3	4.5	5.6	6.7	31.0	37.2	46.5
Ulnar	50	40.0	35.0	3.6	4.5	5.4	32.0	38.4	48.0
Peroneal	41	32.8	28.7	6.6	8.2	9.9	58.0	69.6	87.0
Tibial	41	32.8	28.7	6.0	7.5	9.0	58.0	69.6	87.0

If median CMAP LLN is 4.5 mV, then 80% LLN = 3.6 mV.
If ulnar CMAP LLN is 5.0 mV, then 80% LLN = 4 mV.
If peroneal CMAP LLN is 2.0 mV, then 80% LLN = 1.6 mV.
If tibial CMAP LLN is 4.0 mV, then 80% LLN = 3.2 mV.
Abbreviations: LLN, lower limit of normal; ULN, upper limit of normal.
[a] If amplitude >80% LLN.
[b] If amplitude <80% LLN.

NCS are predicted to be normal in MMN patients. In a retrospective study, significant reduction of at least 1 sensory potential amplitude in a cohort of 21 MMN patients within a follow-up of at least 3 years, defined according to the 2001 ENMC International Workshop Report, was noted in 13 patients (62%), 4 of whom had abnormalities of 2 or more sensory potentials.[33] Comparison of the 13 patients with 8 patients who had no sensory abnormality revealed no significant differences in gender, age at onset, number of involved motor nerves, CSF protein level, presence/absence of anti-GM1 serum antibodies, and response to IVIg.

MMN, by definition, typically involves clinical and electrical abnormalities in more than 1 nerve. However, and intriguing report described 3 patients with an acquired, presumably immune-mediated neuropathy in a single motor nerve (median or peroneal or ulnar) that improved with IVIg therapy.[54] The authors' group reported 9 patients with the phenotype of MMN who had only axonal features on electrodiagnostic studies,[55] and termed this phenotype multifocal acquired motor axonopathy (MAMA). Three of 6 treated patients showed improvement. Recently, another group confirmed these observations by demonstrating that 5 of 6 MAMA patients responded to IVIg.[56]

Pathology

Sensory nerve biopsies from patients with MMN are usually unrevealing,[57,58] and this is not a routine test in the evaluation of MMN. Whereas one study has shown evidence for demyelination without inflammatory cell infiltrates at the site of motor conduction block,[59] another pathologic study of 7 patients has demonstrated multifocal axonal degeneration without any overt signs of demyelination.[60] These findings suggest that an antibody-mediated attack directed against components of axolemma at nodes of Ranvier could cause transient conduction block that is rapidly reversible with IVIg and axonal degeneration and regeneration. T2-weighted magnetic resonance imaging scans of the brachial plexus may show increased signal intensity associated with a diffuse nerve swelling of the brachial plexus.[61,62]

Therapy

Although corticosteroids (CS) and plasma exchange (PE) may rarely improve MMN patients, other MMN patients have deteriorated with these treatments.[63,64] Several studies have demonstrated the efficacy of IVIg in MMN, including 2 small randomized controlled trials.[65,66] IVIg, a pooled gammaglobulin product from several thousand blood donors, has a complex immunomodulatory mechanism of action. It is thought to involve pathogenic autoantibody production modulation and binding inhibition, proinflammatory cytokine suppression, Fc-receptor blockade, macrophage colony–stimulating factor and monocyte chemotactant protein–1 increase, alteration in T-cell function, decrease in circulating CD54 lymphocytes, and inhibition of cell transmigration into the muscle. More recently, investigators from the Rockefeller found that Fc core polysaccharide sialylation mediates the anti-inflammatory properties of IVIg,[67] and also determined the precise immunoglobulin G (IgG) Fc-fragment N-linked glycan requirements for this anti-inflammatory activity. In vitro the anti-inflammatory property of IVIg in a 2,6-sialylated IgG Fc-recombinant molecule was recapitulated at a much reduced dose.[68] These sialylated Fcs were shown to require a specific C-type lectin, SIGN-R1 (specific ICAM-3 grabbing non–integrin-related 1), which is expressed on macrophages in the splenic marginal zone.[69] Anthony and colleagues[70] found that in transgenic mice, IVIg suppresses inflammation through a novel T-helper 2 (Th2) pathway. Administration of Fc fragments with glycans terminating in α2,6-sialic acids resulted in the production of interleukin (IL)-33 which, in turn, induces expansion of

IL-4–producing basophils that promote increased expression of the inhibitory Fc-receptor FcγRIIB on effector macrophages. Systemic administration of the Th2 cytokines IL-33 or IL-4 upregulated FcγRIIB in macrophages. In untreated CIDP patients these FcγRIIB receptors have lower expression levels on naïve B cells, compared with demographically matched healthy controls.[71] Following clinically effective IVIg therapy, FcγRIIB protein expression is upregulated and partially restored on B cells and monocytes. Therefore, modulating FcγRIIB function might be another promising therapeutic approach in CADP.

Most MMN patients respond to IVIg, with improvement typically beginning within several days and lasting several weeks to months. Most responders show improvement after the first treatment, and will have a long-term response to IVIg.[72–74] However, over time axon loss and disability may accrue.[75] In a detailed study looking at the effect of IVIg in 11 MMN patients given regularly for 4 to 8 years, most of the improvement was noted in the first several months. Also, strength tended to decrease slightly over time, although patients were still significantly better at the last follow-up in comparison with pretreatment.[76] Conduction block in some nerves resolved, but in other nerves, despite treatment, conduction block or evidence of axonal loss appeared. Another group reported their experience treating 10 MMN patients with IVIg for 5 to 12 years.[77] Only 2 patients maintained maximal improvement; 8 worsened despite IVIg treatment. The decline started between 3 and 7 years into the therapy. Therefore, although IVIg often has a significant benefit initially, the response declines over time.

In a cross-sectional descriptive study of 88 MMN patients, 94% responded to IVIg therapy. Nonresponders had longer disease duration before the first treatment.[78] Over the 6-year median IVIg maintenance duration, the median IVIg dose increased from 12 to 17 g per week. Independent determinants of worse weakness and disability were axon loss and longer disease duration without IVIg. Early IVIg treatment may postpone axonal degeneration and permanent deficits. Most recently, a large 15-month multicenter crossover trial of 10% IVIg for the treatment of MMN was concluded (http://clinicaltrials.gov/ct2/show/NCT00666263?term=motor+neuropathy&rank=2). The 44 enrolled patients from 17 sites had 3 stabilization phases on IVIg with 2 blinded phases on 10% IVIg or placebo, and 41 completed the study. In an accelerated switch to open-label IVIg, 10% was allowed if grip strength decreased by at least 50% in the more affected hand or intolerable functional deterioration was objectified. The preliminary results of this study were presented at the 2012 American Academy of Neurology annual meeting.[79] There was a substantially greater decline from baseline (34%) in the mean grip strength in the more affected hand following placebo administration, compared with IVIg ($P = .005$). A greater proportion of subjects had a 30% or greater decline in grip strength of the more affected hand (43% vs 5%; $P<.001$), as well as the less affected hand (31% vs 0%; $P<.001$), following placebo versus IVIg treatment. Sixty-nine percent of subjects required accelerated switch while on placebo, compared with only 1 accelerated switch (2.4%) on blinded IVIg. Therefore, IVIg was demonstrated to be a safe, well-tolerated, and effective treatment for MMN in this phase III study.

The authors closely monitor patients with the first infusion, starting at a very slow rate of 25 to 50 mL/h for 30 minutes and increasing it progressively by 50 mL/h every 15 to 20 minutes up to 150 to 200 mL/h. Mild reactions (headache, nausea, chills, myalgia, chest discomfort, back pain) occur in 10% and are improved with slowing the infusion rate, and are preventable with premedication with acetaminophen, benadryl and, if necessary, intravenous methylprednisolone. Moderate (rare) reactions include chemical meningitis and delayed red, macular skin reaction of the palms, soles, and trunk, with desquamation. Acute renal failure is uncommon, and related to patient dehydration and the sucrose or maltose diluent. Other severe and rare reactions are anaphylaxis, stroke, myocardial infarction, or pulmonary emboli due to hyperviscosity syndrome. The latter is more likely to occur in concert with old age, immobility, diabetes, thrombocythemia, hypercholesterolemia, hypergammaglobulinemia, and cryoglobulinemia. The authors avoid using IVIg in patients with several of these risk factors, and place IVIg recipients on low-dose aspirin prophylactically. Two articles discussed stroke as a complication of IVIg. In the report by Caress and colleagues,[80] all but 1 of the 16 patients had risk factors for stroke. Okuda and colleagues[81] successfully treated 3 of 4 patients who had a vascular complication from IVIg (3 strokes; 1 leg ischemia) with tissue plasminogen activator, and recommend using only 5% solutions and limiting the maximum infusion rate to 15 g/h to minimize the viscosity changes. The extremely rare patients with total immunoglobulin A (IgA) deficiency should not be receiving IVIg. The authors generally infuse IVIg no faster than 150 to 200 mL/h, although a recent report described infusion rates of up to 800 mL/h in 50 patients, which was reasonably well tolerated.[82] In this study the complication rate was 26%, but most of these consisted of headaches, malaise, or nausea, and all patients recovered without sequelae. Patients were premedicated with acetaminophen and diphenhydramine.

Although there are no data from prospective randomized controlled trials,[83] there are several reports of benefit from rituximab, a monoclonal anti-CD20 antibody.[84–88] The largest published case series is a 2-year open-label study of rituximab in 14 MMN patients, with the control group consisting of 13 patients who were not treated as a result of patient choice, lack of insurance coverage, or evaluation and follow-up before rituximab.[85] Quantitative strength measures improved by 13% to 22% in the rituximab group at 1 and 2 years, and remained essentially unchanged in the control subjects. This improvement was associated with a 45% reduction in anti-GM1 antibody titers at 2 years. However, most patients with initial benefit developed recurrent weakness at 3 to 9 months after treatment, and received a second treatment then one infusion every 10 weeks to maintain benefit. Clearly not all patients with MMN neuropathy will respond to this novel therapeutic approach, and further study of rituximab in MMN is needed. Intravenous cyclophosphamide is effective in more than 70% of MMN patients.[20,30,41] In patients with significant deficits who are unresponsive to IVIg or rituximab, the authors consider monthly pulses of intravenous cyclophosphamide, 0.5 to 1.0 gm/m^2 with or without PE, for 6 months.

Lee and colleagues[89] treated 2 CIDP patients with subcutaneous infusion of immunoglobulins (SCIg) after IVIg therapy was shown to be effective. Application of SCIg was well tolerated and led to stabilization of the disease course. In a recent study of 9 patients with MMN, short-term infusion of SCIg preserved muscle strength for a few months of treatment. Five patients preferred to continue SCIg after the trial and another patient chose to start SCIg. These 6 patients were enrolled in a long-term SCIg maintenance therapy study for 2 years.[90] Side effects consisted of mild and transient local skin reactions. The neuropathy impairment and disability scores remained unchanged, and isokinetic muscle strength was stable. In another study,[91] 4 of 5 patients treated with a SCIg dose equivalent to the IVIg maintenance dose had stable muscle strength over the 6 months of follow-up. Besides local adverse events, mild systemic adverse events were reported, mostly in the first week of treatment. Finally,[92] an open-label multicenter study assessed the efficacy, safety, and convenience of SCIg in 8 MMN patients over 6 months, as an alternative to IVIg. Although 1 patient deteriorated and was withdrawn, muscle strength, disability, motor function, and health status were unchanged in all 7 who completed the study. Despite these encouraging data, the role of SCIg in MMN is uncertain. A large, prospective randomized controlled trial of SCIg in MMN has yet to be done.

In a randomized controlled trial,[93] 28 MMN patients responding to IVIg treatment were eligible for randomization to mycophenolate mofetil (MMF) or placebo for 12 months. After 12 months, IVIg reduction did not differ significantly between the 2 treatment groups and anti-GM1 antibody titers did not change. Adjunctive treatment of MMN patients with MMF at a dose of 1 g twice daily was found to be safe but did not allow significant reduction of IVIg doses.

MULTIFOCAL ACQUIRED DEMYELINATING SENSORY AND MOTOR NEUROPATHY
Clinical Presentation

In 1982, Lewis and colleagues[94] described several patients with chronic demyelinating sensorimotor neuropathy, mononeuritis multiplex, and persistent multifocal conduction block on electrophysiologic studies; all had a generally favorable response to CS. This report is erroneously cited as the first description of MMN. However, these patients had objective sensory abnormalities that set them apart from MMN. Oh and colleagues[95] were the first to point out the important clinical differences between patients with MMN and those with multifocal demyelinating sensory and motor neuropathy. To distinguish it from MMN, the authors proposed the descriptive term "multifocal acquired demyelinating sensory and motor (MADSAM) neuropathy" (see **Table 1**).[11] Other terms describing identical patients include focal upper limb demyelinating neuropathy, upper limb predominant, multifocal chronic inflammatory demyelinating polyneuropathy, and multifocal inflammatory demyelinating neuropathy.[62,96,97] It is apparent that MADSAM neuropathy is a multifocal variant of CIDP, and that both diseases are distinct from MMN.

MADSAM patients have a chronic sensorimotor mononeuritis multiplex with, typically, an insidious onset and slow progression. Initial involvement is usually in the arms, with later spread to the distal legs. Patients can present initially with involvement of single nerves that progress to confluent and symmetric involvement.[94,98] In up to one-half of patients MADSAM may evolve into a typical pattern of generalized CIDP.[12] Many patients experience pain and paresthesias. Cranial neuropathies have been reported, including optic neuritis and oculomotor, trigeminal, and facial palsies.[11,94,95] Muscle-stretch reflexes are reduced or absent in a multifocal pattern, with progression to areflexia late in the disease.

Laboratory and Electrodiagnostic Testing

CSF protein is elevated in up to 82% of patients with MADSAM neuropathy.[11] Unlike MMN, MADSAM neuropathy is not associated with anti-GM1 antibodies.[11,95–97] As in MMN and CIDP, NCS in MADSAM neuropathy show conduction block, temporal dispersion, prolonged distal latencies, slow conduction velocities, and delayed or absent F-waves in 1 or more motor nerves (see **Table 2**). In contrast to MMN, sensory NCS are also abnormal at the outset. These clinical and laboratory features overlap with hereditary neuropathy with liability to pressure palsies, which should be considered, especially if there is history of recurrent compressive palsies, foot deformities, or family history of compression or generalized neuropathies.

Pathology

In general, sensory cutaneous nerve biopsies show prominent demyelinating features with many thinly myelinated large-diameter fibers, scattered demyelinating fibers, and onion bulbs, similar to the findings in CIDP.[11,94–97] Teased-fiber preparations reveal evidence of demyelination or remyelination,[11] with asymmetric pathologic findings within and between fascicles.[99,100]

Therapy

Although prospective randomized controlled studies have not been performed, retrospective series have demonstrated improvement in response to IVIg treatment in more than 70% of patients with MADSAM neuropathy.[11,62,94–97,99,100] In contrast to MMN, most patients with MADSAM neuropathy have also shown a response to CS treatment. Therefore, it is important to distinguish MADSAM neuropathy from MMN because the former is steroid-responsive whereas the latter is not. Prednisone therapy is initiated with 100 mg orally once daily in the morning. When improvement begins, usually within 2 to 4 weeks, patients can be switched to alternate-day therapy. When strength has returned to normal or improvement has plateaued, usually within 3 to 6 months, the prednisone dose is slowly tapered by 5 mg every 2 to 3 weeks. Although a minority of patients can eventually be tapered completely off prednisone, many patients relapse. It is important for both the patient and the physician to realize that MADSAM neuropathy is a chronic disorder that may require immunosuppressive therapy for 1 or more years. Some patients will require a steroid-sparing agent to facilitate a downward prednisone taper (see later discussion).

Because the risks of long-term therapy with CS are numerous, discussing such risks with the patient as well as establishing a monitoring plan in collaboration with the primary care physician is integral to the management plan. Before CS initiation, the authors perform a PPD skin test to identify the need for isoniazid in previously exposed patients. As CS therapy is started, a baseline bone dual-energy x-ray absorptiometry scan is obtained and the patient is requested to seek an ophthalmologic examination, with yearly follow-up for both. Patients are maintained on oral calcium, 500 to 600 mg 2 to 3 times daily, with vitamin D 400 to 800 IU daily. If there is osteopenia or osteoporosis, or there are fractures, starting an antiresorptive agent such as alendronate is recommended. If patients develop gastric irritation, they are instructed to use H2 blockers or proton-pump inhibitors. Patients and their families are asked to be alert about personality changes and psychiatric side effects, are requested to reduce the salt and carbohydrate in their diet, and are advised to visit their primary care physician regularly for blood pressure, serum glucose, and potassium measurements. The authors advocate the pneumococcal vaccine and yearly flu shots, but caution against live vaccines, which are contraindicated.

A recent retrospective chart review from the Washington University neuromuscular group suggests that intravenous, high-dose methylprednisolone may be an effective treatment for CIDP and that this may be an option for MADSAM neuropathy.[101] One gram of methylprednisolone was administered daily for 3 to 5 days, weekly for 4 to 8 weeks, and then monthly based on clinical course. Treatment of patients with CIDP using high-dose intermittent intravenous methylprednisolone resulted in improved strength equal to that with IVIg and oral prednisone. This favorable response was observed in 13 of 16 patients at 6-month follow-up. In addition, patients treated with intravenous methylprednisolone had less weight gain and fewer cushingoid features when compared with those treated with daily oral prednisone. To further investigate the potential to reduce CS side effects, an open-label prospective study of pulsed oral weekly methylprednisolone was recently conducted.[102] All 10 CIDP patients were started on oral methylprednisolone, 500 mg once a week for 3 months, and the dose was adjusted every 3 months by 50 to 100 mg. All patients improved and off-treatment remission occurred in 60% of patients. Treatment was fairly well tolerated, with many side effects being short lasting following methylprednisolone ingestion (1–2 days), although steroid-induced osteoporosis remained a problem in 5 of 9 patients.

PE was demonstrated to be more effective than "sham" pheresis for CIDP in 2 important studies.[103,104] PE is typically used if patients are severely weak, if they relapse on prednisone or IVIg, or if they are unresponsive to these therapies, thus suggesting that PE would be a viable option for MADSAM neuropathy. However, IVIg may also be effective in severely weak patients. Risks of PE include those of central venous indwelling catheter, hypotension, allergic reaction to albumin, hypocalcemia, anemia, thrombocytopenia, and citrate toxicity. The response obtained with PE is faster than that from prednisone or IVIg. Five to 10 treatments are usually performed over 2 to 4 weeks at the initiation of therapy. Unlike the situation in Guillain-Barré syndrome, there is no benchmark goal of how much total fluid to remove. The effects of PE are transient, usually lasting 4 to 8 weeks, but sometimes only 1 to 2 weeks. Therefore, unless another immunomodulatory treatment such as prednisone is given, PE will need to be performed indefinitely, something not typically pursued because of cost, risk to the patient, and often the need for a long-term indwelling vascular access device. When initiating PE in a patient already on prednisone but who has worsened, the authors usually increase the steroid dose or add a second oral immunosuppressive agent; otherwise, the patient may relapse once the effect of PE has worn off.

When a patient does not respond to or cannot tolerate first-line agents (IVIg, CS, PE), other medications may be beneficial. Azathioprine, cyclophosphamide, cyclosporine, interferon-α, interferon-β, MMF, and methotrexate have all been reported to be beneficial in CIDP patients not responsive to initial therapies.[42,105–120] For the most part, however, these studies were not prospective, randomized, or blinded. In a small controlled trial, patients randomly assigned to azathioprine, 2 mg/kg, and prednisone did no better than those assigned to glucocorticoids alone.[105] Besides azathioprine, MMF, cyclosporine, and methotrexate are often used as steroid-sparing agents.

In a retrospective review of the efficacy of MMF, 3 patients with CIDP (30%) improved, allowing the reduction of steroid or IVIg therapy.[113] In another retrospective case series of 8 CIDP patients, the average Neuropathy Impairment Score improved from baseline after MMF therapy.[121] Six of these 8 patients were either able to stop CS or IVIg or reduce their doses and frequency by at least 50%. Caution in using MMF with CS is important, because 3 of 10 treated patients with dermatomyositis are reported to have had associated opportunistic infections, leading to death in 1 patient.[122]

More recently, a negative randomized controlled trial of oral methotrexate, 15 mg weekly, was reported in CIDP.[123] Fifty-two percent of those taking methotrexate and 44% of those on placebo had a greater than 20% reduction in mean weekly dose of CS or IVIg (adjusted odds ratio 1.21, 95% confidence interval 0.40–3.70). Perhaps a higher methotrexate weekly dose would have been more effective. A recent study evaluated whether treatment with intramuscular interferon-β1a (Avonex) at low (30 μg weekly), intermediate (30 μg twice weekly or 60 μg weekly), and high dosage (60 μg twice weekly) would permit the discontinuation of IVIg in CIDP patients receiving regular IVIg maintenance therapy.[124] Participants were maintained on IVIg through week 16, when IVIg was discontinued, and patients who worsened were restarted on IVIg. The primary outcome was total IVIg dose (g/kg) administered from weeks 16 to 32. Because of a greater than 20% patient dropout rate, this randomized controlled Class I study by design trial was downgraded to Class II evidence. Unfortunately, adding intramuscular interferon-β1a to IVIg for CIDP did not show a significant benefit. In patients with progressive demyelinating neuropathy with IgM monoclonal gammopathy of unknown significance (MGUS), oral treatment with fludar-abine was well tolerated, and induced stabilization and improvement in the modified Rankin scale at 1-year follow-up in 5 of 16 patients.[125]

In comparison with the 2006 report from the European Federation of Neurological Societies/Peripheral Nerve Society (EFNS/PNS) joint task force,[126] the most recent treatment recommendation upgrades the use of IVIg in CIDP to a Level A recommen-dation, while downgrading CS therapy in sensory and motor CIDP to Level C and retain-ing the Level A recommendation for PE when IVIg and CS are ineffective.[127] Good practice points include IVIg as the initial treatment in pure motor CIDP, as well as combi-nation therapy or adding an immunosuppressant drug if the therapeutic response is inadequate or if the maintenance dose of the initial treatment is high. This recommen-dation is in addition to symptomatic treatment and multidisciplinary management.

DISTAL ACQUIRED DEMYELINATING SYMMETRIC NEUROPATHY
Clinical Presentation

This entity is characterized by a distal, symmetric demyelinating neuropathy pheno-type. DADS neuropathy is a slowly progressive disorder that is typically sensory and ataxic, with frequent tremor. Features distinguishing DADS neuropathy from classic CIDP are listed in **Table 1**. The majority (two-thirds) of patients with DADS neuropathy phenotype will have an MGUS, which is almost exclusively IgM-κ and is labeled DADS-M.[10] Many of these cases have been reported in the literature under such names as CIDP-MGUS or IgM-MGUS neuropathy.[128–132] More than 90% of DADS-M patients are men, with onset in the sixth decade or later. When motor signs are present they are usually confined to the distal (toes, ankles, fingers, wrists) limb musculature. Mild ankle dorsiflexion and plantarflexion weakness is present in 60% of patients. DADS-M patients typically have predominantly sensory symptoms and signs despite prominent demyelination on motor NCS. Because of profound sensory involvement, gait unsteadiness and tremor are frequent findings.

Laboratory and Electrodiagnostic Testing

Serum antibodies reactive against MAG are frequently present, in one study in 10 of 15 patients with DADS-M neuropathy.[10] However, the clinical phenotype and treat-ment response are dictated by the presence of IgM-κ monoclonal gammopathy regardless of MAG status. Therefore, it remains uncertain whether there are any prac-tical differences with regard to management, prognosis, or pathophysiology between MAG-positive and MAG-negative IgM-MGUS neuropathy cases.[10,132–135] CSF protein is elevated in most patients.

Motor NCS demonstrate widespread symmetric slowing, most accentuated in distal sensory and motor nerves (see **Table 2**). Conduction block is uncommon. In most cases distal latencies are dramatically prolonged, resulting in a short terminal latency index (TLI), which has been suggested as an electrodiagnostic hallmark of anti-MAG neuropathy.[136,137] Some,[136] but not all[10] reports have found that a short TLI can reli-ably distinguish anti-MAG neuropathy patients from those with other chronic demye-linating neuropathies.

Pathology

Nerve biopsies have a characteristic finding, consisting of widely spaced myelin outer lamellae, which is only seen on electron microscopy. In addition to deposits of IgM and complement on sural nerve myelinated fibers, skin biopsies from patients with anti-MAG neuropathy have demonstrated IgM deposits on dermal myelinated fibers in all cases, with a greater prevalence at the distal site of the extremities and a decrease in epidermal nerve fiber density, reflecting associated axonal loss.[138]

Therapy

Patients with DADS-M neuropathy respond poorly to immunomodulatory therapy. Despite treatment with prednisone, IVIg, PE, and cyclophosphamide, none demonstrate objective improvement. In the authors series[10] only 30% showed any improvement. Most had only sensory manifestations, making objective assessments of treatment responses difficult. In the literature, IgM-MGUS polyneuropathies are not categorized by clinical phenotype or evidence of demyelination but by the presence of an antibody and its type. However, there is general consensus that IgM-MGUS and MAG-positive patients either do not respond or respond poorly to immunomodulatory therapy.[139–143] Most of these cases correspond to the DADS phenotype.

There have been only 3 randomized placebo-controlled trials assessing immunomodulatory therapies in IgM-MGUS polyneuropathy. PE was no better than sham PE in patients with IgM-MGUS polyneuropathy, whereas active treatment produced a superior response among IgG-MGUS and IgA-MGUS patients.[141] Dalakas and colleagues[144] found a response rate of 18% for IVIg in IgM-MGUS patients. In a placebo-controlled trial, no benefit of interferon-α was detected.[145]

Despite other investigators reporting a response to open-label use,[83,84,146–148] the authors' experience with rituximab in DADS-M has not been positive.[149] Rituximab is a chimeric monoclonal antibody that specifically binds to CD20 antigen, expressed from pre–B-cell stage to a mature B-cell stage, on normal and malignant B lymphocytes. It reduces peripheral B-lymphocyte counts by approximately 90% within 3 days, and cell counts begin to recover within 90 days. Another proposed mechanism of action of rituximab concerns its role as a cellular decoy.[150] This mechanism acts through binding of tens of thousands of rituximab-IgG molecules to B cells, generating cellular immune complexes that efficiently attract and bind Fcγ-receptor–expressing effector cells. In turn this reduces effector-cell recruitment at sites of immune-complex deposition, thereby reducing tissue inflammation. Benedetti and colleagues[151] found that improvement in the mean inflammatory neuropathy cause and treatment (INCAT) sensory sum score was significant at 12 months in anti-MAG neuropathy, and correlated with lower anti-MAG antibody at both entry and follow-up. Investigators from Utrecht studied the effect of rituximab in 17 patients with polyneuropathy and IgM monoclonal gammopathy.[152] Rituximab induced an improvement of 1 point or more on the Overall Disability Sum Score in 2 of 17 patients, an improvement of 5% or more in the distal Medical Research Council sum score in 4 of 17 patients, and a similar improvement in the sensory sum score in 9 of 17 patients. The presence of antibodies to MAG and a disease duration shorter than 10 years predicted treatment response.

More recently, a randomized controlled trial compared rituximab with placebo in 26 patients with anti-MAG neuropathy.[153] The primary end-point measure was a change of 1 or more points in the INCAT leg disability scale score at month 8. There was no statistically significant difference between placebo response (0 of 13 patients) and that to rituximab (4 of 13 patients). After excluding a rituximab patient who in retrospect may have had an INCAT score of 0 rather than 1 at entry, this difference became significant. The time to walk 10 m was reduced in the rituximab group from 8.3 ± 3.2 seconds at baseline to 7.4 ± 2.5 seconds after treatment. However, identifying the minority of anti-MAG patients who may respond to rituximab remains a challenge.

Because the clinical deficit in most patients with IgM-MGUS polyneuropathy is primarily sensory and significant progression over time may be minimal, even without treatment, the risks of aggressive management should be weighed against this relatively benign course.[142] Recent guidelines jointly issued by the EFNS/PNS advocate withholding immunomodulatory therapy from DADS-M patients who do not have significant disability,[154] because potential benefit should be balanced against possible side effects and the usually slow disease progression.

Other groups continue to show that patients with IgG or IgA monoclonal gammopathy and neuropathy are different from those with IgM monoclonals. Magy and colleagues[155] found that patients with IgM monoclonals were more likely to have predominantly sensory clinical manifestations, including ataxia, and were more likely to have evidence of distal demyelination on motor NCS, essentially confirming the DADS phenotype. The IgA/IgG group was in general much more heterogeneous, with some axonal and some demyelinating cases. Isoardo and colleagues[156] again showed that patients with MAG antibodies are more likely to have a sensory phenotype despite severe demyelination findings on motor NCS, particularly distally.

The remaining one-third of patients with the DADS phenotype do not have an M-protein and are referred to as idiopathic DADS neuropathy (DADS-I). These patients do not have the striking older age and male preponderance of DADS-M patients. Individuals classified as DADS-I are heterogeneous and show a response to treatment that is intermediate between DADS-M and CIDP.[10] Patients corresponding to DADS-I have been labeled in the literature as "sensory CIDP," because they have only sensory symptoms or signs even though there is electrodiagnostic evidence of motor demyelination.[157–159] These patients may respond to immunomodulatory therapy, but this can be difficult to measure if there are only sensory manifestations.

LESS COMMON CADP VARIANTS

Other less common variants include chronic inflammatory sensory polyradiculopathy (CISP), with normal NCS but abnormal somatosensory evoked potentials,[160] and chronic ataxic neuropathy with ophthalmoparesis, M-protein, cold agglutinins, and disialosyl ganglioside antibodies (CANOMAD).[161] In the Mayo Clinic series of 15 CISP[160] patients, 3 were confined to a wheelchair and 5 relied on a cane. CSF protein was increased in 13 of 14 patients. Despite normal NCS in all, 12 of 12 patients had abnormal SSEP: 7 of 12 had prolonged median nerve N13 latencies or N9-N13 interpeak latencies, 9 of 12 had delayed tibial nerve scalp responses (with absent cervical and lumbar responses), and 2 had absent tibial responses. Of 5 patients with radiologic evidence of thickening of the lumbar nerve root, 3 did not have an evoked potential study. Lumbar sensory rootlet biopsies in 3 patients showed thickened rootlets, decreased density of large myelinated fibers, segmental demyelination, onion-bulb formation, and endoneurial inflammation. All 6 patients requiring aided ambulation responded markedly, within a few months, to intravenous steroids (n = 2) or IVIg (n = 4).

CANOMAD is another rare ataxic variant with a heterogeneous mode of presentation.[161] In addition to weakness in 14 of 18 patients, 16 had variable degrees of ophthalmoparesis, 15 had gait and limb ataxia, and 1 had ataxia confined to limbs. Less commonly, the facial and trigeminal nerves were affected. One patient presented only with limb paresthesia and bulbar dysfunction. The course was slowly progressive, with 13 of 18 patients experiencing relapses in ocular (n = 10), sensory (n = 9), bulbar (n = 8), or motor (n = 4) symptoms. One had a respiratory relapse requiring temporary mechanically assisted ventilation. Some degree of demyelination on NCS was ultimately present in 12 of 18 patients. CSF protein was elevated in 11 of 16 patients, and 2 of 8 imaged patients had multifocal brain white matter lesions without any oligoclonal band. An M-protein was found in 17 of 18 patients, and 8 had cold agglutinins.

A variety of IgM antiganglioside antibodies were detected in all 18 patients, with 17 having identifiable GD1b (n = 16) and/or GQ1b (n = 17) antibodies. A single patient had isolated GD3 antibody elevation. At last assessment, 5 patients were wheelchair bound and only 3 walked unaided. Patients may respond to IVIg or PE. To avoid agglutination in the extracorporeal arm, the replacement fluid temperatures of PE should be controlled carefully.

Case report

A 52 year-old man developed progressive weakness in his right hand over the last 2 years. He loss of dexterity and cramps. He denies any numbness.

Examination showed normal reflexes, pinprick. light touch and proprioception. Vibration was mildly reduced at the toes. Right arm was 3/5 at finger extension, and 4/5 at little and right finger flexion with fasciculations and mild hand atrophy. Otherwise strength is preserved in the rest of the right arm muscles as well as the left arm and bilateral legs. Cranial nerves and gait testing were normal.

Laboratory studies including vitamin B12 level and 2 hour glucose tolerance test were normal and there was no serum monoclonal protein. IgM GMI antibody titers were normal. Nerve conduction studies showed 35% reduction of right peroneal and ulnar motor conduction velocities. There was 60% reduction in the radial motor amplitude recording from the extensor indicis proprius muscle between the forearm and elbow stimulation sites.

He was started on intravenous gammaglobulin for the diagnosis of MMN with improvement in strength. Over the next two years numbness developed on the dorsum of the right hand.

REFERENCES

1. Eichhorst H. Beitrage zur pathologie der nerven und muskeln. Cor Kl Schweiz Aertze 1890;20:59–71.
2. Austin JH. Recurrent polyneuropathies and their corticosteroids treatment. Brain 1958;8:157–92.
3. Dyck PJ, Lais AC, Otha M, et al. Chronic inflammatory polyradiculoneuropathy. Mayo Clin Proc 1975;50:621–37.
4. Dyck PJ, Arnason BG. Chronic inflammatory demyelinating polyradiculoneuropathy. In: Dyck PJ, Thomas PK, Lambert EH, et al, editors. Peripheral neuropathy. 2nd edition. Philadelphia: WB Saunders; 1984. p. 2101–14.
5. Dyck PJ, Oviatt KF, Lambert EH. Intensive evaluation of referred unclassified neuropathies yields improved diagnosis. Ann Neurol 1981;10(3):222–6.
6. Barohn RJ. Approach to peripheral neuropathy and neuronopathy. Semin Neurol 1998;18(1):7–18.
7. Khan S, Wolfe G, Nascimento O, et al. North America and South America (NA-SA). Neurology 2006;66:A84.
8. Saperstein DS, Katz JS, Amato AA, et al. Clinical spectrum of chronic acquired demyelinating polyneuropathies. Muscle Nerve 2001;24:311–24.
9. Koller H, Kieseier BC, Jander S, et al. Chronic inflammatory demyelinating polyneuropathy. N Engl J Med 2005;352:1343–56.
10. Katz JS, Saperstein DS, Gronseth G, et al. Distal acquired demyelinating symmetric (DADS) neuropathy. Neurology 2000;54:615–20.
11. Saperstein DS, Amato AA, Wolfe GI, et al. Multifocal acquired demyelinating sensory and motor neuropathy: the Lewis-Sumner syndrome. Muscle Nerve 1999;22:560–6.

12. Viala K, Renié L, Maisonobe T, et al. Follow-up study and response to treatment in 23 patients with Lewis-Sumner syndrome. Brain 2004;127:2010–7.

13. Verschueren A, Azulay JP, Attarian S, et al. Lewis-Sumner syndrome and multifocal motor neuropathy. Muscle Nerve 2004;31:88–94.

14. Alaedini A, Sanders HW, Hays AP, et al. Antiganglioside antibodies in multifocal acquired sensory and motor neuropathy. Arch Neurol 2003;60:42–6.

15. Viala K, Maisonobe T, Stojkovic T, et al. A current view of the diagnosis, clinical variants, response to treatment and prognosis of chronic inflammatory demyelinating polyradiculoneuropathy. J Peripher Nerv Syst 2010;15(1):50–6.

16. Parry GJ, Clarke S. Multifocal acquired demyelinating neuropathy masquerading as motor neuron disease. Muscle Nerve 1988;11:103–7.

17. Chad DA, Hammer K, Sargent J. Slow resolution of multifocal weakness and fasciculation: a reversible motor neuron syndrome. Neurology 1986;36:1260–3.

18. Kaji R, Shibasaki H, Kimura J. Multifocal demyelinating motor neuropathy: cranial nerve involvement and immunoglobulin therapy. Neurology 1992;42: 506–9.

19. Krarup C, Stewart JD, Sumner AJ, et al. A syndrome of asymmetric limb weakness with motor conduction block. Neurology 1990;40:118–27.

20. Pestronk A, Cornblath DR, Ilyas AA, et al. A treatable multifocal motor neuropathy with antibodies to GM1 ganglioside. Ann Neurol 1988;24:73–8.

21. Roth G, Rohr J, Magistris MR, et al. Motor neuropathy with proximal multifocal persistent conduction block, fasciculations and myokymia. Evolution to tetraplegia. Eur Neurol 1986;25:416–23.

22. Katz JS, Wolfe GI, Bryan WW, et al. Electrophysiologic findings in multifocal motor neuropathy. Neurology 1997;48:700–7.

23. Azulay JP, Attarian S, Pouget J. Effect of cyclophosphamide in multifocal motor neuropathies with or without conduction block. Neurology 1999;52(Suppl 2): A550–1.

24. Ellis CM, Leary S, Shaw J, et al. Use of human intravenous immunoglobulin in lower motor neuron syndromes. J Neurol Neurosurg Psychiatry 1999;67:15–9.

25. Pakiam AS, Parry GJ. Multifocal motor neuropathy without overt conduction block. Muscle Nerve 1998;21:243–5.

26. Auer RN, Bell RB, Lee MA. Neuropathy with onion bulb formations and pure motor manifestations. Can J Neurol Sci 1989;16:194–7.

27. Chaudhry V. Multifocal motor neuropathy. Semin Neurol 1998;18:73–81.

28. Chaudhry V, Corse AM, Cornblath DR, et al. Multifocal motor neuropathy: response to human immune globulin. Ann Neurol 1993;33:237–42.

29. Chaudhry V, Corse AM, Cornblath DR, et al. Multifocal motor neuropathy: electrodiagnostic features. Muscle Nerve 1994;17:198–205.

30. Feldman EL, Bromberg MB, Albers JW, et al. Immunosuppressive treatment in multifocal motor neuropathy. Ann Neurol 1991;30:397–401.

31. Parry GJ, Sumner AJ. Multifocal motor neuropathy. Neurol Clin 1992;10:671–84.

32. Lambrecq V, Krim E, Rouanet-Larrivière M, et al. Sensory loss in multifocal motor neuropathy: a clinical and electrophysiological study. Muscle Nerve 2009;39(2): 131–6.

33. Lievens I, Fournier E, Viala K, et al. Multifocal motor neuropathy: a retrospective study of sensory nerve conduction velocities in long-term follow-up of 21 patients. Rev Neurol (Paris) 2009;165(3):243–8 [in French].

34. Joint Task Force of the EFNS and the PNS. European Federation of Neurological Societies/Peripheral Nerve Society guideline on management of multifocal motor neuropathy. Report of a joint task force of the European Federation of

Neurological Societies and the Peripheral Nerve Society—first revision. J Peripher Nerv Syst 2010;15(4):295–301.

35. Joint Task Force of the EFNS and the PNS. European Federation of Neurological Societies/Peripheral Nerve Society Guideline on management of multifocal motor neuropathy. Report of a joint task force of the European Federation of Neurological Societies and the Peripheral Nerve Society. J Peripher Nerv Syst 2006;11:1–8.

36. Kaji R, Hirota N, Oka N, et al. Anti-GM1 antibodies and impaired blood-nerve barrier may interfere with remyelination in multifocal motor neuropathy. Muscle Nerve 1994;17:108–10.

37. Kornberg AJ, Pestronk A. The clinical and diagnostic role of anti-GM1 antibody testing. Muscle Nerve 1994;17:100–4.

38. Lange DJ, Trojaborg W, Latov N, et al. Multifocal motor neuropathy with conduction block: is it a distinct clinical entity? Neurology 1992;42:497–505.

39. Parry GJ. Antiganglioside antibodies do not necessarily play a role in multifocal motor neuropathy. Muscle Nerve 1994;17:97–9.

40. Sadiq SA, Thomas FP, Kilidireas K, et al. The spectrum of neurologic disease associated with anti-GM1 antibodies. Neurology 1990;40:1067–72.

41. Tan E, Lynn DJ, Amato AA, et al. Immunosuppressive treatment of motor neuron syndromes. Attempts to distinguish a treatable disorder. Arch Neurol 1994;51:194–200.

42. Mowzoon N, Sussman A, Bradley WG. Mycophenolate (CellCept) treatment of myasthenia gravis, chronic inflammatory polyneuropathy and inclusion body myositis. J Neurol Sci 2001;185(2):119–22.

43. Taylor BV, Gross L, Windebank AJ. The sensitivity and specificity of anti-GM1 antibody testing. Neurology 1996;47:951–5.

44. Van Schaik IN, Bossuyt PM, Brand A, et al. Diagnostic value of GM1 antibodies in motor neuron disorders and neuropathies: a meta-analysis. Neurology 1995;45:1570–7.

45. Pestronk A, Chaudhry V, Feldman EL, et al. Lower motor neuron syndromes defined by patterns of weakness, nerve conduction abnormalities, and high titers of antiglycolipid antibodies. Ann Neurol 1990;27:316–26.

46. Pestronk A, Choksi R. Multifocal motor neuropathy. Serum IgM anti-GM1 ganglioside antibodies in most patients detected using covalent linkage of GM1 to ELISA plates. Neurology 1997;49:1289–92.

47. Carpo M, Allaria S, Scarlato G, et al. Marginally improved detection of GM1 antibodies by Covalink ELISA in multifocal motor neuropathy. Neurology 1999;53:2206–7.

48. Pestronk A, Chuquilin M, Choksi R. Motor neuropathies and serum IgM binding to NS6S heparin disaccharide or GM1 ganglioside. J Neurol Neurosurg Psychiatry 2010;81(7):726–30.

49. Laughlin RS, Dyck PJ, Melton LJ 3rd, et al. Incidence and prevalence of CIDP and the association of diabetes mellitus. Neurology 2009;73(1):39–45.

50. McCombe PA, Pollard JD, McLeod JG. Chronic inflammatory demyelinating polyradiculoneuropathy. A clinical and electrophysiological study of 92 cases. Brain 1987;110:1617–30.

51. Holzbauer SM, DeVries AS, Sejvar JJ, et al. Epidemiologic investigation of immune-mediated polyradiculoneuropathy among abattoir workers exposed to porcine brain. PLoS One 2010;5(3):e9782.

52. Gorson KC, Allam G, Ropper AH. Chronic inflammatory demyelinating polyneuropathy: clinical features and response to treatment in 67 consecutive patients with and without a monoclonal gammopathy. Neurology 1997;48:321–8.

53. Vucic S, Black K, Siao Tick Chong P, et al. Cervical nerve root stimulation. Part II: findings in primary demyelinating neuropathies and motor neuron disease. Clin Neurophysiol 2006;117(2):398–404.
54. Felice KJ, Goldstein J. Monofocal motor neuropathy: improvement with intravenous immunoglobulin. Muscle Nerve 2002;25:674–8.
55. Katz JS, Barohn RJ, Kojan S, et al. Axonal multifocal motor neuropathy without conduction block or other features of demyelination. Neurology 2002;58:615–20.
56. Fisher D, Grothe C, Schmidt S, et al. On the early diagnosis of IVIg-responsive chronic multifocal acquired motor axonopathy. J Neurol 2004;251:1204–7.
57. Bouche P, Moulonguet A, Younes-Chennoufi AB, et al. Multifocal motor neuropathy with conduction block: a study of 24 patients. J Neurol Neurosurg Psychiatry 1995;59:38–44.
58. Corse AM, Chaudhry V, Crawford TO, et al. Sensory nerve pathology in multifocal motor neuropathy. Ann Neurol 1996;39:319–25.
59. Kaji R, Oka N, Tsuji T, et al. Pathological findings at the site of conduction block in multifocal motor neuropathy. Ann Neurol 1993;33:152–8.
60. Taylor BV, Pyck PJ, Engelstad J, et al. Multifocal motor neuropathy; pathologic alterations at the site of conduction block. J Neuropathol Exp Neurol 2004;63:129–37.
61. Van Es HW, Van den Berg LH, Franssen H, et al. Magnetic resonance imaging of the brachial plexus in patients with multifocal motor neuropathy. Neurology 1997;48:1218–24.
62. Van den Berg-Vos RM, Van den Berg LH, Franssen H, et al. Multifocal inflammatory demyelinating neuropathy: a distinct clinical; entity? Neurology 2000;54:26–32.
63. Carpo M, Cappellari A, Mora G, et al. Deterioration of multifocal motor neuropathy after plasma exchange. Neurology 1998;50(5):1480–2.
64. Donaghy M, Mills KR, Boniface SJ, et al. Pure motor demyelinating neuropathy: deterioration after steroid treatment and improvement with intravenous immunoglobulin. J Neurol Neurosurg Psychiatry 1994;57:778–83.
65. Azulay JP, Blin O, Pouget J, et al. Intravenous immunoglobulin treatment in patients with motor neuron syndromes associated with anti-GM1 antibodies: a double-blind, placebo-controlled study. Neurology 1994;44:429–32.
66. Van den Berg LH, Kerkhoff H, Oey PL, et al. Treatment of multifocal motor neuropathy with high dose intravenous immunoglobulins: a double blind, placebo controlled study. J Neurol Neurosurg Psychiatry 1995;59:248–52.
67. Sabatelli M, Madia F, Mignogna T, et al. Pure motor chronic inflammatory demyelinating polyneuropathy. J Neurol 2001;248:772–7.
68. Dionne A, Nicolle MW, Hahn AF. Clinical and electrophysiological parameters distinguishing acute-onset chronic inflammatory demyelinating polyneuropathy from acute inflammatory demyelinating polyneuropathy. Muscle Nerve 2010;41(2):202–7.
69. Ruts L, Drenthen J, Jacobs BC, et al, Dutch GBS Study Group. Distinguishing acute-onset CIDP from fluctuating Guillain-Barre syndrome: a prospective study. Neurology 2010;74(21):1680–6.
70. Anthony RM, Kobayashi T, Wermeling F, et al. Intravenous gammaglobulin suppresses inflammation through a novel T(H)2 pathway. Nature 2011;475(7354):110–3.
71. Steck AJ. Inflammatory neuropathy: pathogenesis and clinical features. Curr Opin Neurol Neurosurg 1992;5(5):633–7.

72. Chaudhry V, Corse A, Cornblath D, et al. Maintenance immune globulin therapy for multifocal motor neuropathy: results of long-term follow-up. Ann Neurol 1996; 40:513–4.

73. Azulay JP, Rihet P, Pouget J, et al. Long term follow up of multifocal motor neuropathy with conduction block under treatment. J Neurol Neurosurg Psychiatry 1997;62:391–4.

74. Biessels GJ, Franssen H, Van den Berg LH, et al. Multifocal motor neuropathy. J Neurol 1997;244:143–52.

75. Taylor BV, Wright RA, Harper CM, et al. Natural history of 46 patients with multifocal motor neuropathy with conduction block. Muscle Nerve 2000;23:900–8.

76. Van den Berg-Vos RM, Franssen H, Wokke JH, et al. Multifocal motor neuropathy: long-term clinical and electrophysiological assessment of intravenous immunoglobulin maintenance treatment. Brain 2002;125:1875–86.

77. Terenghi F, Cappellari A, Bersano A, et al. How long is IVIg effective in multifocal motor neuropathy? Neurology 2004;62:666–8.

78. Cats EA, van der Pol WL, Piepers S, et al. Correlates of outcome and response to IVIg in 88 patients with multifocal motor neuropathy. Neurology 2010;75(9):818–25.

79. Koski C, Beydoun S, Schiff R, et al, MMN Study Group. Efficacy, safety, and tolerability of intravenous gammaglobulin (IGIV, 10%) in a phase 3, randomized, placebo-controlled, cross-over trial for the treatment of multifocal motor neuropathy (MMN). Neurology 2012;78(Suppl 1):PL02.002.

80. Hodgkinson SJ, Pollard JD, McLeod JG. Cyclosporine A in the treatment of chronic demyelinating polyradiculopathy. J Neurol Neurosurg Psychiatry 1990; 53:327–30.

81. Barnett MH, Pollard JD, Davies L, et al. Cyclosporin A in resistant chronic inflammatory demyelinating polyradiculoneuropathy. Muscle Nerve 1998;21(4):454–60.

82. Anthony RM, Kobayashi T, Wermeling F, et al. Intravenous gammaglobulin suppresses inflammation through a novel T(H)2 pathway. Nature 2011; 475(7354):110–3.

83. Ibrahim H, Dimachkie MM, Shaibani A. A review: the use of rituximab in neuromuscular diseases. J Clin Neuromuscul Dis 2010;12(2):91–102.

84. Levine TD, Pestronk A. IgM antibody-related polyneuropathies: B-cell depletion chemotherapy using Rituximab. Neurology 1999;52:1701–4.

85. Pestronk A, Florence J, Miller T, et al. Treatment of IgM antibody associated polyneuropathies using rituximab. J Neurol Neurosurg Psychiatry 2003;74:485–9.

86. Ruegg SJ, Fuhr P, Steck AJ. Rituximab stabilizes multifocal motor neuropathy increasingly less responsive to IVIg. Neurology 2004;63:2178–9.

87. Gorson TG, Natarajan N, Ropper AH, et al. Rituximab treatment in patients with IVIg-dependent immune polyneuropathy: a prospective pilot trial. Muscle Nerve 2007;35:66–9.

88. Stieglbauer K, Topakian R, Hinterberger G, et al. Effect of rituximab monotherapy in multifocal motor neuropathy. Neuromuscul Disord 2009;19:473–5.

89. Lee DH, Linker RA, Paulus W, et al. Subcutaneous immunoglobulin infusion: a new therapeutic option in chronic inflammatory demyelinating polyneuropathy. Muscle Nerve 2008;37(3):406–9.

90. Harbo T, Andersen H, Jakobsen J. Long-term therapy with high doses of subcutaneous immunoglobulin in multifocal motor neuropathy. Neurology 2010;75(15): 1377–80.

91. Eftimov F, Vermeulen M, de Haan RJ, et al. Subcutaneous immunoglobulin therapy for multifocal motor neuropathy. J Peripher Nerv Syst 2009;14(2): 93–100.

92. Misbah SA, Baumann A, Fazio R, et al. A smooth transition protocol for patients with multifocal motor neuropathy going from intravenous to subcutaneous immunoglobulin therapy: an open-label proof-of-concept study. J Peripher Nerv Syst 2011;16(2):92–7.

93. Piepers S, Van den Berg-Vos R, Van der Pol WL, et al. Mycophenolate mofetil as adjunctive therapy for MMN patients: a randomized, controlled trial. Brain 2007; 130(Pt 8):2004–10.

94. Lewis RA, Sumner AJ, Brown MJ, et al. Multifocal demyelinating neuropathy with persistent conduction block. Neurology 1982;32:958–64.

95. Oh SJ, Claussen GC, Dae SK. Motor and sensory demyelinating mononeuropathy multiplex (multifocal motor and sensory demyelinating neuropathy): a separate variant of chronic inflammatory demyelinating polyneuropathy. J Peripher Nerv Syst 1997;2:362–9.

96. Gorson KC, Ropper AH, Weinberg DH. Upper limb predominant, multifocal chronic inflammatory demyelinating polyneuropathy. Muscle Nerve 1999;22: 758–65.

97. Thomas PK, Claus D, Jaspert A, et al. Focal upper limb demyelinating neuropathy. Brain 1996;119:765–74.

98. Verma A, Tandan R, Adesina AM, et al. Focal neuropathy preceding chronic inflammatory demyelinating polyradiculoneuropathy by several years. Acta Neurol Scand 1990;81(6):516–21.

99. Gibbels E, Behse F, Kentenich M, et al. Chronic multifocal neuropathy with persistent conduction block (Lewis- Sumner syndrome). A clinico-morphologic study of two further cases with review of the literature. Clin Neuropathol 1993; 12:343–52.

100. Nukada H, Pollock M, Haas LF. Is ischemia implicated in chronic multifocal demyelinating neuropathy? Neurology 1989;39:106–10.

101. Caress JB, Cartwright MS, Donofrio PD, et al. The Clinical features of 16 cases of stroke associated with administration of IVIg. Neurology 2003;60:1822–4.

102. Okuda D, Flaster M, Frey J, et al. Arterial thrombosis induced by IVIg and its treatment with tPA. Neurology 2003;60:1825–6.

103. Kaneko Y, Nimmerjahn F, Ravetch JV. Anti-inflammatory activity of immunoglobulin G resulting from Fc sialylation. Science 2006;313(5787):670–3.

104. Anthony RM, Nimmerjahn F, Ashline DJ, et al. Recapitulation of IVIG anti-inflammatory activity with a recombinant IgG Fc. Science 2008;320(5874):373–6.

105. Good JL, Chehrenama M, Mayer RF, et al. Pulsed cyclophosphamide in chronic inflammatory demyelinating polyneuropathy. Neurology 1998;51:1735–8.

106. Brannagan TH, Pradham A, Heiman-Patterson T, et al. High-dose cyclophosphamide without stem-cell rescue for refractory CIDP. Neurology 2002;58: 1856–8.

107. Chaudhry V, Cornblath DR, Griffin JW, et al. Mycophenolate mofetil: a safe and promising immunosuppressant in neuromuscular diseases. Neurology 2001;56: 94–6.

108. Gorson KC, Amato AA, Ropper AH. Efficacy of mycophenolate mofetil in patients with chronic immune demyelinating polyneuropathy. Neurology 2004;63:715–7.

109. Sabatelli M, Mignona T, Lippi G, et al. Interferon-alpha may benefit steroid unresponsive chronic inflammatory demyelinating polyneuropathy. J Neurol Neurosurg Psychiatry 1995;58:638–9.

110. Choudhary PP, Thompson N, Hughes RA. Improvement following interferon beta in chronic inflammatory demyelinating polyradiculoneuropathy. J Neurol 1995; 242:252–3.

111. Gorson KC, Ropper AH, Clark BD, et al. Treatment of chronic inflammatory demyelinating polyneuropathy with interferon alpha 2a. Neurology 1998;50:84–7.
112. Hadden RD, Sharrack B, Bensa S, et al. Randomized trial of interferon B-1a in chronic inflammatory demyelinating polyradiculoneuropathy. Neurology 1999; 53:57–61.
113. Kuntzer T, Radziwill AJ, Lettry-Trouillat R, et al. Interferon-B1a in chronic inflammatory demyelinating polyneuropathy. Neurology 1999;53:1364–5.
114. Pavesi G, Cattaneo L, Marbini A, et al. Long-term efficacy of interferon-alpha in chronic inflammatory demyelinating neuropathy. J Neurol 2002;249:777–9.
115. Vallat JM, Hahn AF, Leger JM, et al. Interferon beta 1a as an investigational treatment for CIDP. Neurology 2003;60(Suppl 3):S23–8.
116. Fialho D, Chan YC, Allen DC, et al. Treatment of chronic inflammatory demyelinating polyradiculoneuropathy with methotrexate. J Neurol Neurosurg Psychiatry 2006;77:544–7.
117. Bedi G, Brown A, Tong T, et al. Chronic inflammatory demyelinating polyneuropathy responsive to mycophenolate mofetil therapy. J Neurol Neurosurg Psychiatry 2010;81(6):634–6.
118. Rowin J, Amato AA, Deisher N, et al. Mycophenolate mofetil in dermatomyositis: is it safe? Neurology 2006;66(8):1245–7.
119. RMC Trial Group. Randomised controlled trial of methotrexate for chronic inflammatory demyelinating polyradiculoneuropathy (RMC trial): a pilot, multicentre study. Lancet Neurol 2009;8(2):158–64.
120. Hughes RA, Gorson KC, Cros D, et al, Avonex CIDP Study Group. Intramuscular interferon beta-1a in chronic inflammatory demyelinating polyradiculoneuropathy. Neurology 2010;74(8):651–7.
121. Niermeijer JM, Eurelings M, Lokhorst H, et al. Neurologic and hematologic response to fludarabine treatment in IgM MGUS polyneuropathy. Neurology 2006;67(11):2076–9.
122. Vermeulen M, Van Oers MH. Successful autologous stem cell transplantation in a patient with chronic inflammatory demyelinating polyneuropathy. J Neurol Neurosurg Psychiatry 2002;72:127–8.
123. Oyama MD, Sufit R, Loh Y, et al. Nonmyeloablative autologous hematopoietic stem cell transplantation for refractory CIDP. Neurology 2007;69:1802–3.
124. Gladstone DE, Prestrud AA, Brannagan TH III. High-dose cyclophosphamide results in long-term disease remission with restoration of a normal quality of life in patients with severe refractory chronic inflammatory demyelinating polyneuropathy. J Peripher Nerv Syst 2005;10(1):11–6.
125. Taylor RP, Lindorfer MA. Drug insight: the mechanism of action of rituximab in autoimmune disease–the immune complex decoy hypothesis. Nat Clin Pract Rheumatol 2007;3(2):86–95.
126. Comi G, Amadio S, Galardi G, et al. Clinical and neurophysiological assessment of immunoglobulin therapy in five patients with multifocal motor neuropathy. J Neurol Neurosurg Psychiatry 1994;57(Suppl):35–7.
127. Bosboom WM, Van den Berg LH, Franssen H, et al. Diagnostic value of sural demyelination in chronic inflammatory demyelinating polyneuropathy. Brain 2001;124:2427–38.
128. Dalakas M, Houff SA, Engel WK, et al. CSF "monoclonal" bands in chronic relapsing polyneuropathy. Neurology 1980;30:864–7.
129. Nobile-Orazio E, Manfredini E, Carpo M, et al. Frequency and clinical correlates of anti-neural IgM antibodies in neuropathy associated with IgM monoclonal gammopathy. Ann Neurol 1994;36:416–24.

130. Notermans NC, Franssen H, Eurerlings M, et al. Diagnostic criteria for demyelinating polyneuropathy associated with monoclonal gammopathy. Muscle Nerve 2000;23:73–9.
131. Smith IS. The natural history of chronic demyelinating neuropathy associated with benign IgM paraproteinaemia. A clinical and neurophysiological study. Brain 1994;117:949–57.
132. Suarez GA, Kelly JJ Jr. Polyneuropathy associated with monoclonal gammopathy of undetermined significance: further evidence that IgM-MGUS neuropathies are different than IgG-MGUS. Neurology 1993;43:1304–8.
133. Chassande B, Leger JM, Younes-Chennoufi AB, et al. Peripheral neuropathy associated with IgM monoclonal gammopathy: correlations between M-protein antibody activity and clinical/electrophysiological features in 40 cases. Muscle Nerve 1998;21:55–62.
134. Gosselin S, Kyle RA, Dyck PJ. Neuropathy associated with monoclonal gammopathies of undetermined significance. Ann Neurol 1991;30:54–61.
135. Simovic D, Gorson KC, Ropper AH. Comparison of IgM-MGUS and IgG-MGUS polyneuropathy. Acta Neurol Scand 1998;97:194–200.
136. Kaku DA, England JD, Sumner AJ. Distal accentuation of conduction slowing in polyneuropathy associated with antibodies to myelin-associated glycoprotein and sulphated glucuronyl paragloboside. Brain 1994;117:941–7.
137. Trojaborg W, Hays AP, van den BL, et al. Motor conduction parameters in neuropathies associated with anti-MAG antibodies and other types of demyelinating and axonal neuropathies. Muscle Nerve 1995;18:730–5.
138. Lombardi R, Erne B, Lauria G, et al. IgM deposits on skin nerves in anti-myelin-associated glycoprotein neuropathy. Ann Neurol 2005;57(2):180–7.
139. Kissel JT, Mendell JR. Neuropathies associated with monoclonal proteins. Neuromuscul Disord 1995;6:3–18.
140. Yeung KB, Thomas PK, King RH, et al. The clinical spectrum of peripheral neuropathies associated with benign monoclonal IgM, IgG and IgA paraproteinaemia. Comparative clinical, immunological and nerve biopsy findings. J Neurol 1991;238:383–91.
141. Dyck PJ, Low PA, Windebank AJ, et al. Plasma exchange in polyneuropathy associated with monoclonal gammopathy of undetermined significance. N Engl J Med 1991;325:1482–6.
142. Nobile-Orazio E, Meucci N, Baldini L, et al. Long-term prognosis of neuropathy associated with anti-MAG IgM M-proteins and its relationship to immune therapies. Brain 2000;123:710–7.
143. Pollard JD, Young GA. Neurology and the bone marrow. J Neurol Neurosurg Psychiatry 1997;63:706–18.
144. Dalakas MC, Quarles RH, Farrer RG, et al. A controlled study of intravenous immunoglobulin in demyelinating neuropathy with IgM gammopathy. Ann Neurol 1996;40:792–5.
145. Mariette X, Brouet JC, Chevret S, et al. A randomised double blind trial versus placebo does not confirm the benefit of alpha-interferon in polyneuropathy associated with monoclonal IgM. J Neurol Neurosurg Psychiatry 2000;69(2):279–80.
146. Briani C, Zara G, Zambello R, et al. Rituximab-responsive CIDP. Eur J Neurol 2004;11(11):788.
147. Renaud S, Gregor M, Fuhr P, et al. Rituximab in the treatment of polyneuropathy associated with anti-MAG antibodies. Muscle Nerve 2003;27:611–5.
148. Renaud S, Fuhr P, Gregor M, et al. High-dose rituximab and anti-MAG-associated polyneuropathy. Neurology 2006;66:742–4.

149. Dimachkie MM, Herbelin L, Pasnoor M, et al. Efficacy of rituximab in DADS-M neuropathy. J Peripher Nerv Syst 2008;13:166a.
150. Iijima M, Tomita M, Morozumi S, et al. Single nucleotide polymorphism of TAG-1 influences IVIg responsiveness of Japanese patients with CIDP. Neurology 2009;73(17):1348–52.
151. Benedetti L, Briani C, Grandis M, et al. Predictors of response to rituximab in patients with neuropathy and anti-myelin associated glycoprotein immunoglobulin. J Peripher Nerv Syst 2007;12(2):102–7.
152. Niermeijer JM, Eurelings M, Lokhorst HL, et al. Rituximab for polyneuropathy with IgM monoclonal gammopathy. J Neurol Neurosurg Psychiatry 2009;80(9):1036–9.
153. Dalakas MC, Rakocevic G, Salajegheh M, et al. Placebo-controlled trial of rituximab in IgM anti-myelin-associated glycoprotein antibody demyelinating neuropathy. Ann Neurol 2009;65(3):286–93.
154. Joint Task Force of the EFNS and the PNS. European Federation of Neurological Societies/Peripheral Nerve Society Guideline on management of paraproteinemic demyelinating neuropathies. Report of a joint task force of the European Federation of Neurological Societies and the Peripheral Nerve Society. J Peripher Nerv Syst 2006;11:9–19.
155. Magy L, Chassande B, Maisonobe T, et al. Polyneuropathy associated with IgG/IgA monoclonal gammopathy: a clinical and electrophysiological study of 15 cases. Eur J Neurol 2003;10:677–85.
156. Isoardo G, Migiaretti G, Ciaramitaro P, et al. Differential diagnosis of chronic dysimmune demyelinating polyneuropathies with and without anti-MAG antibodies. Muscle Nerve 2005;31:52–8.
157. Oh SJ, Joy JL, Kuruoglu R. "Chronic sensory demyelinating neuropathy": chronic inflammatory demyelinating polyneuropathy presenting as a pure sensory neuropathy. J Neurol Neurosurg Psychiatry 1992;55:677–80.
158. Oh SJ, Joy JL, Sunwoo I, et al. A case of chronic sensory demyelinating neuropathy responding to immunotherapies. Muscle Nerve 1992;15:255–6.
159. Simmons Z, Tivakaran S. Acquired demyelinating polyneuropathy presenting as a pure clinical sensory syndrome. Muscle Nerve 1996;19:1174–6.
160. Sinnreich M, Klein CJ, Daube JR, et al. Chronic immune sensory polyradiculopathy: a possibly treatable sensory ataxia. Neurology 2004;63(9):1662–9.
161. Willison HJ, O'Leary CP, Veitch J, et al. The clinical and laboratory features of chronic sensory ataxic neuropathy with anti-disialosyl IgM antibodies. Brain 2001;124(Pt 10):1968–77.

The Neuropathies of Vasculitis

Michael P. Collins, MD[a],*, William David Arnold, MD[b],
John T. Kissel, MD[c]

KEYWORDS

- Vasculitis • Neuropathy • Nerve biopsy • Antineutrophil cytoplasmic antibodies
- Treatment

KEY POINTS

- Vasculitic neuropathy is an uncommon but important cause of axonal neuropathy due to potential treatment implications.
- The diagnosis should always be considered in patients presenting with a painful, asymmetric neuropathy.
- Vasculitis rarely may be associated with symmetric clinical and electrodiagnostic features.
- Corticosteroid (CS) therapy and other immune therapies are effective in vasculitis, but patients should be carefully monitored for short-term and long-term side effects.
- It is important to be mindful that clinical recovery, despite aggressive treatment, is typically slow and may be incomplete in severely affected nerves.

INTRODUCTION/CLASSIFICATION

The vasculitides are clinically, pathogenically, and etiologically diverse disorders sharing a predilection for inflammatory destruction of vessel walls, ischemic injury to involved organs, and corresponding clinical symptoms.[1] Vasculitis usually affects multiple tissues simultaneously or sequentially. Clinical features of these systemic vasculitides are determined by the location and size of the affected vessels, severity of the inflammatory process, and comorbid conditions. When the peripheral nervous system (PNS) is affected, a vasculitic neuropathy ensues. In some patients, vasculitis is restricted to vessels in a single organ, tissue, or body region.[2] These localized or nonsystemic vasculitides have been described for almost all organs, including the

Funding Sources: Dr Collins and Dr Arnold: None; Dr Kissel received drugs from Abbott Pharmaceuticals for a clinical trial in SMA, is a paid consultant for Alexion Pharmaceuticals and Cytokinetics, and is funded by NIH grant U10 NS77382-2 for NeuroNEXT.
Conflict of Interest: None.
[a] Medical College of Wisconsin, 9200 West Wisconsin Avenue, Milwaukee, WI 52366, USA; [b] The Ohio State University, 395 West 12th Avenue, Columbus, OH 43210, USA; [c] Division of Neuromuscular Medicine, The Ohio State University, 395 West 12th Avenue, Columbus, OH 43210, USA
* Corresponding author.
E-mail address: mcollins@mcw.edu

neurologic.theclinics.com

PNS, a condition known as nonsystemic vasculitic neuropathy (NSVN).[3] Vasculitic neuropathy is classically acute or subacute in onset and multifocal in distribution, but in many patients, progression is slower with overlapping asymmetric or symmetric deficits. Vasculitis, therefore, needs to be considered in almost any patient with a progressive axonal neuropathy.

A Peripheral Nerve Society task force classified the vasculitides associated with neuropathy into 3 groups: primary systemic, secondary systemic, and nonsystemic (**Box 1**).[4] Primary systemic vasculitis includes disorders with no known underlying cause. Secondary systemic vasculitis refers to immune-mediated vessel injury triggered by infections, drugs, or a preexisting autoimmune inflammatory condition, such as a connective tissue disease (CTD). The most widely used classification criteria for the primary systemic vasculitides are those published by the American College of Rheumatology (ACR) in 1990.[5] Although useful for classifying already diagnosed patients for clinical studies, these criteria are not appropriate for diagnosis because they do not distinguish vasculitic from nonvasculitic conditions. In 1994, the Chapel Hill Consensus Conference (CHCC1994) proposed a vasculitis nomenclature based on the size and histopathology of the involved vessels.[6] Giant cell arteritis (GCA) and Takayasu arteritis primarily target large vessels; polyarteritis nodosa (PAN) and Kawasaki disease involve small to medium-sized arteries; and Wegener granulomatosis, Churg-Strauss syndrome, microscopic polyangiitis (MPA), Henoch-Schönlein purpura, cryoglobulinemic vasculitis, and cutaneuous leukocytoclastic angiitis all predominantly affect the microvasculature (with small and medium-sized arteries less commonly involved).

The CHCC1994 and ACR systems have various limitations. When applied to the same cohort of patients, the criteria are often discordant.[7] Neither system functions well as diagnostic criteria for de novo patients, and neither uses ANCAs.[8] ANCAs are antibodies directed against cytoplasmic protein antigens in neutrophils and monocytes.[8–10] They are classified as perinuclear (pANCAs) or cytoplasmic (cANCAs) based on their immunofluorescent staining pattern on alcohol-fixed neutrophils. cANCAs are usually directed against proteinase 3 (PR3) and pANCAs against myeloperoxidase (MPO). MPO-ANCAs and PR3-ANCAs are highly specific for primary systemic vasculitides affecting small to medium-sized vessels and exhibiting few vascular immune deposits in biopsy material. There is abundant evidence that ANCAs may participate in the pathogenesis of small-vessel vasculitis.[9,10] Moreover, recent analyses have shown that ANCA specificity is a better predictor of outcome (especially relapse rate) than the clinical syndrome.[11,12] Furthermore, the first genome-wide association study of ANCA-associated vasculitides (AAV) revealed Wegener granulomatosis and MPA to be genetically distinct entities, with the genetic associations determined more by PR3 versus MPO-ANCA antigen specificity than the clinical syndrome itself.[13] A major effort is now under way to use data-driven consensus methodology to derive new classification and diagnostic criteria for the vasculitides that will highlight ANCA status and specificity, sponsored by the ACR and European League Against Rheumatism.[14]

The 2012 Revised International Chapel Hill Consensus Conference (CHCC2012) convened for the purpose of changing nomenclature for the previously defined vasculitides and adding categories of vasculitis not included in CHCC1994, given improved understanding of the vasculitides (**Fig. 1**).[15] Eponyms were phased out except for disorders with poorly understood pathogeneses. The nomenclature maintained focus on the noninfectious vasculitides, which were categorized by integrating knowledge about etiology, pathogenesis, pathology, demographics, and clinical markers. The first level of categorization was still size of predominantly involved vessels. There

---

Box 1
Classification of vasculitides associated with neuropathy

I. Primary systemic vasculitides

  1. Predominantly small-vessel vasculitis

    a. Microscopic polyangiitis[a]

    b. Eosinophilic granulomatosis with polyangiitis (EGPA) (Churg-Strauss syndrome)[a]

    c. Granulomatosis with polyangiitis (GPA) (Wegener granulomatosis)[a]

    d. Essential mixed cryoglobulinemia (non–hepatitis C virus [HCV])

    e. IgA vasculitis (Henoch-Schönlein purpura)

  2. Predominantly medium-vessel vasculitis

    a. PAN

  3. Predominantly large-vessel vasculitis

    a. GCA

II. Secondary systemic vasculitides associated with one of the following:

  1. Connective tissue diseases

    a. Rheumatoid arthritis

    b. Systemic lupus erythematosus

    c. Sjögren syndrome

    d. Systemic sclerosis

    e. Dermatomyositis

    f. Mixed connective tissue disease

  2. Sarcoidosis

  3. Behçet disease

  4. Infection (such as hepatitis B virus [HBV], HCV, HIV, cytomegalovirus [CMV], leprosy, Lyme disease, and human T-lymphotropic virus 1)

  5. Drugs

  6. Malignancy

  7. Inflammatory bowel disease

  8. Hypocomplementemic urticarial vasculitis syndrome

III. Nonsystemic/localized vasculitis

  1. NSVN

    a. Includes non–diabetic radiculoplexus neuropathy (non-DRPN)

    b. Includes some cases of Wartenberg migrant sensory neuritis

  2. DRPN

  3. Localized cutaneous/neuropathic vasculitis

    a. Cutaneous PAN

    b. Others

[a] Antineutrophil cytoplasmic antibody (ANCA)-associated vasculitides.
From Collins MP, Dyck PJ, Gronseth GS, et al. Peripheral Nerve Society guideline on the classification, diagnosis, investigation, and immunosuppressive therapy of non-systemic vasculitic neuropathy: executive summary. J Peripher Nerv Syst 2010;15:176–84; with permission.

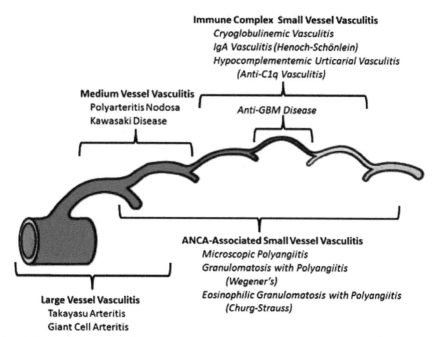

Fig. 1. Revised international CHCC2012 nomenclature of vasculitides. GBM, glomerular basement membrane. (*From* Jennette J, Falk R, Bacon P, et al. 2012 revised international Chapel Hill consensus conference nomenclature of vasculitides. Arthritis Rheum 2013;65:1; with permission.)

were no major changes in the large-vessel (GCA and Takayasu arteritis) group. PAN and Kawasaki disease were still categorized as medium-vessel vasculitides, and PAN was still restricted to cases with no microvascular involvement, but ANCAs were newly listed as an exclusionary feature for PAN. The small-vessel vasculitis category was divided into vasculitides associated with sparse versus prominent vascular wall deposits of immunoglobulin and complement. The pauci-immune group was labeled the AAV, including MPA, Wegener granulomatosis, and Churg-Strauss syndrome. Wegener was renamed GPA, whereas Churg-Strauss was renamed EGPA. Patients matching these definitions but lacking in ANCAs were designated ANCA-negative AAV. Patients with moderate to marked deposits of immunoglobulin and complement in small vessels were defined a having immune complex small-vessel vasculitis. This group included antiglomerular basement disease (Goodpasture syndrome), cryoglobulinemic vasculitis, IgA vasculitis (Henoch-Schönlein purpura), and hyopcomplementemic urticarial vasculitis or anti-C1q vasculitis. The new definition of cryoglobulinemic vasculitis emphasized PNS involvement. Neuropathies occur rarely in the other 3 immune complex vasculitides.

CHCC2012 was more expansive than CHCC1994 and included several new categories. First, Behçet disease and Cogan syndrome were labeled variable vessel vasculitides. These vasculitides affect vessels of all sizes nonpreferentially. Vasculitic neuropathies are rare in these diseases. Second, single-organ vasculitis was the consensus designation for vasculitis restricted to vessels in a single organ with no signs of an underlying systemic vasculitis. The conferees highlighted isolated CNS vasculitis, but NSVN should also be included in this group. Third, the many secondary causes of vasculitis were incorporated into vasculitis associated with systemic disease (eg, rheumatoid arthritis and lupus) and vasculitis associated with a probable etiology (eg, drug-associated, hepatitis B–associated PAN, hepatitis C–associated cryoglobulinemic vasculitis, and cancer-associated vasculitis).

Neuropathy is a common feature in both primary and secondary systemic vasculitides that affect small arteries and arterioles. The primary systemic vasculitides most likely to produce a neuropathy are EGPA, PAN, and MPA.[16–18] Of the secondary systemic vasculitides, nerves are most commonly affected in HBV-associated PAN, HCV-related cryoglobulinemic vasculitis, and rheumatoid vasculitis.[17,19,20] Alternatively, neuropathies are uncommon in GCA, unreported in Takayasu arteritis and Kawasaki disease, and rare in the noncryoglobulinemic immune complex small-vessel vasculitides. All of the systemic vasculitic neuropathies (SVNs) are accompanied by other-organ involvement. In contrast, vasculitis in NSVN is predominantly confined to the blood supply of the PNS. Most patients with NSVN do not develop systemic symptoms during follow-up, but many exhibit subclinical involvement of regional muscles and skin.[21–24]

In terms of prevalence, GCA and the primarily cutaneous vasculitides are the most common systemic vasculitides, followed by rheumatoid vasculitis, GPA, and MPA.[25,26] No study has determined the incidence or prevalence of any vasculitic neuropathy, but the relative frequency of these disorders can be derived from nerve biopsy series.[24,27,28] The 5 most common vasculitic neuropathies in these series are NSVN and those associated with PAN, MPA, rheumatoid arthritis, and EGPA. In the primary small-vessel to medium-vessel systemic vasculitides, vasculitic neuropathy is not a risk factor for death or relapse,[29–31] but it does impair quality of life.[32]

PATHOLOGY AND PATHOGENIC MECHANISMS

Nerve biopsies in patients with SVNs and NSVNs reveal changes consistent with an axonal neuropathy (**Fig. 2**), including decreased myelinated nerve fiber density, wallerian-like degeneration, and regenerating axonal clusters.[33–38] Axon loss tends to be centrofascicular in proximal watershed areas but becomes multifocal in distal nerves due to intermingling of descending fibers.[35,39,40] Peripheral nerve vasculitis affects mainly epineurial vessels with diameters of 50 μm to 300 μm.[3,22,33,34,38] NSVN tends to involve smaller vessels (<100 μm) but is not limited to the

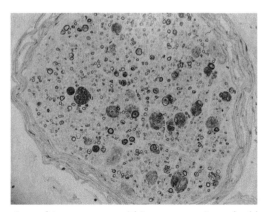

Fig. 2. Low-power view of transverse, semithin, epoxy resin–embedded, toluidine blue–stained section of sural nerve biopsy in a patient with necrotizing vasculitis showing abundant wallerian-like degeneration, a characteristic feature of active vasculitic neuropathies. (Original magnification ×20).

microvasculature.[38,41] Vasculitic lesions are characterized by epineurial T cells and macrophages invading vessel walls, producing fibrinoid necrosis and other signs of vascular damage; B cells are uncommon and natural killer cells and polymorphonuclear leukocytes rare.[38,42–44] Direct immunofluorescence shows immune deposits of IgM, fibrinogen, C3, or complement terminal membrane attack complex in epineurial vessel walls in 55% to 80% of patients.[34,36,45]

Although ANCAs seem to play a key pathogenic role in the AAV, their involvement in the pathogenesis of vasculitic neuropathies is questionable. Nerve biopsies in patients with vasculitic neuropathy only rarely reveal neutrophils, the key effector cells in AAV. In addition, whereas AAV are pauci-immune (ie, few vascular immunoglobulin and complement deposits in tissues), immune deposits are common in nerve biopsies of patients with vasculitic neuropathy.[45] Furthermore, neuropathies occur in more than 60% of patients with ANCA-negative EGPA.[46] Finally, in the most common vasculitic neuropathy – NSVN – ANCAs are rarely present.[4]

Available evidence suggests that NSVNs and most SVNs are mediated primarily by cellular mechanisms (T-cell cytotoxicity and chronic delayed–type hypersensitivity).[42–44] One analysis of patients with vasculitic neuropathy revealed many genes involved in T-cell and macrophage inflammatory responses to be differentially up-regulated.[47] Analysis of mRNA expression in nerve biopsies of patients with PAN and HCV-related cryoglobulinemia revealed a type 1 helper T-cell cytokine profile and up-regulation of chemokines and chemokine receptors involved in the migration and activation of T cells and macrophages.[48] Sural nerve biopsies in patients with vasculitic neuropathy demonstrate a marked predominance of CD4$^+$ or CD8$^+$ T cells and macrophages,[38,42,44,49] and many of the T cells express markers characteristic of cytotoxic T lymphocytes.[44,49] Antigen-presenting cells (APCs) are also increased in the epineurium and endoneurium.[42,50,51] Costimulatory molecule inducible costimulator, which is expressed preferentially by effector memory CD4$^+$/CD8$^+$ cells, is up-regulated on epineurial T cells, whereas inducible costimulator ligand is up-regulated on epineurial macrophages, suggesting that macrophages act as APCs to restimulate activated T cells.[52] These and other observations support a pathogenic model wherein autoreactive T cells are recruited to the PNS; recognize self-glycolipid or peptide antigens presented by macrophages, Schwann cells, and/or endothelial cells; undergo activation; and then mature into or recruit cytotoxic T cells that damage epineurial vessels.

Humoral mechanisms may also be operative in vasculitic neuropathy. As discussed previously, epineurial vessel walls often contain deposits of immunoglobulin and complement.[45] An analysis of differential gene expression in patients with vasculitic neuropathy revealed immunoglobulin genes to be maximally up-regulated.[47] Therefore, immune complex deposition or in situ formation with subsequent activation of complement and recruitment of phagocytes might constitute another mechanism of vascular damage in vasculitic neuropathy.

CLINICAL FINDINGS

The clinical presentation of vasculitic neuropathy depends on the distribution and severity of blood vessel involvement.[3,4,21,24,27,30,33–38,41,53–64] In primary and secondary systemic vasculitis, signs and symptoms related to renal, gastrointestinal (GI), or other-organ dysfunction usually are predominant, but neuropathy may be a heralding feature in up to 25% of patients with PAN or AAV.[65] By definition, NSVN is not accompanied by symptoms indicative of non-PNS tissue involvement, but constitutional symptoms, such as fatigue, weight loss, myalgias, and arthralgias, occur in 30% of patients and fevers in 10%.[4]

Vasculitic neuropathy, whether systemic or nonsystemic, has a characteristic clinical presentation, but SVN tends to be more severe than NSVN.[38,63] Symptoms usually develop over weeks to months, with median delay from onset to diagnosis ranging from 2 to 8 months.[21,34,36–38,55,63] Whereas some patients present fulminantly,[66] others exhibit indolent progression and are not diagnosed for years.[21,67] Most patients experience one or more acute attacks, but one-third have a chronic, slowly progressive course.[3,24,37,63] As elegantly demonstrated by Morozumi and colleagues,[40] PNS vasculitis generally affects peripheral nerves rather than anterior horn cells or sensory/autonomic ganglia. As such, most patients develop both sensory and motor deficits, but 15% have predominantly sensory symptoms due to cutaneous nerve involvement.[19] The sensory disturbance usually involves all modalities; small fiber neuropathies are only rarely vasculitic.[63] Pure motor or autonomic presentations are exceptional. Eighty percent of vasculitic neuropathies are painful.[4]

The signature phenotype is a multifocal neuropathy or multiple mononeuropathy, produced by sequential ischemic insults to individual nerves. In other patients, individual mononeuropathies overlap, yielding an asymmetric polyneuropathy. The least common and least distinctive pattern is a distal, symmetric polyneuropathy. The reported frequency of these patterns is 45% multifocal neuropathy, 35% asymmetric polyneuropathy, and 20% distal symmetric polyneuropathy, but the symmetric phenotype is rare if minor asymmetries are not discounted.[4] A patient who presents with a chronic, slowly progressive, distal, symmetric polyneuropathy for years is unlikely to be suffering from vasculitis. Certain nerves have a propensity for vasculitic involvement, probably due to their poor collateral vessel supply, but at presentation, many patients exhibit diffuse involvement of multiple nerves derived from the lumbosacral plexus.[21] The most frequently affected individual nerve is the common peroneal or peroneal division of the distal sciatic nerve.[3,21,63,68] In the arms, the ulnar nerve proximal to the elbow is most commonly involved. Cranial neuropathies occur in only 10% of patients.[21,38,63]

TYPES OF VASCULITIC NEUROPATHY
Primary Small-vessel and Medium-vessel Systemic Vasculitides

The small-vessel and medium-vessel primary systemic vasculitides are potentially life-threatening diseases characterized by vasculitic involvement of multiple organs (**Table 1**).[69] They include PAN, MPA, EGPA, GPA, IgA vasculitis, antiglomerular basement membrane disease, and hypocomplementemic urticarial vasculitis (see **Fig. 1**).[15] Their annual incidence is approximately 10 to 20 per million.[26,70] The AAVs (ie, GPA, MPA, and EGPA) share a predilection for small vessels, paucity of immune deposits in vascular lesions, and potential for rapidly progressive glomerulonephritis and pulmonary capillaritis.[71] PAN and the AAV are often accompanied by a SVN.

Polyarteritis nodosa

PAN is a systemic vasculitis that affects small and medium-sized arteries, characterized by renal arteritis (renal infarcts and hypertension), occasional hepatitis B surface antigenemia, and angiographically demonstrated visceral microaneurysms.[17,72] It has traditionally represented the most common small-vessel to medium-vessel systemic vasculitis and the most common cause of vasculitic neuropathy. Its incidence, however, as a diagnostic entity has been severely reduced by the CHCC nomenclature, which mandates that any pathologically proved microvessel involvement exclude the diagnosis, making MPA the more prevalent disease.[15] It is also excluded by pulmonary vasculitis, glomerulonephritis, cryoglobulins, or ANCAs.[15,17] PAN usually develops between the ages of 40 and 70 years.[1,17,72–74] Onset is typically subacute,

Table 1
Clinical and pathologic features of primary vasculitides associated with neuropathy

Disorder	Histopathology	Vessels Affected	Other Clinically Involved Organs (%)	Laboratory Studies (%)	PNS, CNS Changes
PAN	Necrotizing vasculitis; mixed infiltrate; sparse immune deposits	Small and medium arteries	Skin 55–60 Joints ~50 Kidneys 40–50 GI ~30 Testes 2–29 Heart 10–15 ENT—rare Lung—rare	↑ESR ~85 ↑WBC ~70 ↓Hgb ~60 ↑Platelets ~60 RF ~30 Hep B 20–30 ↓Comp ~25 ANA ~15 Hep C 5–10 ANCA <10 Angio 70 (aneurysm)	PNS 65–70 CrN <5 CNS ~5
MPA	Necrotizing vasculitis; mixed infiltrate; sparse immune deposits; LCV in skin	Arterioles, capillaries, venules, veins > small and medium arteries	Kidney 75–90 Joints 40–60 Skin 30–60 Lungs 35–50 GI 30–40 ENT 20–30 Heart 10–20 Testes—rare	↑ESR >90 ANCA 75–85 (MPO >PR3) RF 25–50 ANA 20–30 ↓Comp—rare Hep B/C (−) Angio—rare	PNS 40–50 CNS 10–15

Disease	Pathology	Vessels	Organ involvement	Laboratory	Neurologic
EGPA (Churg-Strauss syndrome)	Necrotizing vasculitis; mixed infiltrate with eosinophils; granulomas; sparse immune deposits; LCV in skin	Small and medium arteries, arterioles, capillaries, venules, veins	Lungs 100 (asthma) 40–75 (infiltrates) ENT (sinusitis, rhinitis) 60–80 Skin 50–70 GI 35–50 Joints 30–50 Heart 30–50 60 by MRI Kidney 15–30	↑Eos 100 ↑ESR ~85 ↑IgE ~75 ANCA 30–40 (MPO >PR3) RF 40–50 ANA ~10 ↓Comp—rare Hep B/C (−) Angio 30	PNS 65 CrN <5 CNS 10–15
GPA (Wegener granulomatosis)	Necrotizing vasculitis; granulomas; collagen necrosis; sparse immune deposits; LCV in skin	Small and medium arteries, arterioles, capillaries, venules, veins	ENT 90–95 Lungs 85 Kidney 60–75 Eyes 50–60 Skin 25–50 Joints 65–75 Heart 5–20 GI 5–10	ANCA 80–90 (PR3 >MPO) ↑ESR ~85 ↓Hgb ~75 ↑Platelets 55 RF 50–60 ↑WBC ~35 ANA ~25	PNS 20–25 CNS 5–10 CrN 15
IgA vasculitis (Henoch-Schönlein purpura)	LCV in skin; IgA vascular deposits	Arterioles, capillaries, venules	Skin 100 Joints 65–70 GI ~60 GN ~40 children, ~70 adults Testes ~15 Lungs—rare	↑ESR 50–60 ↑IgA ~50 ↑WBC ~50 ↑ASO 20–50 Cryos 20–25 ↓Comp 10–20 ↓Hgb 5–15 RF ~5 ANA ~5 ANCA <5	PNS—rare CNS—rare

(continued on next page)

Table 1
(continued)

Disorder	Histopathology	Vessels Affected	Other Clinically Involved Organs (%)	Laboratory Studies (%)	PNS, CNS Changes
Cryoglobulinemic vasculitis	Necrotizing vasculitis; microangiopathy; non-IgA immune deposits; LCV in skin	Small arteries, arterioles, capillaries, venules	Skin ~95 Joints 70–90 GN ~30 Salivary glands (sicca) ~30 Raynaud 25–50 GI (pain) 10–20	Hep C 80–90 ↓Comp 70–90 RF 70–90 ↑ESR ~70 ↓Hgb ~70 ANA ~55 Hep B ~5 ANCA <5 Angio—infreq	PNS ~65 CNS—rare
GCA	Necrotizing vasculitis; mononuclear infiltrate; granulomas and giant cells ~50%	Medium-large arteries	PMR ~50 Liver ~30 (abnormal LFTs) Subclavian-axillary-brachial 6–8 Aorta 15–20 Superficial femoral-popliteal 2–7 GN ~10	↑CRP 98–100 ↑ESR 85–100 ↓Hgb 55–60 ↑WBC 20–30 ANCA–rare RF (−) ANA (−) Angio—infreq	Otologic 60–90 Optic nerve 15–20 PNS ~5 CNS ~5
NSVN	Necrotizing vasculitis in epineurium/perineurium >> endoneurium; mononuclear infiltrate; immune deposits	Small arteries, arterioles, capillaries, venules	Muscle 25	↑ESR ~50 ANA ~25 ↓Hgb ~20 ↑WBC ~15 RF ~10 ↓Comp ~5	PNS 100 CNS 0

Abbreviations: Angio, abdominal angiographically-demonstrated microaneurysms; CNS, central nervous system; comp, circulating complement factors; CrN, cranial nerve involvement; cryos, cryoglobulins; ENT, upper respiratory tract involvement; Eos, eosinophils; GN, glomerulonephritis; Hep B, hepatitis B surface antigenemia; Hep C, hepatitis C antibodies or RNA; Hgb, hemoglobin; Infreq, infrequent; LCV, leukocytoclastic vasculitis; LFTs, liver function tests; PMR, polymyalgia rheumatica; WBC, white blood cell count.

characterized by emerging constitutional symptoms over weeks to months. Fevers and weight loss occur in 60% to 70% of patients. The most commonly affected tissues are the PNS, joints, skin, kidneys, muscles, GI tract, and testes. Neuropathies occur in 60% to 70% of patients.[17,75] Cranial neuropathies are uncommon. Up to 28% of patients relapse.[17] Death most commonly ensues from mesenteric vasculitis.

Laboratory studies in PAN reveal a highly elevated erythrocyte sedimentation rate (ESR), leukocytosis, anemia, and thrombocytosis. Antinuclear antibodies (ANAs), rheumatoid factors (RFs), and hypocomplementemia occur uncommonly. Visceral angiography shows microaneurysms in renal, hepatic, and mesenteric arteries in two-thirds of patients and nonspecific occlusive changes in 98%.[76] Pathologically, PAN is a focal, segmental, necrotizing vasculitis of small and medium-sized arteries. Granulomas and eosinophilic infiltrates are rarely observed.

Microscopic polyangiitis
MPA is a microscopic form of PAN that primarily affects arterioles, capillaries, and venules.[16,71,77–81] In contrast to GPA and EGPA, there are no granulomas. Unlike the immune complex vasculitides, immune deposits are inconspicuous. The annual incidence of MPA in Europe ranges from 3 to 10 per million.[70] The mean or median age at diagnosis ranges from 60 to 71 years.[82,83] Clinically, MPA is similar to PAN, but distinguishing features include rapidly progressive glomerulonephritis in approximately 80% of patients, occasional pulmonary involvement (20% with alveolar hemorrhage), ANCAs, and the absence of hepatitis B surface antigenemia and visceral aneurysms. MPO-pANCAs are positive in 50% to 70% of patients and PR3-cANCAs in another 20% to 30%.[8,9] The reported incidence of neuropathy in MPA is highly variable but averages approximately 45% in recent series.[16,60,79,81,84,85] MPA relapses in about one-third of patients.[86] Death ensues most commonly from renal failure, pulmonary hemorrhage, or infection.

Eosinophilic granulomatosis with polyangiitis (Churg-Strauss syndrome)
EGPA is another AAV, but ANCAs only occur in 30% to 40% of patients (usually anti–MPO-pANCAs).[18,71,87–93] Its salient histopathologic alterations are (1) eosinophilic tissue infiltration, (2) extravascular granulomas, and (3) vasculitis.[87] The Lanham clinical diagnostic criteria require (1) asthma, (2) eosinophilia (>1500/mm³), and (3) vasculitis involving 2 or more nonpulmonary sites.[87] EGPA develops at a younger age than MPA, with a mean age at diagnosis of 48 to 52 years.[88–90,92,93] EGPA is the least common AAV with annual incidence rates of 1 to 3 per million.[70] The disease usually begins with atopic manifestations, such as asthma and allergic rhinosinusitis, and later transitions into peripheral blood eosinophilia with eosinophilic tissue infiltration (eg, eosinophilic pneumonia). The third phase is characterized by systemic vasculitis, which is typically delayed 5 to 10 years from the onset of asthma. Clinical features distinguishing EGPA from PAN are (1) asthma (100% of patients); (2) pulmonary infiltrates (50%–75%); (3) allergic rhinosinusitis (60%–80%); (4) glomerulonephritis (15%–30%); and (5) congestive heart failure (25%). In contrast to GPA and MPA, EGPA-related glomerulonephritis only rarely leads to renal failure. Neuropathy develops in 65% of patients,[60,87–94] but cranial neuropathies are uncommon (<5%).[92] Relapses occur in 25% to 30% of patients.[92,93] Up to 50% of deaths are caused by congestive heart failure.[87]

Elevated ESR, leukocytosis, anemia, increased IgE levels, and RFs are characteristic laboratory features.[18,71,87,92] ANAs, hypocomplementemia, and cryoglobulinemia are rarely present. There is no association with hepatitis B or hepatitis C. Visceral angiograms reveal microaneurysms in 30%.[18] Nerve biopsy reveals necrotizing vasculitis in 30% of biopsies, eosinophilic infiltrates in 35%, and granulomas in 10%.[54,59,95,96]

Granulomatosis with polyangiitis (Wegener granulomatosis)

GPA, the third AAV, is defined by the pathologic triad of granulomatous inflammation, necrosis, and vasculitis predominating in the lungs and kidneys.[71,97–100] Vasculitis affects the microvasculature and small to medium-sized arteries and veins. GPA can present at any age but is rare before adolescence; the mean/median age at diagnosis ranges from 50 to 68 years.[82,83] The annual incidence in Europe ranges from 2 to 11 per million.[70] GPA usually begins with a localized phase, characterized by granulomatous inflammation in the respiratory tracts, leading to chronic sinusitis, bloody or purulent nasal drainage, nasal ulceration, nasoseptal perforation, otitis media, saddle nose deformity, and conductive hearing loss.[101] The generalized, vasculitic phase is heralded by constitutional symptoms. Primary vasculitic involvement occurs in the upper respiratory tract, lungs, glomeruli, and eyes. Renal disease may smolder or progress to end-stage failure in 10% to 20%.[99] Neuropathies develop in 20% to 25% of patients.[79,85,97,100,102–105] Cranial neuropathies are more common than in the other AAV, occurring in about 15%.[30,85,103] GPA has the highest relapse rate of the AAV, averaging 50%.[71,97,100] Infections and vasculitis of the kidneys or lungs are the usual causes of death.[97,98,106]

Common laboratory abnormalities include elevated ESR, anemia, thrombocytosis, and RFs. In patients with active, generalized disease, PR3-cANCAs occur in 70% to 80% of patients, whereas MPO-pANCAs are found in 10% to 15%. ANCA positivity drops to 40% to 60% in those with inactive or limited disease.[8,71,101] The diagnostic yield of head, neck, and transbronchial biopsies is low.[107] Open lung biopsies are the most reliable method of diagnosis, yielding vasculitis, necrosis, and granulomas in 90% of specimens.[108]

Predominant Large-vessel Primary Systemic Vasculitides

Giant cell arteritis

GCA is a granulomatous vasculitis involving medium and large arteries, especially branches of the aortic arch and extracranial carotid arteries.[109,110] It almost always develops after age 50. Incidence peaks in the 8th decade.[111] It is the most common primary vasculitis in adults in the United States and Europe, with annual incidence rates of 17 to 29 per 100,000 adults 50 years or age and older[111]; 70% to 80% of patients are women. Typical symptoms are headache, weight loss, fever, jaw claudication, and polymyalgia rheumatica. Vestibular dysfunction occurs in approximately 90% of patients, hearing loss in 60%, and permanent visual loss from acute ischemic optic neuropathy in 15% to 20%.[112] Focal/multifocal neuropathies suspicious for vasculitis occur in only 6% of patients, most commonly involving the distal median nerve, C5/6 nerve roots, or upper brachial plexus.[113–117] Vasculitic neuropathy generally results from larger nutrient artery vasculitis.[113,114] The disease runs a self-limited course, but relapses occur in 40% to 50% of patients, and median duration of treatment is 2 years.[118,119]

ESR and C-reactive protein (CRP) are almost always elevated.[120,121] Interleukin (IL)-6 is another sensitive marker of disease activity.[122] Ultrasonography of the temporal arteries can reveal a characteristic halo sign (dark, hypoechoic, circumferential thickening around the lumen, indicative of edema).[123] Superficial temporal artery biopsy showing granulomatous inflammation, infiltration of macrophages and T cells, and disruption of the internal elastic lamina remains the gold standard for diagnosis.[109]

Secondary Systemic Vasculitides Associated with Neuropathy

Secondary systemic vasculitides are caused by infections, drug, toxins, and diseases predisposing to autoimmune manifestations, such as CTDs, mixed cryoglobulinemia, sarcoidosis, inflammatory bowel diseases, and cancers. Vasculitic neuropathies are estimated to occur in approximately 10% of patients with rheumatoid arthritis, 3% to 4% of those with primary Sjögren syndrome, 2% to 3% of patients with systemic lupus erythematosus, and less than 1% of patients with systemic sclerosis.[19] Apart from a brief discussion of 2 infectious vasculitides commonly associated with neuropathy, review of the remaining causes of a secondary vasculitic neuropathy is beyond the scope of this review.

Virtually any infection can act as an antigenic stimulus for the formation of circulating immune complexes that then induce vasculitis.[124,125] Organisms can also produce vasculitis by direct vascular invasion, release of vascular toxins or toxins acting as superantigens, induction of immune responses against vascular autoantigens via molecular mimicry, or altered immunoregulation. The only organisms known to produce vasculitic neuropathy by direct cytopathic infection of endothelial cells are CMV and varicella zoster virus (VZV).[126,127] Vasculitis associated with bacterial infections only rarely involves the PNS, the primary exception being Lyme disease.[128] Viruses with persistent replication, such as HBV, HCV, HIV, and parvovirus B19 (PB19), have the strongest association with vasculitis and vasculitic neuropathies.[124,125,129,130]

A well-characterized infectious vasculitis is HBV-associated PAN, in which immune complex deposition seems to be the primary mechanism.[124,125,131] Circulating hepatitis B surface antigen is found in 10% to 55% of patients with PAN; conversely, PAN occurs in 1% to 5% of patients with chronic hepatitis B.[132] The clinical features are similar to those in idiopathic PAN, although HBV-related PAN has less frequent cutaneous manifestations and more frequent neuropathy (85%), hypertension, orchitis, and abdominal pain than those with idiopathic PAN.[17] Vasculitis usually develops in the early stages of the HBV infection (first 6 months) and follows a self-limited (but sometimes fatal) course. Relapses are uncommon (10%).[17]

Chronic HCV infection can produce a mixed cryoglobulinic vasculitis.[20,133,134] Cryoglobulins are circulating immunoglobulins that precipitate when cooled below 37°C. Mixed cryoglobulins consist of monoclonal or polyclonal IgM RFs and polyclonal IgG. They can be associated with chronic infections, CTDs, or lymphoproliferative disorders. Most patients with cryoglobulinemia are asymptomatic. The term, *mixed cryoglobulinemic vasculitis*, is reserved for patients with symptoms. Chronic HCV infection accounts for 80% to 90% of otherwise unexplained cases of mixed cryoglobulinemic vasculitis.[20,134] Mixed cryoglobulinemia occurs in 50% of patients with chronic HCV infection, but only 15% develop symptomatic disease, typically many years after the initial infection.[46] Cryoglobulins damage tissues by inducing immune complex-mediated, complement-dependent inflammation of small blood vessels.[134] The clinical syndrome is characterized by palpable purpura, skin ulceration, arthralgias, sicca symptoms, Raynaud phenomenon, neuropathy, glomerulonephritis, and adenopathy. RFs occur in 85% of patients and hypocomplementemia in 70%.[133] The incidence of polyneuropathy in patients with chronic hepatitis C is approximately 10%.[135,136] In patients with HCV-related cryoglobulinemic vasculitis, approximately 65% develop a neuropathy by clinical criteria and 80% by electrodiagnostic findings.[46] Most neuropathies are distal, slowly progressive, and sensory-predominant. Symmetric presentations are as prevalent as asymmetric/multifocal ones. Approximately 50% of neuropathies are painful. Electrodiagnostic studies and nerve biopsies reveal a predominantly axonal process. Biopsies show epineurial perivascular mononuclear inflammation with definite vasculitis in 50%.[46]

Single-Organ Vasculitides

Nonsystemic vasculitic neuropathy

NSVN is the most common PNS vasculitis.[28] Eight large series of NSVN patients have been reported since 1987.[3,21,24,33,36,38,41,63] The diagnosis has generally depended on nerve biopsy evidence of definite or probable vasculitis accompanied by no clinical evidence of systemic involvement despite long-term follow-up. Some groups have found muscle vasculitis in patients with otherwise typical NSVN.[21,22,24,33] A Peripheral Nerve Society guideline group recently derived consensus diagnostic criteria for NSVN.[4] Patients are first required to have pathologically definite or clinically probable vasculitic neuropathy. They are then evaluated for signs, symptoms, or laboratory findings indicative of a systemic vasculitis, which, if present, exclude the diagnosis. Exclusionary features are clinical or laboratory evidence of other-organ involvement, visceral aneurysms, MPO/PR3-ANCAs, ESR greater than or equal to 100 mm/h, cryoglobulins, pathologic evidence of vasculitis in nonneuromuscular tissues, underlying infection, and medical condition/drug predisposing to vasculitis. Constitutional symptoms, diabetes mellitus, and muscle vasculitis are still compatible with NSVN. Recent evidence suggests that NSVN can be associated with subclinical inflammation in adjacent cutaneous tissues that sometimes progresses to vasculitis.[21,23,67,137,138]

NSVN variants/subtypes

Several clinical syndromes described by other names represent variants or subtypes of NSVN.[4] One variant is DRPN, a unique syndrome that occurs in 1% of diabetics, especially men with type 2 diabetes.[139–144] The disease usually commences with acute pain in the hip/thigh, with weakness emerging days to weeks later. Proximal lower limb is more commonly affected than distal, but symptoms generally spread to other segments of the same limb, involving more than nerve. Pain and weakness usually begin unilaterally and spread contralaterally in 80% to 90%. Most patients lose weight. Upper limb involvement occurs in approximately 10%. Laboratory work-up reveals elevated spinal fluid protein in 85%. Symptoms typically progress over several weeks to months and then slowly improve over 1 to 2 years, but 10% to 15% of patients relapse. Nerve biopsies reveal lymphocytic perivascular inflammation involving epineurial and, to a lesser extent, endoneurial microvessels, accompanied by changes suggestive of vasculitis (eg, asymmetric fiber loss, neovascularization, hemosiderin deposition, focal perineural thickening, and complement deposition in vessel walls).[140–144] Necrotizing vasculitis is rare. These findings suggest that DRPN is a PNS microvasculitis, characterized by proximal lower limb involvement and self-limited course. An analogous syndrome is nondiabetic lumbosacral radiculoplexus neuropathy, a proximal subtype of NSVN.[55]

A painless form of DRPN has also been described with slower progression, increased symmetry, greater upper limb involvement (75%), and distal predominance (55%).[145] Upper limb involvement in painful lumbosacral DRPN has been recognized for years, but the existence of a less common cervical variant of DRPN manifesting with pure, predominant, or initial upper limb involvement was recently highlighted.[146] The clinical, laboratory, electrodiagnostic, and pathologic features of these patients are similar to those of lumbosacral DRPN. All of the diabetic radiculoneuropathies seem to be caused by PNS microvasculitis.

Another recent addition to the list of NSVN subtypes is postsurgical inflammatory neuropathy.[147] This a self-limited, monophasic, acute, focal or multifocal, painful neuropathy affecting the lower limbs more commonly than upper limbs that emerges within 30 days of a surgical procedure in which no trauma to the nerves is documented. Nerve biopsies show changes analogous to DRPN (ie, epineurial lymphocytic perivascular inflammation, infiltration of small vessels, infrequent true microvasculitis [vessel wall damage], and pathologic correlates of ischemic nerve injury).

Wartenberg migrant sensory neuritis is defined by episodic, migratory attacks of purely sensory symptoms in the distribution of individual cutaneous nerves.[148–152] Transient pain and tingling is followed by persistent sensory loss. Limb nerves are routinely affected, but in 30% to 40% of patients, the trigeminal or truncal nerves are also involved.[152] Symptoms typically remit after 6 weeks to several months, but, infrequently, numbness persists indefinitely. The clinical course is benign but can extend over years. Nerve biopsy findings suggest that some patients with this phenotype have a benign, purely sensory form of NSVN.[149–151,153]

DIAGNOSTIC MODALITIES

The important first step in diagnosis is to recognize the clinical pattern as one compatible with a vasculitic neuropathy. Acute or subacute multifocal neuropathies are straightforward, but vasculitis should also be considered in patients with slowly progressive, sensory-motor, or sensory polyneuropathies, especially if painful, distal predominant, and asymmetric.

Laboratory Studies

Laboratory evaluation of suspected vasculitic neuropathy routinely includes a complete blood cell count (CBC), metabolic panel, urinalysis, ESR, CRP, ANA, ANCAs, RF, angiotensin-converting enzyme, serum protein immunofixation electrophoresis, glucose tolerance test and/or glycosylated hemoglobin, cryoglobulins, complement, hepatitis B surface antigen, hepatitis C antibodies, and chest radiograph.[4] Testing for other inflammatory, genetic, or infectious disorders (eg, HIV, PB19, CMV, VZV, Lyme disease, porphyria, and transthyretin amyloidosis) should be considered in select cases. Vascular endothelial growth factor (VEGF) and β_2-microglobulin levels might also be predictive of biopsy-confirmed vasculitic neuropathy.[154,155] In NSVN, a mildly to moderately elevated ESR is found in 50% of patients, but severe elevation (>100 mm/h) is concerning for a systemic condition.[4] ANAs occur in 25% of patients with NSVN. Approximately 20% of patients are anemic and 15% have leukocytosis. RFs and hypocomplementemia occur in less than 10%.[24,28,64] ANCAs are rare and, if present, exclude the diagnosis.[4] For patients with SVN, laboratory abnormalities are more common: elevated ESR 85%, leukocytosis 75%, anemia 45% to 50%, RFs 45%, decreased complement 30%, and ANAs 30%.[19] Spinal fluid examination is not usually helpful because CSF pleocytosis is uncommon (5%) and mild-to-moderate CSF protein elevation occurs in only 30% of patients with both NSVN and SVN,[19] but lumbar puncture should be considered in patients with (1) proximal signs and symptoms suggestive of root involvement; (2) electrodiagnostic evidence of demyelinating or mixed axonal/demyelinating features; or (3) clinically suspected sarcoidosis, cancer, or meningeal infection.[4]

Electrodiagnostic Testing

Electromyography and nerve conduction studies help to define the distribution of nerve involvement (focal, multifocal, or length dependent), identify involved functional modalities (sensory and/or motor), characterize the probable nerve pathology (axon loss vs demyelination), and select an appropriate nerve to biopsy.[62,156] Nerve conduction studies in vasculitic neuropathy usually demonstrate reduced sensory and motor amplitudes with normal or mildly reduced conduction velocities, indicative of axon loss. H reflexes and F waves are often impersistent with normal or mildly prolonged latencies.

Needle electromyography demonstrates active denervation (fibrillation potentials) in approximately 70% of patients, decreased recruitment in clinically weak muscles, and motor unit potential remodeling consistent with chronic reinnervation in those with sufficiently longstanding disease or preexisting neurogenic disorders.[4] Findings of axon loss in an asymmetric pattern or in the distribution of multiple nerves are supportive of a vasculitic neuropathy.[62] Conversely, symmetric findings reduce the likelihood of vasculitis. "Pseudo" or "axon noncontinuity" conduction blocks occur in approximately 15% of patients, resulting from ongoing, ischemia-induced, wallerian-like degeneration.[3,21,58,63] If nerve conductions are repeated in 2 weeks, pseudo-conduction blocks disappear due to degeneration of the distal stumps.[157] True demyelinating partial motor conduction blocks are rare.[158] Significantly reduced conduction velocities or other findings of demyelination, such as abnormal temporal dispersion or persistent conduction block, should prompt clinicians to look for an alternative diagnosis, such as Lewis-Sumner syndrome.

Nerve Biopsy and Pathologic Diagnosis

Because of the serious risks associated with long-term immunosuppressive therapy, nerve biopsy for definitive diagnosis is crucial to the evaluation of a patient with suspected vasculitic neuropathy. One possible exception is a patient with an established diagnosis of systemic vasculitis who develops a multifocal neuropathy, with the understanding that vasculitis is only one of many causes of a multiple mononeuropathy. Alternatively, not all patients with an idiopathic axonal neuropathy require nerve biopsy for vasculitis. In patients with an unexplained, chronic, distal, symmetric polyneuropathy, the yield of nerve biopsy for definite vasculitis is only 4%, contrasting with approximately 20% in patients with a phenotype more typical of vasculitis.[53,156,159–161] This low yield must be weighed against the risks of permanent sensory loss, post-biopsy pain, delayed wound healing, and wound infection. The likelihood of identifying vasculitis is enhanced if a patient has an asymmetric/multifocal neuropathy,[43,62,155,159] acute-onset,[155] subacutely progressive clinical course,[162] ANCAs,[163] elevated ESR/CRP,[155,162] elevated β_2-microglobulin,[155] or increased VEGF.[154]

Commonly biopsied nerves are the sural, superficial peroneal, and superficial radial, but clinical and electrodiagnostic examinations should guide the selection of biopsy site. Superficial peroneal nerve biopsy is usually combined with a peroneus brevis muscle biopsy, using a single incision in the distal lateral leg.[24,33,37] Sural nerve biopsy can be combined with a gastrocnemius, anterior tibialis, or quadriceps muscle biopsy.[56,63,156] Although nerve is more commonly diagnostic than muscle in cases of vasculitic neuropathy, especially NSVN, concomitant muscle biopsy may reveal vasculitis not found in the nerve biopsy due to sampling error. One meta-analysis showed that muscle biopsy increased the yield for definite vasculitis by 15% in patients with a final diagnosis of vasculitic neuropathy.[164] In the only study, however, in which a proximal muscle was biopsied (quadriceps), yield was not increased, suggesting that this conclusion pertains only to distal leg muscles.[63] In patients with NSVN, biopsies of distal leg muscles (peroneus brevis muscle, gastrocnemius, and anterior tibialis) have revealed definite vasculitis in 25% of patients.[21,22,24,58]

A histologic diagnosis of definite vasculitic neuropathy requires inflammation within the vessel wall and signs of active or chronic vascular damage (**Fig. 3**).[4] Perivascular or mural inflammation alone is nonspecific. A diagnosis of pathologically probable vasculitic neuropathy can be made if (1) perivascular inflammation occurs in combination with signs of vascular damage or (2) perivascular/vascular inflammation unassociated with vascular injury is accompanied by one or more changes predictive of definite vasculitis (ie, vascular immune deposits of IgM, complement, or fibrinogen by direct

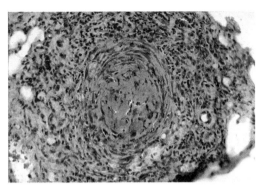

Fig. 3. High-power view of a frozen cross section of nerve biopsy showing definite vasculitis involving an epineurial arteriole with luminal occlusion, intimal destruction, fibrinoid necrosis, relatively preserved tunica media, and surrounding intense mononuclear inflammatory infiltrate (hematoxylin and eosin). (Original magnification ×40).

immunofluorescence; prominent wallerian-like degeneration; asymmetric nerve fiber loss; hemosiderin deposits; or myofiber necrosis in peroneus brevis muscle biopsy) (see **Fig. 2**; **Fig. 4**).[24,37,45,162,165,166] Focal perineurial damage, injury neuroma with microfasciculation, endoneurial hemorrhage, neovascularization, and experimentally demonstrated axonal changes typical of acute ischemia are also suggestive features but their specificity for vasculitis is not established (**Fig. 5**).[22,35,39,144] The Peripheral Nerve Society guideline on NSVN includes consensus diagnostic criteria for pathologically definite and probable vasculitic neuropathy (**Boxes 2** and **3**).[4]

In the absence of an independent gold standard, the true sensitivity of nerve or nerve/muscle biopsy for vasculitic neuropathy cannot be determined. In patients lacking nerve biopsy evidence of definite vasculitis, however, clinically probable vasculitic neuropathy can be diagnosed by resort to clinical and pathologic criteria (eg, consensus criteria found in Peripheral Nerve Society guideline on NSVN).[4]

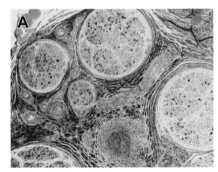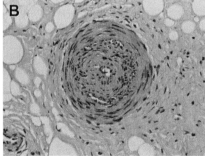

Fig. 4. (*A*) Low-power view of cross-section through epoxy resin–embedded, toluidine blue–stained nerve biopsy in patient with necrotizing vasculitis showing variation in myelinated nerve fiber density between and within fascicles. This finding is supportive of vasculitis in biopsies lacking manifest necrotizing vasculitis. (Original magnification ×10). (*B*) Transverse section through paraffin-embedded sural nerve biopsy stained with hematoxylin-eosin in a patient with probable vasculitic neuropathy demonstrating small epineurial arteriole featuring intimal proliferation and recanalized thrombus without inflammation. Perivascular inflammation was noted elsewhere in the biopsy. (Original magnification ×40).

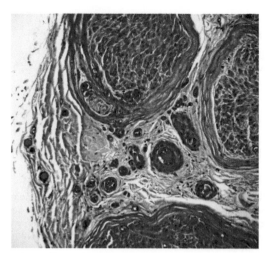

Fig. 5. Cross-section of paraffin-embedded superficial peroneal nerve biopsy in patient with probable NSVN europathy showing fascicle with focal perineurial thickening associated with mild microfasciculation and neovascularization extending from subperineurial endoneurium through perineurium into adjacent epineurium (hematoxylin-eosin). (Original magnification ×20).

Assuming these clinically or pathologically probable cases truly have vasculitic neuropathy, estimated diagnostic sensitivities can be derived. By combining data from multiple studies, the estimated sensitivity for a finding of definite vasculitis in sural nerve biopsy alone is 50% to 55%,[21,36,38,56,57,61,63,95,156] whereas that for combined superficial peroneal nerve/peroneus brevis muscle or sural nerve/distal leg muscle biopsy is approximately 60%.[21,22,24,27,37,53,56,62,92] A nerve or nerve/muscle biopsy finding of definite vasculitis is more common in SVN than NSVN.[3,22,24,38,63]

DIAGNOSTIC DILEMMAS

The differential diagnosis of vasculitic neuropathy includes other etiologies for a sensory-motor or sensory asymmetric/multifocal neuropathy. Among the many conditions to be considered are multifocal acquired sensory and motor demyelinating neuropathy (Lewis-Sumner syndrome), neuralgic amyotrophy, sarcoidosis, chronic graft-versus-host disease, sensory perineuritis, paraneoplastic or primary Sjögren syndrome-associated sensory neuronopathy, paraneoplastic asymmetric sensory-motor neuropathies or polyradiculoneuropathies, Lyme disease, leprosy, VZV infection, HIV infection (complicated by diffuse infiltrative lymphomatosis syndrome or CMV infection of the PNS), hereditary neuropathy with liability to pressure palsies (HNPP), non–HNPP–related multiple nerve entrapments, porphyria, primary or familial amyloidosis, mitochondrial disorders, motor neuron disease with sensory involvement, neoplastic meningitis or PNS infiltration, and intraneural hemorrhage.

For patients with pathologic evidence of definite/probable vasculitic neuropathy, the differential diagnosis includes all conditions associated with vasculitis of the PNS (eg, DRPN, the primary systemic vasculitides, cutaneous PAN, CTDs [especially rheumatoid arthritis], hepatitis B, hepatitis C, HIV infection, CMV infection, VZV infection, human T-lymphotropic virus 1, erythema nodosum leprosum, mixed cryoglobulinemia, sarcoidosis, cancers, and—rarely—other infections or drugs) (see **Box 1**). Diagnosis of a systemic vasculitis syndrome relies on recognition of the characteristic

---

Box 2

Diagnostic criteria for pathologically definite vasculitic neuropathy[a]

Active lesion: nerve biopsy showing collection of inflammatory cells in vessel wall AND one or more signs of acute vascular damage:

1. Fibrinoid necrosis

2. Loss/disruption of endothelium

3. Loss/fragmentation of internal elastic lamina

4. Loss/fragmentation of smooth muscle cells in media (can be highlighted with anti–smooth muscle actin staining)

5. Acute thrombosis

6. Vascular/perivascular hemorrhage

OR

7. Leukocytoclasia

Chronic lesion with signs of healing/repair: nerve biopsy showing collection of mononuclear inflammatory cells in vessel wall AND one or more signs of chronic vascular damage with repair:

1. Intimal hyperplasia

2. Fibrosis of media

3. Adventitial/periadventitial fibrosis

OR

4. Chronic thrombosis with recanalization

No evidence of another primary disease process that can mimic vasculitis pathologically, such as lymphoma, lymphomatoid granulomatosis, or amyloidosis.

[a] Presence of a chronic lesion does not exclude active vasculitis (vasculitides are usually segmental and multifocal, producing lesions of different ages in the same tissue or end-organ).
  From Collins MP, Dyck PJ, Gronseth GS, et al. Peripheral Nerve Society guideline on the classification, diagnosis, investigation, and immunosuppressive therapy of non-systemic vasculitic neuropathy: executive summary. Peripher Nerv Syst 2010;15:176–84; with permission.

---

clinical, laboratory, and pathologic features of the disease. Key factors include the spectrum of clinical involvement, presence or absence of ANCAs, autoantibodies associated with CTDs, granulomatous inflammation, and vascular immune deposits.

The differential diagnosis for a rapidly progressive, symmetric, axonal, sensory-motor, or sensory presentation of vasculitis includes but is not limited to the acute inflammatory demyelinating, acute sensory, and acute motor-sensory axonal variants of Guillain-Barré syndrome; critical illness neuropathy; acute alcohol-nutritional deficiency neuropathies; other causes of nutritional deficiency, such as inadequate dietary intake, repeated vomiting after gastric reduction surgery, other GI disorders, beriberi, and emesis gravidarum; acute exposures to certain drugs or toxins; the acute painful diabetic neuropathy; and high-grade neoplastic infiltrative neuropathies.

MANAGEMENT

Treatment of vasculitis begins with a search for precipitating factors, such as drugs, infections, or cancers. If found, the triggering condition is eliminated or treated. No inciting antigen can be identified in most vasculitides, however, necessitating the use of nonspecific immunomodulation.

Box 3
Diagnostic criteria for pathologically probable vasculitic neuropathy

I. Pathologically probable vasculitic neuropathy

1. Pathologic criteria for definite vasculitic neuropathy not satisfied (see **Box 2**)

   AND

2. Predominantly axonal changes

   AND

3. Perivascular inflammation accompanied by signs of active or chronic vascular damage (as defined in **Box 2**) OR perivascular/vascular inflammation plus at least one additional class II or III pathologic predictor of definite vasculitic neuropathy:[a]

   a. Vascular deposition of complement, IgM, or fibrinogen by direct immunofluorescence

   b. Hemosiderin deposits (Perls stain for iron)

   c. Asymmetric nerve fiber loss or degeneration

   d. Prominent active axonal degeneration or

   e. Myofiber necrosis, regeneration, or infarcts in peroneus brevis muscle biopsy (not explained by underlying myopathy)

[a] Additional alterations used by some authorities as supportive of vasculitis but lacking in adequate evidence (more study required):

1. Neovascularization (class II/III evidence suggests that this finding is probably not a predictor of vasculitis)

2. Endoneurial purpura (one negative class II study; one positive class III study)

3. Focal perineurial inflammation, degeneration, thickening (only class IV evidence)

4. Injury neuroma, microfasciculation (only class IV evidence) and

5. Swollen axons filled with organelles (one negative but nonconvincing class II study) and other experimentally demonstrated axonal changes of acute ischemia, such as attenuated axons, flattened myelin profiles, tubular profiles, and axonal cytolysis.

From Collins MP, Dyck PJ, Gronseth GS, et al. Peripheral Nerve Society guideline on the classification, diagnosis, investigation, and immunosuppressive therapy of non-systemic vasculitic neuropathy: executive summary. J Peripher Nerv Syst 2010;15:176–84; with permission.

Goals

Vasculitic neuropathy is associated with axon loss. Despite aggressive immunomodulatory treatment, reinnervation and clinical recovery of sensory and motor function are typically slow and may be incomplete in severely affected nerves. The short-term goal of therapy is thus to stabilize (not reverse) preexisting deficits and prevent the development of new PNS lesions. During the initial weeks of therapy, caution must be exercised to avoid overtreatment if ongoing disease activity is not apparent. The long-term goal of therapy (ie, approximately 6 months) is to achieve an improvement in the pretreatment neurologic deficits, understanding that complete recovery from any severe axonal neuropathy is uncommon.

Pharmacologic Strategies: Infectious Vasculitides

Antigen removal is especially important for vasculitides caused by a chronic viral infection because immunosuppressive therapy may worsen the underlying infection.[124] An infectious diseases consultant or hepatologist should always direct therapy in these patients. Concerning HBV-related PAN, many studies have shown that CS therapy in patients with chronic hepatitis B activates viral replication, increases HBV-DNA viremia, amplifies expression of HBV genome and gene products, predisposes to chronic active hepatitis, and accelerates hepatic damage.[124,167,168] The cornerstone of treatment of HBV-PAN involves antiviral agents, with the understanding that complete eradication of HBV in chronically infected patients is rarely possible. Instead, therapeutic efficacy is gauged by normalization of transaminases, sustained suppression of serum HBV-DNA, hepatitis B e antigen seroconversion, and improved liver histology.[169] Currently approved treatments for chronic hepatitis B include standard interferon-α, pegylated interferon-α, and 5 oral nucleoside/nucleotide analogs (lamivudine, adefivor, entecavir, telbivudine, and tenofovir).[169,170] In a protocol designed by the French Vasculitis Study Group, patients with HBV-related PAN are treated with antiviral agents, plasma exchanges (PE) to remove circulating immune complexes, and a 2-week course of CS to control severe disease manifestations.[124,131] This protocol induces complete remission in 80% to 90% of patients, with a 50% hepatitis B e antigen seroconversion rate. There are no data on pegylated interferon-α or the newer nucleos(t)ide analogs for HBV-PAN, apart from a few case reports documenting responses to entecavir.[171]

Antiviral therapy (pegylated interferon-α and ribavirin) has also been successfully applied to HCV-related mixed cryglobulinemia,[46,134] but rituximab, a humanized murine monoclonal antibody against CD20 that selectively depletes B cells, may be more effective in patients with severe cryoglobulinemic vasculitis.[172,173] For mild HCV-related cryglobulinemic neuropathies, antiviral therapy alone should be instituted, but for more severe neuropathies, rituximab combined with antiviral therapy is emerging as a regimen of choice.[46] Vasculitis associated with HIV infection may arise from HIV infection of the vessel wall, immune complex deposition, altered immune responses, or opportunistic agents, such as CMV.[130] For CMV-related vasculitic neuropathy, treatment is directed at the CMV infection, using ganciclovir, valganciclovir, foscarnet, or cidofovir.[174] For non–CMV-related vasculitis, treatment patterned after that in HBV-associated PAN has been proposed, using antiviral therapy combined with PE, but the mainstay of treatment is still prednisone.[75,130]

Pharmacologic Strategies: Noninfectious Vasculitides

Primary small-vessel/medium-vessel systemic vasculitides

Treatment recommendations for the primary small-vessel to medium-vessel systemic vasculitides (PAN, MPA, EGPA, and GPA) are derived from studies compared with natural history controls, retrospective cohort surveys, open randomized controlled trials (RCTs), and a few blinded RCTs.[175] The standard immunosuppressive regimen consists of CS combined with cyclophosphamide (CYC).[176] Prednisone is started at 1.0 mg/kg/d for 2 to 4 weeks, tapered to 60 mg every other day over 1 to 2 months, and then tapered more gradually over 12 months. CYC is used at a dose of 2 mg/kg/d continued for 1 year after complete remission and then tapered by 25 mg every 2 to 3 months. Although effective in inducing remission in most vasculitides, long-term follow-up studies revealed standard therapy-treated GPA to be a chronic, relapsing disease with considerable drug-related morbidity, including a 33-fold increase in bladder cancers and 11-fold increase in lymphomas.[97,98]

These and other studies have provided impetus to more rapidly taper CS and reduce patient exposure to CYC by replacing CYC in the induction phase for patients with non-severe disease or using non–CYC-based maintenance regimens for patients with severe disease.[175,177,178] As proposed in 2 consensus guidelines on treatment of systemic small-vessel to medium-vessel vasculitides, patients with localized or mild, generalized disease characterized by no organ-threatening manifestations should be treated with high-dose CS and methotrexate (MTX) 15 mg/wk to 25 mg/wk, with the caveat that induction therapy with MTX is associated with a higher relapse rate than CYC.[177–179] Prednisone is started at 1.0 mg/kg/d for 1 month, tapered to 10 mg/d by 6 months, and then stopped or continued at 5.0 mg to 7.5 mg daily. A meta-analysis concluded that continuation of low-dose CS might reduce relapses.[180] MTX is stopped after 18 to 24 months. Patients with moderate-to-severe, generalized disease characterized by poor prognostic factors or threatened organ involvement (including progressive neuropathies) are treated with CYC and CS. CYC is administered orally at 2.0 mg/kg/d or in intravenous (IV) pulses (eg, 15 mg/kg or 0.60–0.70 g/m^2 every 2–3 weeks). The dose is reduced in the elderly and those with chronic kidney disease. CYC is stopped once the patient remits, generally in 3 to 6 months, replaced by an agent to maintain remission, usually azathioprine (AZA), 1.5 mg/kg/d to 2.0 mg/kg/d, or MTX, 20 mg/wk to 25 mg/wk. In an open RCT, mycophenolate mofetil (MMF) was inferior to AZA in preventing relapses in AAV.[181] Maintenance therapy is continued for at least 18 to 24 months. In patients with severe renal disease (creatinine >5.6 mg/dL) or alveolar hemorrhage, CS/CYC is augmented with PE.[182]

Since these consensus guidelines were published, 2 RCTs comparing rituximab plus CS to CYC plus CS in AAV showed that rituximab/CS is not inferior to CYC/CS for induction of remission and might be superior in relapsing disease.[183,184] Hence, rituximab is now a first-line option for induction of remission in MPA/GPA, but there are safety concerns, given the severe adverse effects (primarily infections) that developed in 22% to 42% of rituximab-treated patients. There were also high relapse rates of 44% to 57% in 2 retrospective studies after median delays of 12 to 14 months.[185,186] A recent retrospective cohort study showed that a 2-year fixed-interval (every 6 months) rituximab retreatment regimen was associated with a significant reduction in relapse rate.[187] Therefore, routine rituximab retreatment might be an effective strategy for remission maintenance. In uncontrolled series, almost 90% of neuropathies improved with rituximab in treatment-refractory AAV.[46]

SVN and NSVN

Most patients with vasculitic neuropathy require treatment, exceptions being those with clearly improving clinical courses or prolonged clinical stability who lack active involvement of other organs. Four major questions need to be addressed: (1) Should treatment be initiated with CS alone or CS combined with a cytotoxic agent? (2) How long should the induction regimen be continued before transitioning to a maintenance program with a less toxic agent or lower dose? (3) What agents should be used for maintenance of remission? (4) How long should maintenance therapy be continued? For an SVN with active multiorgan disease, these questions are usually answered by a rheumatologist, nephrologist, or pulmonologist with input from a neurologist. For NSVN, alternatively, these treatment decisions are best handled by a neurologist.

There are no RCTs of treatment of vasculitic neuropathy associated with any type of vasculitis. Although lacking in evidence-based support, vasculitic neuropathies occurring in the primary small-vessel to medium-vessel systemic vasculitides are generally managed in the same manner as the underlying systemic vasculitis (discussed previously). Although none of the controlled trials in these vasculitides had primary neuropathic endpoints, data in these studies suggest that SVNs typically improve hand in hand with the non-neurologic manifestations.[4]

Several studies have shown that NSVN is clinically and pathologically milder than an SVN, suggesting that less-aggressive therapy may be required.[22,38,63] Although no RCTs of therapy in NSVN have been performed, 2 class III retrospective cohort surveys demonstrated that combination therapy is possibly more effective than CS monotherapy in inducing sustained remission and improving disability in NSVN.[21,36] Nonetheless, the Peripheral Nerve Society task force recommended starting with CS monotherapy unless the neuropathy is rapidly progressive (**Fig. 6**).[4] The initial prednisone dose is 1.0 mg/kg/d, tapered to 25 mg at 3 months, 15 mg to 20 mg at 4 months, and 10 mg at 6 months if symptom control permits. Continuation of low-dose prednisone (5–7.5 mg/d) from 6 to 18 months might further reduce relapses.[180] Pulse IV methylprednisolone is often used in patients with severe, rapidly progressive NSVN but showed no benefit in one class III study.[21] Combination therapy is recommended for rapidly progressive NSVN and for patients who progress on CS monotherapy. First-line options for CS adjuncts are CYC, MTX, and AZA, with CYC preferred for severe neuropathies. CYC is generally administrated in IV pulses to decrease the cumulative dose. One protocol is 0.6 g/m^2 every 2 weeks for 3 doses, then 0.7 g/m^2 every 3 weeks for 3 to 6 doses. The dose should be decreased in elderly patients and those with kidney failure (eg, 0.5 g/m^2). Patients should also receive mesna or IV hydration to reduce the risk of bladder toxicity. MTX is started at 15 mg/wk and titrated to 25 mg/wk over 1 to 2 months. A standard AZA dose is 2.0 mg/kg/d to 2.5 mg/kg/d. Once clinical remission is achieved in those receiving combination therapy, experience in the systemic vasculitides supports the use of maintenance therapy with AZA 1.0 mg/kg/d to 2.0 mg/kg/d or MTX 20 mg/wk to 25 mg/wk to reduce relapses. Clinical remission can be inferred when there is no evidence of worsening by any objective measure and some improvement by at least one objective measure after 6 months of observation.

Nonpharmacologic Strategies

Effective management of patients with vasculitic neuropathy also incorporates supportive care, including pain management, rehabilitation, counseling, and education. High-dose CSs are often effective in reducing the neuropathic pain associated with nerve ischemia, but for many patients, pain control is a fundamental issue, mandating the use of tricyclic antidepressants, gabapentin, pregabalin, serotonin-norepinephrine reuptake inhibitors, carbamazepine, valproate, tramadol, topical lidocaine, topical capsaicin, and scheduled narcotics.[188] In general, continued pain in the absence of progressive neurologic deficits is not an indication to continue high-dose CS.

There is limited research regarding rehabilitation interventions, but physical and occupational therapy should be initiated as soon as severe pain has subsided. Physical therapy helps to maintain strength and range of motion, prevent contractures, limit osteoporosis, and limit or prevent CS myopathy. Occupational therapy serves to maximize function, especially for activities of daily living, sometimes facilitated by appropriate bracing. Walking aids or a wheelchair may be required to maintain mobility. Functional recovery ensues from the combined influences of pain management, rehabilitation efforts, and neurologic recovery dependent on axonal regeneration.

The value of counseling and psychological support cannot be overemphasized. Because of chronic pain, physical limitations, exposure to CS, prolonged recovery, and uncertain prognosis, patients with vasculitic neuropathy are at high risk for depression and other psychological reactions.[189] Elderly patients treated with high doses of CS are particularly susceptible. Treating physicians must maintain a high index of suspicion and provide pharmacologic support or psychiatric referral for patients who develop depression or other psychiatric issues.

Treatment resistance

Treatment-resistant or refractory disease is defined as unchanged or increased disease activity after 4 to 6 weeks of CYC/CS therapy or improved but persistent

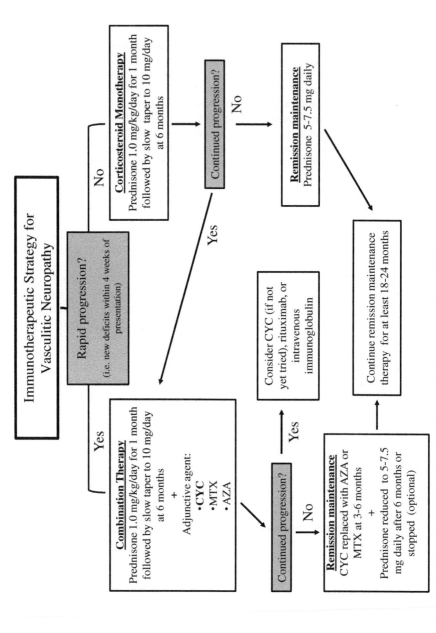

Fig. 6. Treatment algorithm for NSVN and neuropathy-predominant systemic vasculitis.

disease activity after 8 weeks of therapy.[190] The Peripheral Nerve Society guideline group on NSVN reviewed 16 studies addressing treatment of refractory disease in patients with small-vessel to medium-vessel primary systemic vasculitis.[4] One study was class I and the rest were uncontrolled studies of 10 or more patients (class III compared with natural history controls). The class I study was a double-blind RCT of IV immunoglobulin (IVIG) in refractory GPA or MPA.[191] Patients were randomized to IVIG 0.4 g/kg/d for 5 days versus placebo added to unchanged doses of immuno-suppressive drugs. Significantly more patients responded to IVIG (82%) than placebo (35%); 5 of 7 patients with neuropathy remitted with IVIG. Hence, add-on therapy with IVIG is effective in improving disease activity in patients with refractory AAV. The agents investigated in the uncontrolled studies were IVIG, MMF, rituximab, anti–human thymocyte globulin, 15-deoxyspergualin, infliximab, and alemtuzumab. Of these agents, the group concluded that (1) IVIG and rituximab seemed the safest; (2) survival over 1 to 2 years was high with all drugs but reduced with MMF and alem-tuzumab; (3) complete remission rates were lowest with 15-deoxyspergualin and anti–human thymocyte globulin; and (4) relapse rates were greatest with MMF, anti–human thymocyte globulin, and alemtuzumab. More recent uncontrolled trials of rituximab in AAV have revealed higher relapse rates, suggesting a need for scheduled retreatment (discussed previously).[185,186] More recent uncontrolled trials of infliximab in AAV have yielded disappointing results.[192,193] In summary, rituximab and IVIG seem to be the most promising agents for refractory patients with systemic disease.

For patients with refractory NSVN not already treated with CYC, pulse IV or contin-uous oral CYC should be tried. In patients refractory to CYC, the diagnosis should first be reconsidered. Patients with confirmed diagnoses should be enrolled in a clinical trial. If no trial is available, first-line but unproved treatment options are IVIG and ritux-imab. For responders to either of these agents, retreatment may be necessary to prevent relapse. Plasma exchange, MMF, alemtuzumab, infliximab, antithymocyte globulin, and calcineurin inhibitors require more study.

Complications of Treatment

Control of the multiple toxic effects of immunomodulatory therapy is another and often neglected aspect to managing patients with vasculitic neuropathy.[194] All patients on CS should be placed on a low-calorie, low-salt diet and monitored closely for blood pressure and ocular (eg, cataracts) and hyperglycemic side effects (**Table 2**).[195] *Pneumocystis jirovecii* pneumonia prophylaxis (ie, trimethoprim-sulfamethoxazole, dapsone, aerosolized pentamidine, or atovaquone) should be considered, especially if patients are treated with more than one immunosuppressive agent. Patients should undergo tuberculin skin or QuantiFERON-TB testing before therapy is begun, with positive responders referred to an infectious disease specialist for antituberculous therapy. All patients receiving CS and other immunosuppressive therapy should receive pneumococcal and influenza vaccination. Antidepressants and sedative/hypnotics can help to manage mood swings and insomnia, which, if severe enough, interfere with patient compliance or result in suicidal ideation. Glucocorticoid-induced osteoporosis (GIOP) is one of the most serious complications of CS treat-ment. Bone loss commences within 3 months of therapy, develops rapidly in the first year (6%–12%), and then continues at a slower annual rate of approximately 3% with chronic treatment.[196] It predisposes to a high rate of fractures (30%–50%) in patients on chronic CS. Vertebral fractures are most common. There is a strong correlation between daily dose and risk of fracture and cumulative dose and loss of bone mineral density.[197] The minimum prednisone dose that increases the fracture risk is 5 mg daily. Bone mineral density should be determined at baseline and at least yearly as

Table 2
Corticosteroid adverse effects and management

Side Effects	
Common (>10%)	Uncommon (<10%)
Acne	Accelerated atherosclerosis (?)
Cataracts	Avascular necrosis of hips and other joints
Facial plethora	Bowel perforation
Fat redistribution	Confusion
Moon facies	Epidural lipomatosis
Truncal adiposity	Gastric ulcers
Fluid retention/edema	Glaucoma
Growth suppression	Hypokalemia
Hirsutism	Myopathy
Hyperglycemia	Pancreatitis
Hypertension	Tendon rupture
Impaired wound healing	
Increased appetite; weight gain	
Insomnia	
Menstrual irregularities	
Nausea	
Osteoporosis/fractures	
Psychiatric reactions	
Skin atrophy; bruising	
Suppression of hypothalamic-pituitary-adrenal axis	
Susceptibility to infections	

Monitoring	
Baseline	Surveillance
CBC, electrolytes, glucose, glycosylated hemoglobin	CBC, electrolytes, glucose
Blood pressure	Blood pressure
Eye examination	Weight
QuantiFERON-TB, chest radiograph, hepatitis B, hepatitis C, HIV	25-OH vitamin D (at least annual)
Height and weight	Bone mineral densitometry (annual)
Osteoporosis risk assessment	Height (annual)
• CBC, ESR, calcium, phosphorus, creatinine, blood urea nitrogen, alkaline phosphatase, liver functions, 25-OH vitamin D, testosterone, thyrotropin, serum protein electrophoresis/immunofixation, celiac disease antibodies	Eye examination (annual)
• Bone mineral densitometry	
• Assess fall risk	
• Assess incident fragility fractures	
• Consider spine radiographs	

Preventative Measures

Diet	Osteoporosis Prophylaxis	Infections
Calorie-restricted, low-sodium, low simple sugar	Regular weight-bearing, resistance exercises	No live vaccines
Adequate calcium	Calcium 1200–1500 mg/d	Give influenza and pneumococcal vaccines
Eliminate tobacco and alcohol	Vitamin D 800–1000 units/d or calcitriol 0.25–0.50 ug/d (maintain optimal 25-OH vitamin D levels)	*Pneumocystis jirovecii* prophylaxis
	Consider testosterone replacement in hypogonadal men	• With concomitant immunosuppressives
	Consider bisphosphonates	• First-line: trimethoprim/sulfamethoxazole 160/800 mg tiw or 80/400 mg daily
	• Alendronate 5–10 mg/d (or 35–70 mg/wk) or	• Second line: dapsone 100 mg daily, atovaquone 1500 mg daily, or nebulized pentamidine 300 mg monthly
	• Risedronate 5 mg/d or	
	• Zoledronic acid 5 mg IV q 12 mo or	
	• Etidronate 400 mg/d × 2 wk q 3 mo	
	Consider teriparatide 20 μg/d SC	
	Consider denosumab 60 mg SC q 6 mo	

Abbreviations: OH, hydroxy; SC, subcutaneous.

long as therapy continues. If bone loss occurs at a rate greater than 3% per year, osteoporosis treatment needs to be augmented by an endocrinologist specializing in osteoporosis. Laboratory tests to exclude secondary causes of osteoporosis should be obtained (see **Table 2**). Consideration should be given to periodic radiographic imaging of the spine.[198]

The ACR 2010 recommendations for the prevention and treatment of GIOP stratify patients into low-risk, medium-risk, and high-risk categories, guided in part on the FRAX risk assessment tool.[198] The specific recommendations of this and other guidelines are beyond the scope of this review, but basic principles can be summarized.[198,199] All patients starting CS at any dose for an anticipated duration greater than 3 months should receive counseling on weight-bearing exercise, smoking cessation, avoidance of excessive alcohol intake, and adequate calcium and vitamin D intake. Total calcium intake by diet and supplementation should be 1200 mg to 1500 mg daily. Vitamin D should be supplemented at 800 units to 1000 units per day or at a dose sufficient to maintain therapeutic levels of 25-hydroxyvitamin D. Testosterone replacement should be implemented in hypogonadal men, assuming no prostate cancer or other contraindication. Postmenopausal women and men age older than 50 years falling in a medium-risk or high-risk category or receiving greater than or equal to 7.5 mg of prednisone daily should be treated with antiosteoporotic agents with established efficacy in GIOP, such as alendronate, residronate, zoledronic acid, or teriparatide. For younger men and women, the evidence is more limited.

The side effects of the other immunosuppressive agents must be managed equally aggressively.[68]

Evaluation of Outcome

A major difficulty in treating patients with vasculitic neuropathy is that there is no easy way to monitor disease activity and remission (eg, by resort to a laboratory study or radiographic procedure). Subjective responses are important to consider, but immediate improvements in pain, fatigue, and malaise more often reflect improvements in mood and overall sense of well being than true PNS function. Objective monitoring is crucial and depends on multimodality monitoring of such measures as manual muscle testing–quantified weakness, sensory loss to all modalities, maximized compound muscle and sensory nerve action potential amplitudes, needle electromyography findings (fibrillation potentials), ESR/CRP if elevated, neuropathy impairment scores, and disability scales (eg, Overall Neuropathy Limitations Scale). In patients with vasculitic neuropathy with no other evidence of ongoing vasculitis, worsening pain may be a clue of re-emerging disease activity, but it is not generally an indication to intensify immunosuppression unless concomitant neurologic deficits emerge.

Treatment of vasculitic neuropathy usually continues for more than 1 year. During this time, a clinician needs to frequently (ie, every 4–8 weeks) assess motor, sensory, and functional findings to ensure that patients are not developing new deficits as a result of continued ischemic nerve injury. Surveillance electrodiagnostic studies are usually not necessary but can be helpful in equivocal situations, especially for patients with painful, sensory-predominant neuropathies. New motor or sensory deficits emerging during treatment are an indication to increase the doses of the current drug regimen or change to a new agent. Stable deficits, alternatively, do not necessarily signify treatment failure, because recovery depends largely on axonal regeneration, a slow process. It is unusual to observe any objective improvement in the first few weeks or months of therapy. More commonly, patients initially stop progressing, with true improvement not evident until months later. During this early phase of treatment, the prescribed regimen should not be altered unless deficits consistent with new or progression lesions appear.

Case report

A 74 year-old woman with type 2 diabetes mellitus and hypothyroidism presented with a 3-month history of numbness, paresthesias, and pain in her left foot. An electrodiagnostic study revealed findings suggestive of a length-dependent, axonal neuropathy, except for a mild asymmetry that was discounted due to lower limb edema. Her symptoms were attributed to a diabetic polyneuropathy, but over the next 2 months, left lower limb symptoms continued to progress, and she developed new symptoms of pain and weakness in her left hand. Her progressive symptoms prompted a neurology consultation. Additional history was then elicited for malaise and low-grade fevers for a few weeks, but there were no signs or symptoms to suggest other-organ involvement. Her only medications were those for diabetes and hypothyroidism. Examination revealed symmetric, distally accentuated weakness and sensory loss in the lower limbs and superimposed focal weakness and sensory loss in the distributions of the left common peroneal and ulnar nerves. Laboratory testing revealed a moderately elevated ESR (83 mm/hr) and was otherwise normal. There were no ANCAs. Repeat electrodiagnostic testing showed evidence of a progressive axonal polyneuropathy with features of subacute, asymmetric axon-loss in the left common peroneal and ulnar nerve distributions. Left sural nerve biopsy was consistent with definite vasculitis. The patient was diagnosed with NSVN and started on prednisone monotherapy. Her symptoms stabilized and gradually improved over several months.

This patient satisfied Peripheral Nerve Society consensus criteria for NSVN. She presented with a phenotype suggestive of a vasculitic neuropathy (subacutely progressive, asymmetric/multifocal, distal-predominant, and axonal), with confirmatory nerve biopsy findings. She had no clinical features to suggest the presence of a SVN, such as signs, symptoms, or laboratory abnormalities indicative of extra-neurologic involvement; ANCAs; ESR ≥ 100 mm/hr; cryoglobulins; or medical condition, infection, or drug predisposing to vasculitis. She did have constitutional symptoms and diabetes mellitus, but neither excludes a diagnosis of NSVN. This case highlights the importance of considering vasculitis in any patient with a progressive, asymmetric, axonal neuropathy. Asymmetry is key. The asymmetry in this patient's initial EMG was discounted for technical issues, but in retrospect, it comported with the asymmetry in her symptoms and was probably non-artifactual. When evaluating neuropathies, a bilateral electrodiagnostic study should be performed to assess for asymmetries and avoid the mistake of diagnosing a length-dependent process in a patient with a distal-predominant but multifocal neuropathy. The initial restriction of this patient's symptoms to one foot should have raised a "red flag" against the diagnosis of diabetic polyneuropathy, a prototypical distal symmetric neuropathy.

REFERENCES

1. Langford CA, Fauci AS. Chapter 326. The vasculitis syndromes. In: Longo DL, editor. Harrison's principles of internal medicine. 18th edition. New York: McGraw-Hill; 2012. Available at: http://www.accessmedicine.com/content.aspx?aID=9138083. Accessed December 27, 2012.
2. Hernández-Rodríguez J, Hoffman GS. Updating single-organ vasculitis. Curr Opin Rheumatol 2012;24:38–45.
3. Dyck PJ, Benstead TJ, Conn DL, et al. Nonsystemic vasculitic neuropathy. Brain 1987;110:843–53.
4. Collins MP, Dyck PJ, Gronseth GS, et al. Peripheral nerve society guideline on the classification, diagnosis, investigation, and immunosuppressive therapy of non-systemic vasculitic neuropathy: executive summary. J Peripher Nerv Syst 2010;15:176–84.
5. Fries JF, Hunder GG, Bloch DA, et al. The American College of Rheumatology 1990 criteria for the classification of vasculitis. Summary. Arthritis Rheum 1990;33:1135–6.
6. Jennette JC, Falk RJ, Andrassy K, et al. Nomenclature of systemic vasculitides. Proposal of an international consensus conference. Arthritis Rheum 1994;37:187–92.

7. Bruce IN, Bell AL. A comparison of two nomenclature systems for primary systemic vasculitis. Br J Rheumatol 1997;36:453–8.
8. Wiik AS. Autoantibodies in ANCA-associated vasculitis. Rheum Dis Clin North Am 2010;36:479–89.
9. Kallenberg CG. Pathogenesis of ANCA-associated vasculitis, an update. Clin Rev Allergy Immunol 2011;41:224–31.
10. Cartin-Ceba R, Peikert T, Specks U. Pathogenesis of ANCA-associated vasculitis. Curr Rheumatol Rep 2012;14:481–93.
11. Lionaki S, Blyth ER, Hogan SL, et al. Classification of antineutrophil cytoplasmic autoantibody vasculitides: the role of antineutrophil cytoplasmic autoantibody specificity for myeloperoxidase or proteinase 3 in disease recognition and prognosis. Arthritis Rheum 2012;64:3452–62.
12. Mahr A, Katsahian S, Varet H, et al. Revisiting the classification of clinical phenotypes of anti-neutrophil cytoplasmic antibody-associated vasculitis: a cluster analysis. Ann Rheum Dis 2012. http://dx.doi.org/10.1136/annrheumdis-2012-201750.
13. Lyons PA, Rayner TF, Trivedi S, et al. Genetically distinct subsets within ANCA-associated vasculitis. N Engl J Med 2012;367:214–23.
14. Watts RA, Suppiah R, Merkel PA, et al. Systemic vasculitis—is it time to reclassify? Rheumatology 2011;50:643–5.
15. Jennette J, Falk R, Bacon P, et al. 2012 revised international Chapel Hill consensus conference nomenclature of vasculitides. Arthritis Rheum 2013;65:1–11.
16. Guillevin L, Durand-Gasselin B, Cevallos R, et al. Microscopic polyangiitis: clinical and laboratory findings in eighty-five patients. Arthritis Rheum 1999;42:421–30.
17. Pagnoux C, Seror R, Henegar C, et al. Clinical features and outcomes in 348 patients with polyarteritis nodosa: a systematic retrospective study of patients diagnosed between 1963 and 2005 and entered into the French Vasculitis Study Group Database. Arthritis Rheum 2010;62:616–26.
18. Dunogué B, Pagnoux C, Guillevin L. Churg-strauss syndrome: clinical symptoms, complementary investigations, prognosis and outcome, and treatment. Semin Respir Crit Care Med 2011;32:298–309.
19. Collins MP, Kissel JT. Vasculitic neuropathies and neuropathies of connective tissue diseases. In: Katirji B, Kaminski HJ, Ruff RL, editors. Neuromuscular disorders in clinical practice. 2nd edition. New York: Springer, in press.
20. Terrier B, Cacoub P. Cryoglobulinemia vasculitis: an update. Curr Opin Rheumatol 2013;25:10–8.
21. Collins MP, Periquet MI, Mendell JR, et al. Nonsystemic vasculitic neuropathy: insights from a clinical cohort. Neurology 2003;61:623–30.
22. Vital C, Vital A, Canron MH, et al. Combined nerve and muscle biopsy in the diagnosis of vasculitic neuropathy. A 16-year retrospective study of 202 cases. J Peripher Nerv Syst 2006;11:20–9.
23. Uçeyler N, Devigili G, Toyka KV, et al. Skin biopsy as an additional diagnostic tool in non-systemic vasculitic neuropathy. Acta Neuropathol 2010;120:109–16.
24. Agadi JB, Raghav G, Mahadevan A, et al. Usefulness of superficial peroneal nerve/peroneus brevis muscle biopsy in the diagnosis of vasculitic neuropathy. J Clin Neurosci 2012;19:1392–6.
25. Gonzalez-Gay MA, Garcia-Porrua C. Systemic vasculitis in adults in northwestern Spain, 1988-1997. Clinical and epidemiologic aspects. Medicine 1999;78:292–308.
26. Reinhold-Keller E, Herlyn K, Wagner-Bastmeyer R, et al. No difference in the incidences of vasculitides between north and south Germany: first results of the German vasculitis register. Rheumatology 2002;41:540–9.

27. Cartier L, García M, Peñaherrera P, et al. [Multiple mononeuropathy and vasculitis.] Rev Med Chil 1999;127:189–96 [in Spanish].
28. Collins MP, Periquet MI. Isolated vasculitis of the peripheral nervous system. Clin Exp Rheumatol 2008;26:S118–30.
29. Guillevin L, Pagnoux C, Seror R, et al. The Five-Factor Score revisited: assessment of prognoses of systemic necrotizing vasculitides based on the French Vasculitis Study Group (FVSG) cohort. Medicine 2011;90:19–27.
30. Suppiah R, Hadden RD, Batra R, et al. Peripheral neuropathy in ANCA-associated vasculitis: outcomes from the European Vasculitis Study Group trials. Rheumatology 2011;50:2214–22.
31. Walsh M, Flossmann O, Berden A, et al. Risk factors for relapse of antineutrophil cytoplasmic antibody-associated vasculitis. Arthritis Rheum 2012;64:542–8.
32. Walsh M, Mukhtyar C, Mahr A, et al. Health-related quality of life in patients with newly diagnosed antineutrophil cytoplasmic antibody-associated vasculitis. Arthritis Care Res 2011;63:1055–61.
33. Said G, Lacroix-Ciaudo C, Fujimura H, et al. The peripheral neuropathy of necrotizing arteritis: a clinicopathological study. Ann Neurol 1988;23:461–5.
34. Hawke SH, Davies L, Pamphlett R, et al. Vasculitic neuropathy. A clinical and pathological study. Brain 1991;114:2175–90.
35. Midroni G, Bilbao JM. Biopsy diagnosis of peripheral neuropathy. Boston: Butterworth-Heinemann; 1995. p. 241–62.
36. Davies L, Spies JM, Pollard JD, et al. Vasculitis confined to peripheral nerves. Brain 1996;119:1441–8.
37. Collins MP, Mendell JR, Periquet MI, et al. Superficial peroneal nerve/peroneus brevis muscle biopsy in vasculitic neuropathy. Neurology 2000;55:636–43.
38. Sugiura M, Koike H, Iijima M, et al. Clinicopathologic features of nonsystemic vasculitic neuropathy and microscopic polyangiitis-associated neuropathy: a comparative study. J Neurol Sci 2006;241:31–7.
39. Nukada H, Dyck PJ. Microsphere embolization of nerve capillaries and fiber degeneration. Am J Pathol 1984;115:275–87.
40. Morozumi S, Koike H, Tomita M, et al. Spatial distribution of nerve fiber pathology and vasculitis in microscopic polyangiitis-associated neuropathy. J Neuropathol Exp Neurol 2011;70:340–8.
41. Kararizou E, Davaki P, Karandreas N, et al. Nonsystemic vasculitic neuropathy: a clinicopathological study of 22 cases. J Rheumatol 2005;32:853–8.
42. Kissel JT, Riethman JL, Omerza J, et al. Peripheral nerve vasculitis: immune characterization of the vascular lesions. Ann Neurol 1989;25:291–7.
43. Lindenlaub T, Sommer C. Cytokines in sural nerve biopsies from inflammatory and non-inflammatory neuropathies. Acta Neuropathol 2003;105:593–602.
44. Satoi H, Oka N, Kawasaki T, et al. Mechanisms of tissue injury in vasculitic neuropathies. Neurology 1998;50:492–6.
45. Collins MP, Periquet-Collins I, Sahenk Z, et al. Direct immunofluoresence in vasculitic neuropathy: specificity of vascular immune deposits. Muscle Nerve 2010; 42:62–9.
46. Collins MP. The vasculitic neuropathies: an update. Curr Opin Neurol 2012;25: 573–85.
47. Kinter J, Broglio L, Steck AJ, et al. Gene expression profiling in nerve biopsy of vasculitic neuropathy. J Neuroimmunol 2010;225:184–9.
48. Saadoun D, Bieche I, Maisonobe T, et al. Involvement of chemokines and type 1 cytokines in the pathogenesis of hepatitis C virus-associated mixed cryoglobulinemia vasculitis neuropathy. Arthritis Rheum 2005;52:2917–25.

49. Heuss D, Probst-Cousin S, Kayser C, et al. Cell death in vasculitic neuropathy. Muscle Nerve 2000;23:999–1004.
50. Khalili-Shirazi A, Gregson NA, Londei M, et al. The distribution of CD1 molecules in inflammatory neuropathy. J Neurol Sci 1998;158:154–63.
51. Van Rhijn I, Van den Berg LH, Bosboom WM, et al. Expression of accessory molecules for T-cell activation in peripheral nerve of patients with CIDP and vasculitic neuropathy. Brain 2000;123:2020–9.
52. Hu W, Janke A, Ortler S, et al. Expression of CD28-related costimulatory molecule and its ligand in inflammatory neuropathies. Neurology 2007;68:277–82.
53. Chia L, Fernandez A, Lacroix C, et al. Contribution of nerve biopsy findings to the diagnosis of disabling neuropathy in the elderly. A retrospective review of 100 consecutive patients. Brain 1996;119:1091–8.
54. Hattori N, Ichimura M, Nagamatsu M, et al. Clinicopathological features of Churg-Strauss syndrome-associated neuropathy. Brain 1999;122:427–39.
55. Dyck PJ, Norell JE, Dyck PJ. Non-diabetic lumbosacral radiculoplexus neuropathy: natural history, outcome and comparison with the diabetic variety. Brain 2001;124:1197–207.
56. Sanchez J, Coll-Canti J, Ariza A, et al. [Neuropathy due to necrotizing vasculitis: a study of the clinical anatomy, neurophysiological characteristics, and clinical course of the disorder in 27 patients.] Rev Neurol 2001;33:1033–6 [in Spanish].
57. Hattori N, Mori K, Misu K, et al. Mortality and morbidity in peripheral neuropathy associated Churg-Strauss syndrome and microscopic polyangiitis. J Rheumatol 2002;29:1408–14.
58. Seo JH, Ryan HF, Claussen GC, et al. Sensory neuropathy in vasculitis: a clinical, pathologic, and electrophysiologic study. Neurology 2004;63:874–8.
59. Vital A, Vital C, Viallard JF, et al. Neuro-muscular biopsy in Churg-Strauss syndrome: 24 cases. J Neuropathol Exp Neurol 2006;65:187–92.
60. Cattaneo L, Chierici E, Pavone L, et al. Peripheral neuropathy in Wegener's granulomatosis, Churg-Strauss syndrome and microscopic polyangiitis. J Neurol Neurosurg Psychiatry 2007;78:1119–23.
61. Mathew L, Talbot K, Love S, et al. Treatment of vasculitic peripheral neuropathy: a retrospective analysis of outcome. QJM 2007;100:41–51.
62. Zivkovic SA, Ascherman D, Lacomis D. Vasculitic neuropathy—electrodiagnostic findings and association with malignancies. Acta Neurol Scand 2007;115:432–6.
63. Bennett DL, Groves M, Blake J, et al. The use of nerve and muscle biopsy in the diagnosis of vasculitis: a 5 year retrospective study. J Neurol Neurosurg Psychiatry 2008;79:1376–81.
64. Restrepo JF, Rondón F, Matteson EL, et al. Necrotizing lymphocytic vasculitis limited to the peripheral nerves: report of six cases and review. Int J Rheumatol 2009;2009:368032.
65. Wolf J, Schmitt V, Palm F, et al. Peripheral neuropathy as initial manifestation of primary systemic vasculitides. J Neurol 2012. http://dx.doi.org/10.1007/s00415-012-6760-7.
66. De Toni Franceschini L, Amadio S, Scarlato M, et al. A fatal case of Churg-Strauss syndrome presenting with acute polyneuropathy mimicking Guillain-Barré syndrome. Neurol Sci 2011;32:937–40.
67. Cassereau J, Baguenier-Desormeaux C, Letournel F, et al. Necrotizing vasculitis revealed in a case of multiple mononeuropathy after a 14-year course of spontaneous remissions and relapses. Clin Neurol Neurosurg 2012;114:290–3.

68. Collins MP, Periquet-Collins I, Kissel JT. Vasculitis of the peripheral nervous system. In: Noseworthy JH, editor. Neurological therapeutics principles and practice, vol. 2. London: Informa; 2006. p. 2348–82.
69. Langford CA. Vasculitis. J Allergy Clin Immunol 2010;125(2 Suppl 2):S216–25.
70. Ntatsaki E, Watts RA, Scott DG. Epidemiology of ANCA-associated vasculitis. Rheum Dis Clin North Am 2010;36:447–61.
71. Calabrese LH, Molloy ES, Duna G. Antineutrophil cytoplasmic antibody-assocaited vasculitis. In: Firestein GS, Budd RC, Harris ED, et al, editors. Kelley's textbook of rheumatology. 8th edition. Philadelphia: Saunders Elsevier; 2009. p. 1429–51.
72. Stone JH. Polyarteritis nodosa. JAMA 2002;288:1632–9.
73. Lightfoot RW, Michel BA, Bloch DA, et al. The American College of Rheumatology 1990 criteria for the classification of polyarteritis nodosa. Arthritis Rheum 1990;33:1088–93.
74. Ball GV, Bridges SL. Polyarteritis nodosa. In: Koopman WJ, Moreland LW, editors. Arthritis and allied conditions. 15th edition. Philadelphia: Lippincott, Williams & Wilkins; 2005. Accessed December 27, 2012.
75. Collins MP, Kissel JT. Neuropathies with systemic vasculitis. In: Dyck PJ, Thomas PK, editors. Peripheral neuropathy. Philadelphia: Elsevier Saunders; 2005. p. 2335–404.
76. Stanson AW, Friese JL, Johnson CM, et al. Polyarteritis nodosa: spectrum of angiographic findings. Radiographics 2001;21:151–9.
77. Serra A, Cameron JS, Turner DR, et al. Vasculitis affecting the kidney: presentation, histopathology and long-term outcome. QJM 1984;53:181–207.
78. Adu D, Howie AJ, Scott DG, et al. Polyarteritis and the kidney. QJM 1987;62: 221–37.
79. Cisternas M, Soto L, Jacobelli S, et al. [Clinical features of Wegener granulomatosis and microscopic polyangiitis in Chilean patients.] Rev Med Chil 2005;133: 273–8 [in Spanish].
80. Villiger PM, Guillevin L. Microscopic polyangiitis: clinical presentation. Autoimmun Rev 2010;9:812–9.
81. Ahn JK, Hwang JW, Lee J, et al. Clinical features and outcome of microscopic polyangiitis under a new consensus algorithm of ANCA-associated vasculitides in Korea. Rheumatol Int 2012;32:2979–86.
82. Mahr AD. Epidemiological features of Wegener's granulomatosis and microscopic polyangiitis: two diseases or one 'anti-neutrophil cytoplasm antibodies-associated vasculitis' entity? APMIS Suppl 2009;127:41–7.
83. Mohammad AJ, Jacobsson LT, Westman KW, et al. Incidence and survival rates in Wegener's granulomatosis, microscopic polyangiitis, Churg-Strauss syndrome and polyarteritis nodosa. Rheumatology 2009;48:1560–5.
84. Oh JS, Lee CK, Kim YG, et al. Clinical features and outcomes of microscopic polyangiitis in Korea. J Korean Med Sci 2009;24:269–74.
85. Zhang W, Zhou G, Shi Q, et al. Clinical analysis of nervous system involvement in ANCA-associated systemic vasculitides. Clin Exp Rheumatol 2009; 27(Suppl 52):S65–9.
86. Corral-Gudino L, Borao-Cengotita-Bengoa M, Del Pino-Montes J, et al. Overall survival, renal survival and relapse in patients with microscopic polyangiitis: a systematic review of current evidence. Rheumatology 2011;50:1414–23.
87. Lanham JG, Elkon KB, Pusey CD, et al. Systemic vasculitis with asthma and eosinophilia: a clinical approach to the Churg-Strauss syndrome. Medicine 1984;63:65–81.

88. Keogh KA, Specks U. Churg-Strauss syndrome: clinical presentation, antineu-trophil cytoplasmic antibodies, and leukotriene receptor antagonists. Am J Med 2003;115:284–90.

89. Sinico RA, Di Toma L, Maggiore U, et al. Prevalence and clinical significance of antineutrophil cytoplasmic antibodies in Churg-Strauss syndrome. Arthritis Rheum 2005;52:2926–35.

90. Baldini C, Della Rossa A, Grossi S, et al. [Churg-Strauss syndrome: outcome and long-term follow-up of 38 patients from a single Italian centre.] Reumatismo 2009;61:118–24 [in Italian].

91. Vinit J, Muller G, Bielefeld P, et al. Churg-Strauss syndrome: retrospective study in Burgundian population in France in past 10 years. Rheumatol Int 2011;3: 587–93.

92. Comarmond C, Pagnoux C, Khellaf M, et al. Eosinophilic granulomatosis with polyangiitis (Churg-Strauss syndrome)—clinical characteristics and long-term follow-up of the 383 patients enrolled in the FVSG cohort. Arthritis Rheum 2013;65:270–81.

93. Moosig F, Bremer JP, Hellmich B, et al. A vasculitis centre based management strategy leads to improved outcome in eosinophilic granulomatosis and polyan-giitis (Churg-Strauss, EGPA): monocentric experiences in 150 patients. Ann Rheum Dis 2012. http://dx.doi.org/10.1136/annrheumdis-2012-201531.

94. Uchiyama M, Mitsuhashi Y, Yamazaki M, et al. Elderly cases of Churg-Strauss syndrome: case report and review of Japanese cases. J Dermatol 2012;39: 76–9.

95. Oka N, Kawasaki T, Matsui M, et al. Two subtypes of Churg-Strauss syndrome with neuropathy: the roles of eosinophils and ANCA. Mod Rheumatol 2011;21: 290–5.

96. Shimoi T, Shojima K, Murota A, et al. Clinical and pathological features of Churg Strauss syndrome among a Japanese population: a case series of 18 patients. Asian Pac J Allergy Immunol 2012;30:61–70.

97. Hoffman GS, Kerr GS, Leavitt RY, et al. Wegener granulomatosis: an analysis of 158 patients. Ann Intern Med 1992;116:488–96.

98. Reinhold-Keller E, Beuge N, Latza U, et al. An interdisciplinary approach to the care of patients with Wegener's granulomatosis. Long-term outcome in 155 patients. Arthritis Rheum 2000;43:1021–32.

99. Holle JU, Laudien M, Gross WL. Clinical manifestations and treatment of Wegener's granulomatosis. Rheum Dis Clin North Am 2010;36:507–26.

100. Holle JU, Gross WL, Latza U, et al. Improved outcome in 445 patients with Wegener's granulomatosis in a German vasculitis center over four decades. Arthritis Rheum 2011;63:257–66.

101. Holle JU, Gross WL, Holl-Ulrich K, et al. Prospective long-term follow-up of patients with localised Wegener's granulomatosis: does it occur as persistent disease stage? Arthritis Rheum 2011;63:257–66.

102. Anderson JM, Jamieson DG, Jefferson JM. Non-healing granuloma and the nervous system. QJM 1975;44:309–23.

103. Nishino H, Rubino FA, DeRemee RA, et al. Neurological involvement in Wege-ner's granulomatosis: an analysis of 324 consecutive patients at the Mayo Clinic. Ann Neurol 1993;33:4–9.

104. de Groot K, Schmidt DK, Arlt AC, et al. Standardized neurologic evaluations of 128 patients with Wegener granulomatosis. Arch Neurol 2001;58:1215–21.

105. Flores-Suárez LF, Villa AR. Spectrum of Wegener granulomatosis in a Mexican population. Ann N Y Acad Sci 2007;1107:400–9.

106. Luqmani R, Suppiah R, Edwards CJ, et al. Mortality in Wegener's granulomatosis: a bimodal pattern. Rheumatology 2011;50:697–702.
107. Devaney KO, Travis WD, Hoffman G, et al. Interpretation of head and neck biopsies in Wegener's granulomatosis. A pathologic study of 126 biopsies in 70 patients. Am J Surg Pathol 1990;14:555–64.
108. Travis WD, Hoffman GS, Leavitt RY, et al. Surgical pathology of the lung in Wegener's granulomatosis. Review of 87 open lung biopsies from 67 patients. Am J Surg Pathol 1991;15:315–33.
109. Hellman DB. Giant cell arteritis, polymyalgia rheumatica, and Takayasu's arteritis. In: Firestein GS, Budd RC, Harris ED, et al, editors. Kelley's textbook of rheumatology. 8th edition. Philadelphia: Saunders Elsevier; 2009. p. 1409–28.
110. Borchers AT, Gershwin ME. Giant cell arteritis: a review of classification, pathophysiology, geoepidemiology and treatment. Autoimmun Rev 2012;11: A544–54.
111. Gonzalez-Gay MA, Vazquez-Rodriguez TR, Lopez-Diaz MJ, et al. Epidemiology of giant cell arteritis and polymyalgia rheumatic. Arthritis Rheum 2009;61: 1454–61.
112. Amor-Dorado JC, Llorca J, Garcia-Porrua C, et al. Audiovestibular manifestations in giant cell arteritis. A prospective study. Medicine 2003;82:13–26.
113. Caselli RJ, Hunder GG, Whisnant JP. Neurologic disease in biopsy-proven giant cell (temporal) arteritis. Neurology 1988;38:352–9.
114. Burton EA, Winer JB, Barber PC. Giant cell arteritis of the cervical radicular vessels presenting with diaphragmatic weakness. J Neurol Neurosurg Psychiatry 1999;67:223–6.
115. Nesher G. Neurologic manifestations of giant cell arteritis. Clin Exp Rheumatol 2000;18(4 Suppl 20):S24–6.
116. Blaise S, Liozon E, Nadalon S, et al. Horton's disease revealed by brachial C5 plexopathy. Rev Med Interne 2005;26:578–82 [in French].
117. Pfadenhauer K, Roesler A, Golling A. The involvement of the peripheral nervous system in biopsy proven active giant cell arteritis. J Neurol 2007;254:751–5.
118. Proven A, Gabriel SE, Orces C, et al. Glucocorticoid therapy in giant cell arteritis: duration and adverse outcomes. Arthritis Rheum 2003;49:703–8.
119. Martinez-Lado L, Calviño-Díaz C, Piñeiro A, et al. Relapses and recurrences in giant cell arteritis: a population-based study of patients with biopsy-proven disease from northwestern Spain. Medicine 2011;90:186–93.
120. Gonzalez-Gay MA, Lopez-Diaz MJ, Barros S, et al. Giant cell arteritis: laboratory tests at the time of diagnosis in a series of 240 patients. Medicine 2005;84: 277–90.
121. Kermani TA, Schmidt J, Crowson CS, et al. Utility of erythrocyte sedimentation rate and C-reactive protein for the diagnosis of giant cell arteritis. Semin Arthritis Rheum 2012;41:866–71.
122. Weyand CM, Fulbright JW, Hunder GG, et al. Treatment of giant cell arteritis: interleukin-6 as a biologic marker of disease activity. Arthritis Rheum 2000;43: 1041–8.
123. Arida A, Kyprianou M, Kanakis M, et al. The diagnostic value of ultrasonography-derived edema of the temporal artery wall in giant cell arteritis: a second meta-analysis. BMC Musculoskelet Disord 2010;11:44.
124. Pagnoux C, Cohen P, Guillevin L. Vasculitides secondary to infections. Clin Exp Rheumatol 2006;24(2 Suppl 41):S71–81.
125. Lidar M, Lipschitz N, Langevitz P, et al. The infectious etiology of vasculitis. Autoimmunity 2009;42:432–8.

126. Said G, Lacroix C, Chemouilli P, et al. Cytomegalovirus neuropathy in acquired immunodeficiency syndrome: a clinical and pathological study. Ann Neurol 1991;29:139–46.
127. Chretien F, Gray F, Lescs MC, et al. Acute varicella-zoster virus ventriculitis and meningo-myelo-radiculitis in acquired immunodeficiency syndrome. Acta Neuropathol 1993;86:659–65.
128. Schäfers M, Neukirchen S, Toyka KV, et al. Diagnostic value of sural nerve biopsy in patients with suspected Borrelia neuropathy. J Peripher Nerv Syst 2008;13:81–91.
129. Lenglet T, Haroche J, Schnuriger A, et al. Mononeuropathy multiplex associated with acute parvovirus B19 infection: characteristics, treatment and outcome. J Neurol 2011;258:1321–6.
130. Patel N, Patel N, Khan T, et al. HIV infection and clinical spectrum of associated vasculitides. Curr Rheumatol Rep 2011;13:506–12.
131. Guillevin L, Mahr A, Callard P, et al. Hepatitis B virus-associated polyarteritis nodosa: clinical characteristics, outcome, and impact of treatment in 115 patients. Medicine 2005;84:313–22.
132. Han SH. Extrahepatic manifestations of chronic hepatitis B. Clin Liver Dis 2004; 8:403–18.
133. De Vita S, Soldano F, Isola M, et al. Preliminary classification criteria for the cryoglobulinaemic vasculitis. Ann Rheum Dis 2011;70:1183–90.
134. Ramos-Casals M, Stone JH, Cid MC, et al. The cryoglobulinaemias. Lancet 2012;379:348–60.
135. Cacoub P, Renou C, Rosenthal E, et al. Extrahepatic manifestations associated with hepatitis C virus infection. A prospective multicenter study of 321 patients. Medicine 2000;79:47–56.
136. Santoro L, Manganelli F, Briani C, et al. Prevalence and characteristics of peripheral neuropathy in hepatitis C virus population. J Neurol Neurosurg Psychiatry 2006;77:626–9.
137. Yamanaka Y, Hiraga A, Arai K, et al. Leucocytoclastic vasculitic neuropathy diagnosed by biopsy of normal appearing skin. J Neurol Neurosurg Psychiatry 2006;77:706–7.
138. Lee JE, Shun CT, Hsieh SC, et al. Skin denervation in vasculitic neuropathy. Arch Neurol 2005;62:1570–3.
139. Bastron JA, Thomas JE. Diabetic polyradiculopathy: clinical and electromyographic findings in 105 patients. Mayo Clin Proc 1981;56:725–32.
140. Barohn RJ, Sahenk Z, Warmolts JR, et al. The Bruns-Garland syndrome (diabetic amyotrophy). Revisited 100 years later. Arch Neurol 1991;48:1130–5.
141. Said G, Goulon-Goeau C, Lacroix C, et al. Nerve biopsy findings in different patterns of proximal diabetic neuropathy. Ann Neurol 1994;35:559–69.
142. Llewelyn JG, Thomas PK, King RH. Epineurial microvasculitis in proximal diabetic neuropathy. J Neurol 1998;245:159–65.
143. Younger DS, Rosoklija G, Hays AP, et al. Diabetic peripheral neuropathy: a clinicopathologic and immunohistochemical analysis of sural nerve biopsies. Muscle Nerve 1996;19:722–7.
144. Dyck PJ, Norell JE, Dyck PJ. Microvasculitis and ischemia in diabetic lumbosacral radiculoplexus neuropathy. Neurology 1999;53:2113–21.
145. Garces-Sanchez M, Laughlin RS, Dyck PJ, et al. Painless diabetic motor neuropathy: a variant of diabetic lumbosacral radiculoplexus neuropathy? Ann Neurol 2011;69:1043–54.

146. Massie R, Mauermann ML, Staff NP, et al. Diabetic cervical radiculoplexus neuropathy: a distinct syndrome expanding the spectrum of diabetic radiculoplexus neuropathies. Brain 2012;135:3074–88.

147. Staff NP, Engelstad J, Klein CJ, et al. Post-surgical inflammatory neuropathy. Brain 2010;133:2866–80.

148. Wartenberg R. Neuritis, sensory neuritis, neuralgia; a clinical study with review of the literature. New York: Oxford University Press; 1958. p. 233–47.

149. Matthews WB, Esiri M. The migrant sensory neuritis of Wartenberg. J Neurol Neurosurg Psychiatry 1983;46:1–4.

150. Zifko UA, Hahn AF. Migrant sensory neuropathy: report of 5 cases and review of the literature. J Peripher Nerv Syst 1997;2:244–9.

151. Nicolle MW, Barron JR, Watson BV, et al. Wartenberg's migrant sensory neuritis. Muscle Nerve 2001;24:438–43.

152. Stork AC, van der Meulen MF, van der Pol WL, et al. Wartenberg's migrant sensory neuritis: a prospective follow-up study. J Neurol 2010;257:1344–8.

153. Sobue G, Nakao N, Kumazawa K, et al. [Migrating multiple mononeuritis and nonsystemic angitis.] Rinsho Shinkeigaku 1989;29:1210–5 [in Japanese].

154. Sakai K, Komai K, Yanase D, et al. Plasma VEGF as a marker for the diagnosis and treatment of vasculitic neuropathy. J Neurol Neurosurg Psychiatry 2005;76:296.

155. Terrier B, Lacroix C, Guillevin L, et al. Diagnostic and prognostic relevance of neuromuscular biopsy in primary Sjogren's syndrome-related neuropathy. Arthritis Rheum 2007;57:1520–9.

156. Claussen GC, Thomas TD, Goyne C, et al. Diagnostic value of nerve and muscle biopsy in suspected vasculitis cases. J Clin Neuromuscul Dis 2000;1:117–23.

157. McCluskey L, Feinberg D, Cantor C, et al. "Pseudo-conduction block" in vasculitic neuropathy. Muscle Nerve 1999;22:1361–6.

158. Jamieson PW, Giuliani MJ, Martinez AJ. Necrotizing angiopathy presenting with multifocal conduction blocks. Neurology 1991;41:442–4.

159. Deprez M, de Groote CC, Gollogly L, et al. Clinical and neuropathological parameters affecting the diagnostic yield of nerve biopsy. Neuromuscul Disord 2000;10:92–8.

160. Hellmann DB, Laing TJ, Petri M, et al. Mononeuritis multiplex: the yield of evaluations for occult rheumatic diseases. Medicine 1988;67:145–53.

161. Rappaport WD, Valente J, Hunter GC, et al. Clinical utilization and complications of sural nerve biopsy. Am J Surg 1993;166:252–6.

162. Vrancken AF, Notermans NC, Jansen GH, et al. Progressive idiopathic axonal neuropathy—a comparative clinical and histopathological study with vasculitic neuropathy. J Neurol 2004;251:269–78.

163. Chalk CH, Homburger HA, Dyck PJ. Anti-neutrophil cytoplasmic antibodies in vasculitis peripheral neuropathy. Neurology 1993;43:1826–7.

164. Vrancken AF, Gathier CS, Cats EA, et al. The additional yield of combined nerve/muscle biopsy in vasculitic neuropathy. Eur J Neurol 2011;18:49–58.

165. Schenone A, De Martini I, Tabaton M, et al. Direct immunofluorescence in sural nerve biopsies. Eur Neurol 1988;28:262–9.

166. Adams CW, Buk SJ, Hughes RA, et al. Perls' ferrocyanide test for iron in the diagnosis of vasculitic neuropathy. Neuropathol Appl Neurobiol 1989;15:433–9.

167. Lau JY, Bird GL, Alexander GJ, et al. Effects of immunosuppressive therapy on hepatic expression of hepatitis B viral genome and gene products. Clin Invest Med 1993;16:226–36.

168. Lam KC, Lai CL, Trepo C, et al. Deleterious effect of prednisolone in HBsAg-positive chronic active hepatitis. N Engl J Med 1981;304:380–6.

169. Kwon H, Lok AS. Hepatitis B therapy. Nat Rev Gastroenterol Hepatol 2011;8: 275–84.

170. Ayoub WS, Keeffe EB. Review article: current antiviral therapy of chronic hepatitis B. Aliment Pharmacol Ther 2011;34:1145–58.

171. Naniwa T, Maeda T, Shimizu S, et al. Hepatitis B virus-related polyarteritis nodosa presenting with multiple lung nodules and cavitary lesions. Chest 2010;138:195–7.

172. De Vita S, Quartuccio L, Isola M, et al. A randomized controlled trial of rituximab for the treatment of severe cryoglobulinemic vasculitis. Arthritis Rheum 2012;64: 843–53.

173. Sneller MC, Hu Z, Langford CA. A randomized controlled trial of rituximab following failure of antiviral therapy for hepatitis C virus-associated cryoglobulinemic vasculitis. Arthritis Rheum 2012;64:835–42.

174. Ahmed A. Antiviral treatment of cytomegalovirus infection. Infect Disord Drug Targets 2011;11:475–503.

175. Smith RM, Jones RB, Jayne DR. Progress in treatment of ANCA-associated vasculitis. Arthritis Res Ther 2012;14:210.

176. Fauci AS, Haynes BF, Katz P, et al. Wegener's granulomatosis: prospective clinical and therapeutic experience with 85 patients for 21 years. Ann Intern Med 1983;98:76–85.

177. Lapraik C, Watts R, Bacon P, et al. BSR and BHPR guidelines for the management of adults with ANCA associated vasculitis. Rheumatology 2007;46: 1615–6.

178. Mukhtyar C, Guillevin L, Cid MC, et al. EULAR Recommendations for the management of primary small and medium vessel vasculitis. Ann Rheum Dis 2009;68:310–7.

179. Faurschou M, Westman K, Rasmussen N, et al. Brief Report: long-term outcome of a randomized clinical trial comparing methotrexate to cyclophosphamide for remission induction in early systemic antineutrophil cytoplasmic antibody-associated vasculitis. Arthritis Rheum 2012;64:3472–7.

180. Walsh M, Merkel PA, Mahr A, et al. Effects of duration of glucocorticoid therapy on relapse rate in antineutrophil cytoplasmic antibody-associated vasculitis: a meta-analysis. Arthritis Care Res 2010;62:1166–73.

181. Hiemstra TF, Walsh M, Mahr A, et al. Mycophenolate mofetil vs azathioprine for remission maintenance in antineutrophil cytoplasmic antibody-associated vasculitis: a randomized controlled trial. JAMA 2010;304:2381–8.

182. Walsh M, Catapano F, Szpirt W, et al. Plasma exchange for renal vasculitis and idiopathic rapidly progressive glomerulonephritis: a meta-analysis. Am J Kidney Dis 2011;57:566–74.

183. Jones RB, Tervaert JW, Hauser T, et al. Rituximab versus cyclophosphamide in ANCA-associated renal vasculitis. N Engl J Med 2010;363:211–20.

184. Stone JH, Merkel PA, Spiera R, et al. Rituximab versus cyclophosphamide for ANCA-associated vasculitis. N Engl J Med 2010;363:221–32.

185. Jones RB, Ferraro AJ, Chaudhry AN, et al. A multicenter survey of rituximab therapy for refractory antineutrophil cytoplasmic antibody-associated vasculitis. Arthritis Rheum 2009;60:2156–68.

186. Holle JU, Dubrau C, Herlyn K, et al. Rituximab for refractory granulomatosis with polyangiitis (Wegener's granulomatosis): comparison of efficacy in granulomatous versus vasculitic manifestations. Ann Rheum Dis 2012;71:327–33.

187. Smith RM, Jones RB, Guerry MJ, et al. Rituximab for remission maintenance in relapsing antineutrophil cytoplasmic antibody-associated vasculitis. Arthritis Rheum 2012;64:3760–9.
188. Finnerup NB, Sindrup SH, Jensen TS. The evidence for pharmacological treatment of neuropathic pain. Pain 2010;150:573–81.
189. Kenna HA, Poon AW, de los Angeles CP, et al. Psychiatric complications of treatment with corticosteroids: review with case report. Psychiatry Clin Neurosci 2011;65:549–60.
190. Hellmich B, Flossmann O, Gross WL, et al. EULAR recommendations for conducting clinical studies and/or clinical trials in systemic vasculitis: focus on anti-neutrophil cytoplasm antibody-associated vasculitis. Ann Rheum Dis 2007;66:605–17.
191. Jayne DR, Chapel H, Adu D, et al. Intravenous immunoglobulin for ANCA-associated systemic vasculitis with persistent disease activity. QJM 2000;93: 433–9.
192. Morgan MD, Drayson MT, Savage CO, et al. Addition of infliximab to standard therapy for ANCA-associated vasculitis. Nephron Clin Pract 2011;117:c89–97.
193. de Menthon M, Cohen P, Pagnoux C, et al. Infliximab or rituximab for refractory Wegener's granulomatosis: long-term follow up. A prospective randomised multicentre study on 17 patients. Clin Exp Rheumatol 2011;29(1 Suppl 64):S63–71.
194. Wall N, Harper L. Complications of long-term therapy for ANCA-associated systemic vasculitis. Nat Rev Nephrol 2012;8:523–32.
195. Hoes JN, Jacobs JW, Boers M, et al. EULAR evidence-based recommendations on the management of systemic glucocorticoid therapy in rheumatic diseases. Ann Rheum Dis 2007;66:1560–7.
196. Weinstein RS. Clinical practice. Glucocorticoid-induced bone disease. N Engl J Med 2011;365:62–70.
197. van Staa TP, Leufkens HG, Cooper C. The epidemiology of corticosteroid-induced osteoporosis: a meta-analysis. Osteoporos Int 2002;13:777–87.
198. Grossman JM, Gordon R, Ranganath VK, et al. American College of Rheumatology 2010 recommendations for the prevention and treatment of glucocorticoid-induced osteoporosis. Arthritis Care Res 2010;62:1515–26.
199. Lekamwasam S, Adachi JD, Agnusdei D, et al. A framework for the development of guidelines for the management of glucocorticoid-induced osteoporosis. Osteoporos Int 2012;23:2257–76.

Inherited Peripheral Neuropathies

Mario A. Saporta, MD, PhD[a],*, Michael E. Shy, MD[b]

KEYWORDS

- Charcot-Marie-Tooth • Inherited neuropathy • Genetic testing

KEY POINTS

- Identifiable genetic causes of neuropathy elucidate biologic pathways that cause demyelination or axonal loss.
- Charcot-Marie-Tooth (CMT) disease is genetically and clinically heterogeneous with more than 50 genes causing neuropathy that can vary in age of onset and severity.
- Mutations in just four genes (*PMP22*, *GJB1*, *MPZ*, and *MFN2*) cause more than 90% of the genetically identifiable cases of CMT in North America.
- Combining the clinical phenotype and nerve conduction velocities in the arm can further focus genetic testing among these four genes.
- Because CMT can affect family members other than the proband, the authors suggest that genetic counseling be considered for patients and their families.

INTRODUCTION

First described at the end of the nineteenth century by French neurologists Jean Martin Charcot and Pierre Marie and British neurologist Howard Henry Tooth, Charcot-Marie-Tooth (CMT) disease is now identified as the most common inherited neurologic condition, affecting approximately 1 in 2500 people.[1] CMT is frequently the final diagnosis of patients with previously unidentified (idiopathic or cryptogenic) peripheral neuropathies,[2] underscoring the need for better awareness and strategies to help general neurologists navigate through the clinical and molecular diagnosis of this fascinating group of neuropathies. Recent advances in molecular biology have demonstrated that CMT is genetically heterogeneous, with at least 50 genes known to cause CMT when mutated. Most patients have an autosomal dominant form of CMT, though X-linked and autosomal recessive (AR) inheritances are not uncommon. This article describes the characteristics of various forms of CMT, their biologic substrate, as well as the current strategy for genetic testing.

[a] National Laboratory of Embryonic Stem Cells, Biomedical Sciences Department, Federal University of Rio de Janeiro, Rua Republica do Peru 362/602, Rio de Janeiro 22021-040, Brazil;
[b] Department of Neurology, University of Iowa, 200 Hawkins Drive, Iowa City, IA 52242, USA
* Corresponding author.
E-mail address: mariosaporta@gmail.com

Neurol Clin 31 (2013) 597–619
http://dx.doi.org/10.1016/j.ncl.2013.01.009
0733-8619/13/$ – see front matter © 2013 Elsevier Inc. All rights reserved.

neurologic.theclinics.com

THE BIOLOGY OF INHERITED PERIPHERAL NEUROPATHIES

A common feature of most genes mutated in CMT is the role they play in maintaining the structure or function of the two main cellular components of the peripheral nervous system, Schwann cells, and the axons of peripheral neurons (ventral horn spinal motor neurons and dorsal root ganglia sensory neurons) (**Fig. 1**).

The first genes identified to cause CMT express proteins that are essential for compact (peripheral myelin protein 22 [*PMP22*] and myelin protein zero [*MPZ*]) and non-compact (gap junction protein beta 1 [*GJB1*]) myelin structure[3] and their altered expressions cause demyelination or dysmyelination. A novel concept derived from the identification of *PMP22* duplication as the basic pathomechanism in CMT type 1A (CMT1A) is that of gene-protein dosage. It became clear that the correct stoichiometry of *PMP22* is necessary to maintain compact myelin integrity. Too much *PMP22* (duplication) causes CMT1A; too little (haploinsufficiency) causes hereditary neuropathy with liability to pressure palsies (HNPP) (see later discussion).[4] Abnormal expression of *MPZ* also causes demyelination, although in this case it is usually due to point mutations in the *MPZ* gene.

An important biologic feature common to both neurons and Schwann cells are their highly specialized and polarized cellular architecture.[5] Although the polarization of neurons is a well-recognized feature of these cells, with their axons extending more than 1 m in humans, Schwann cells are also very polarized because their membranes have to expand while they concentrically wrap around axons. To overcome the long distances between the cell nucleus and the more distal segments of the membrane, Schwann cells have areas of non-compact myelin rich in gap junctions that provide a radial pathway directly across the layers of the myelin sheath. Connexin 32 (Cx32), the protein expressed by the *GJB1* gene, is the main component of gap junctions in the myelin of Schwann cells and this may explain, at least in part, why *GJB1* mutations cause CMT type 1X (CMT1X).[6] The high polarization of neurons and Schwann cells may also explain why mutations in ubiquitously expressed genes, such as mitofusin 2 (*MFN2*), ganglioside-induced differentiation-associated protein 1 (*GDAP1*), or glycyl-tRNA synthetase (*GARS*), cause preferential dysfunction of the peripheral nervous system. The length-dependent neuropathy commonly found in patients with CMT seems to support the hypothesis that distal peripheral axons are especially susceptible to disruptions in organelle and metabolite axonal transport.

Schwann cells and axons interact at multiple points along the peripheral nerve, including the adaxonal membrane, paranodal myelin loops, microvilli, and

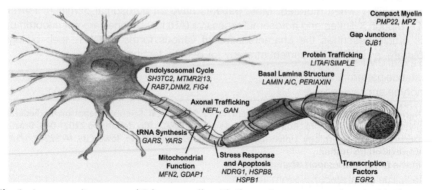

Fig. 1. A neuron: its axon and Schwann cells with the major genes associated with Charcot-Marie-Tooth disease with their respective function and cellular compartment.

juxtaparanodal basal lamina. These interactions are mutually beneficial, providing trophic support to the axon and myelinating cues to the Schwann cell. An example of this important interaction is the occurrence of secondary axonal degeneration in all forms of demyelinating CMT. This axonal degeneration is deemed to occur as a consequence of ineffective Schwann cell support to the axon and is actually more directly related to clinical functional impairment than the demyelination itself.[7]

Several recent studies have demonstrated a specific susceptibility of Schwann cells to mutations yielding misfolded proteins, as seen in certain *PMP22*[8] and *MPZ*[9,10] point mutations. Misfolded proteins accumulate in the endoplasmic reticulum (ER) of Schwann cells inducing a transitory unfolded protein response (UPR), a series of cellular events that help the ER to cope with the increased metabolic demand caused by misfolded protein retention. This, in turn, causes down-regulation of the myelination program genes and dedifferentiation of Schwann cells, a toxic gain of function that worsens the demyelination and is potentially amenable to therapeutic intervention.[11,12]

CLINICAL AND NEUROPHYSIOLOGICAL FEATURES

CMT is clinically, as well as genetically, heterogeneous, with variability in the age of onset, speed of progression, and electrodiagnostic findings. Though both motor and sensory nerves are usually affected, the more prominent phenotypic characteristic is related to motor difficulty in most cases. The classic phenotype includes steppage gait, pes cavus, sensory loss in a stocking or glove distribution, inverted champagne bottle legs, and atrophy in the hands.[13–15] Physical examination also shows decreased or absent deep tendon reflexes, often diffusely but virtually always involving the Achilles tendon. Findings are usually symmetric.[16] Onset is typically in the first to second decade in classic cases, though this may differ depending on the genetic subtype, including early-onset, infantile forms (historically designated Dejerine-Sottas syndrome) and late-onset, adult forms. Symptoms are usually slowly progressive, especially for the classic and late-onset phenotypes, but can be rather severe in early-onset forms. Patients usually have impaired proprioception with balance difficulty. Neuropathic pain affects around 20% of CMT patients.

Nerve conductions allow for classification into demyelinating, axonal, or intermediate groups, based on the motor nerve conduction velocities (MNCV) and compound muscle action potential amplitudes (CMAP). The standard cut off for demyelinating MNCV in the upper extremities is 38 m/s. Velocities between 35 and 45 m/s may be considered intermediately slowed, and greater than 45 m/s are considered axonal if there is a decrease in CMAP. Conduction velocities are performed in the arms because CMAP amplitudes are often unobtainable in the legs, even for demyelinating forms of CMT, due to impaired interactions between abnormal myelin and the underlying axon. CMT can be divided into subtypes based on electrodiagnostic features and inheritance pattern. Patients with autosomal dominant inheritance and a demyelinating phenotype are said to have CMT1. Patients with autosomal dominant inheritance and an axonal phenotype have CMT type 2 (CMT2) and patients with AR inheritance, regardless of the electrodiagnostic features, have CMT type 4 (CMT4). Patients with CMT inherited in an X-linked fashion have CMT type X (CMTX). The subtypes are further divided genetically based on the gene mutated. The gene, or the type of mutation in the gene that causes the condition, defines each genetic subtype, as shown on **Table 1**. The usual electrodiagnostic finding in demyelinating inherited neuropathies is widespread uniform slowing of conduction velocities, as opposed to the multifocal segmental slowing found in demyelinating acquired neuropathies in which temporal

Table 1
Classification of Charcot-Marie-Tooth disease

Type	Gene or Locus	Specific Phenotype
AD CMT1		
CMT1A	Dup 17p (PMP22)	Classic CMT1
	PMP22 (point mutation)	Classic CMT1, DSS, CHN, HNPP
CMT1B	MPZ	CMT1, DSS, CHN, intermediate, CMT2
CMT1C	LITAF	Classic CMT1
CMT1D	EGR2	Classic CMT1, DSS, CHN
CMT1E	NEFL	CMT2 but can have slow MNCVs in CMT1 range ± early-onset severe disease
HNPP		
HNPP	Del 17p (PMP22)	Typical HNPP
	PMP22 (point mutation)	Typical HNPP
X-linked CMT1 (CMT1X)		
CMT1X	GJB1	Intermediate ± patchy MNCVs; male MNCVs less than female MNCVs
AR demyelinating CMT (CMT4)		
CMT4A	GDAP1	Demyelinating or axonal, usually early onset and severe vocal cord and diaphragm paralysis described Rare AD CMT2 families described
CMT4B1	MTMR2	Severe CMT1, facial, bulbar, focally folded myelin
CMT4B2	SBF2	Severe CMT1, glaucoma, focally folded myelin
CMT4C	SH3TC2	Severe CMT1, scoliosis, cytoplasmic expansions
CMT4D (HMSNL)	NDRG1	Severe CMT1, gypsy, deafness, tongue atrophy
CMT4E	EGR2	Classic CMT1, DSS, CHN
CMT4F	PRX	CMT1, more sensory, focally folded myelin
CMT4H	FGD4	CMT1
CMT4J	FIG4	CMT1
CCFDN	CTDP1	CMT1, gypsy, cataracts, dysmorphic features
HMSN-Russe	10q22–q23	CMT1
CMT1	PMP22 (point mutation)	Classic CMT1, DSS, CHN, HNPPs
CMT1	MPZ	CMT1, DSS, CHN, intermediate, CMT2
AD CMT 2		
CMT2A	MFN2	CMT2 Usually severe Optic atrophy
CMT2B	RAB7A	CMT2 with predominant sensory involvement and sensory complications
CMT2C	12q23–q24	CMT2 with vocal cord and respiratory involvement
CMT2D	GARS	CMT2 with predominant hand wasting, weakness, or dHMN V
CMT2E	NEFL	CMT2 but can have slow MNCVs in CMT1 range ± early-onset severe disease

(continued on next page)

Table 1 (continued)		
Type	Gene or Locus	Specific Phenotype
CMT2F	HSPB1 (HSP27)	Classic CMT2 or dHMN II
CMT2G	12q12–q13.3	Classic CMT2
CMT2L	HSPB8 (HSP22)	Classic CMT2 or dHMN II
CMT2	MPZ	CMT1, DSS, CHN, intermediate, CMT2
CMT2 (HMSNP)	3q13.1	CMT2 with proximal involvement
AR CMT2 (also called CMT4)		
AR CMT2A	LMNA	CMT2 proximal involvement and rapid progression described Also causes muscular dystrophy, cardiomyopathy, or lipodystrophy
AR CMT2B	19q13.1–13.3	Typical CMT2
AR CMT2	GDAP1	CMT1 or CMT2 usually early onset and severe Vocal cord and diaphragm paralysis described Rare AD CMT2 families described
DI CMT (DI-CMT)		
DI-CMTA	10q24.1–25.1	Typical CMT
DI-CMTB	DNM2	Typical CMT
DI-CMTC	YARS	Typical CMT
Hereditary neuralgic amyotrophy (HNA)		
HNA	SEPT9	Recurrent neuralgic amyotrophy

Abbreviations: AD, autosomal dominant; CHN, congenital hypomyelinating neuropathy; CTDP1, CTD phosphatase subunit 1; Del, deletion; DMN2, dynamin 2; DSS, Dejerine-Sottas syndrome; Dup, duplication; EGR2, early growth response 2; FGD4, FYVE, RhoGEF, and PH domain containing 4; FIG4, FIG 4 homolog; HSP22, heat shock 22 kDa protein 8; HSP27, heat shock 27 kDa protein 1; KIF1Bb, kinesin family member 1B-b; LITAF, lipopolysaccharide-induced tumor necrosis factor; LMNA, lamin A and C; MCV, motor conduction velocity; MTMR2, myotubularin-related protein 2; MTMR13, myotubularin related protein 13; NDRG1, N-myc downstream regulated gene 1; NEFL, neurofilament, light polypeptide 68 kDa; PRX, periaxin; RAB7, RAB7, member RAS oncogene family; SEPT9, septin 9; SH3TC2, SH3 domain and tetratricopeptide repeats 2; YARS, tyrosyl tRNA synthetase.

From Reilly MM, Shy ME. Diagnosis and new treatments in genetic neuropathies. J Neurol Neurosurg Psychiatry 2009;80(12):1304–14. Copyright 2009, from BMJ Publishing Group Ltd; with permission.

dispersion and conduction block is frequently seen.[17,18] Two exceptions to this rule are men with CMT1X and patients with HNPP. In these cases, focal demyelination with temporal dispersion or conduction block can be seen. In all other cases of demyelinating CMT the finding of focal slowing should raise the possibility of a superimposed inflammatory neuropathy, which can benefit from immunosuppressive therapy.[19]

GENETIC TESTING STRATEGIES

Strategies for focusing genetic testing have been in place since at least 2001, with flow charts to help guide testing.[20] The distribution of causal genes depends, at least in part, on the population tested. For European and North American populations, AR CMT comprises less than 10% of all cases and most patients have dominantly inherited CMT even if their cases are sporadic. Alternatively, populations in which consanguinity is high, such as in North Africa, may have up to 40% of their cases being

AR. Using MNCV and inheritance patterns, several strategies have been published since the 2001 study, mostly based on North American or European populations.[21–23] The authors have recently published testing guidelines which included age of onset of symptoms to help guide testing.[24] Age of onset classifications were infantile (delayed walking), childhood, or adult. These guidelines divided MNCV info four categories: less than or equal to15 m/s (very slow), between 15 and 35 m/s (slow), between 35 and 45 m/s (intermediate), and greater than 45 m/s (axonal). Flow charts were provided using MNCV as the first level of evidence, with age of onset and inheritance patterns guiding the testing strategy within each category (**Figs. 2** and **3**). Of patients who had a genetic diagnosis, 92% were found to have changes in one of four genes: *PMP22*, *GJB1*, *MPZ*, and *MFN2*. Thus, the flow diagrams emphasize testing for these types of CMT, excepting HNPP, which has a distinctive nerve conduction study (NCS) pattern that differs from those of other forms of CMT and should be recognizable.

MNCV Less than or Equal to 15 m/s

All people with very slow MNCV who walked by 15 months of age had CMT1A; thus, genetic testing for the *PMP22* duplication is warranted for these individuals (see **Fig. 2**A). Of those patients who had delayed walking, most had CMT1A but 32% had CMT1B. Genetic testing for CMT1A and CMT1B is appropriate for people in this category. If these tests are negative, genetic testing for more rare forms of CMT may be reasonable.

MNCV Greater than 15 and Less than or Equal to 35 m/s

Approximately 89% of patients with slow MNCV who began walking by 15 months of age had CMT1A; thus, genetic testing should begin with *PMP22* duplication analysis (see **Fig. 2**B). CMT1X was the next most common type of CMT but should only be performed for people who do not have evidence of male-to-male transmission in their pedigree. CMT1B testing is much less likely to be the cause of the CMT for people in this category, but testing may be reasonable if testing if CMT1A and CMT1X are negative or if there is evidence of male-to-male transmission.

MNCV Greater than 35 and Less than or Equal to 45 m/s

Most people who had intermediate conductions had either CMT1X or CMT1B (see **Fig. 3**A). If symptoms began in childhood, and no male-to-male transmission is present in the pedigree, it is most likely for the person to have CMT1X. If this testing is negative, CMT1B testing may be pursued. However, if the symptom onset was in adulthood, testing for CMT1B is more likely to elicit a positive genetic testing result, with CMT1X being a reasonable follow-up test.

MNCV Greater than 45 m/s or Unobtainable CMAP

People with normal velocities or unobtainable CMAP usually present with CMT1X (usually women), CMT1B, or CMT2A (see **Fig. 3**B). People with unobtainable CMAP were usually those with CMT2A, who are often severely affected in infancy and childhood.[25] Thus, for children with early onset or severe CMT, it is proposed to begin genetic testing for CMT2A. For people with axonal CMT who have a classic or adult onset of symptoms, testing should begin with CMT1X in the absence of male-to-male transmission in the pedigree. Testing should begin with CMT1B if male-to-male transmission is present or if CMT1X testing is negative. The authors propose using other clinical findings, such as the upper limbs being more severely affected than the lower limbs, to help guide additional genetic testing if necessary. For these patients, mutations in the *GARS* gene, causing CMT2D may be appropriate.

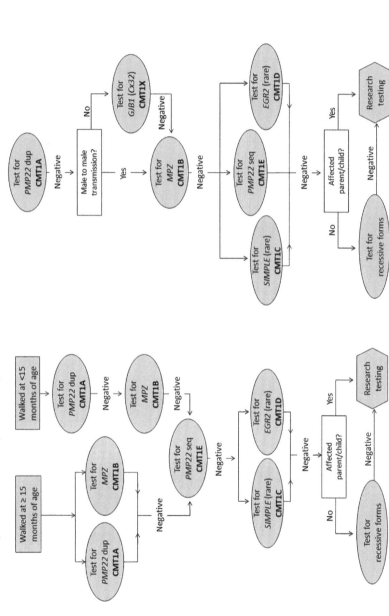

Fig. 2. Algorithm for the genetic diagnosis of patients with Charcot-Marie-Tooth disease and very slow (*A*) or slow (*B*) upper extremity motor nerve conduction velocities. dup, duplication; *EGR2*, early growth response 2; *LITAF*, lipopolysaccharide-induced TNF factor; seq, sequencing. (*From* Saporta AS, Sottile SL, Miller LJ, et al. Charcot-Marie-Tooth disease subtypes and genetic testing strategies. Ann Neurol 2011;69(1):22–33; with permission.)

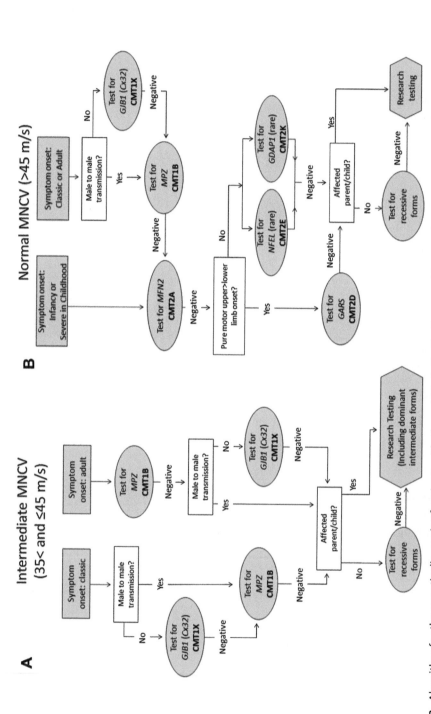

Fig. 3. Algorithm for the genetic diagnosis of patients with Charcot-Marie-Tooth disease and intermediate (A) or normal (B) upper extremity MNCVs. NEFL, neurofilament light polypeptide. (*From* Saporta AS, Sottile SL, Miller LJ, et al. Charcot-Marie-Tooth disease subtypes and genetic testing strategies. Ann Neurol 2011;69(1):22–33; with permission.)

Although a detailed review of the pros and cons for testing is beyond the scope of this article, the authors think it reasonable to provide some information about how we pursue genetic testing.[26] Clearly, not every patient with a genetic neuropathy wants or needs testing to identify the genetic cause of their disease. We believe that the ultimate decision to undergo genetic testing rests with the patient or the patient's parents if a symptomatic child is younger than 18 years of age. Reasons that patients give for obtaining testing include identifying the inheritance pattern of their CMT, making family planning decisions, and obtaining knowledge about the cause and natural history of their form of CMT. Natural history data is available for some forms of CMT such as CMT1A[27] and CMT1X,[28] which can provide guidance for prognosis, recognizing that there can be phenotypic variability in these subtypes. Patients with other forms of CMT frequently choose to undergo genetic testing to contribute to the natural history data collection for other patients with the same subtype. There are also reasons why patients do not want genetic testing. These include the high cost of commercial testing and fears of discrimination in the workplace or in obtaining health insurance. Because there are currently no medications to reverse any form of CMT, many patients decide against testing because their therapies will not depend on the results. We maintain that is always the patient's decision whether or not to pursue genetic testing.

Once a genetic diagnosis has been made in a patient, other family members usually do not need genetic testing but can be identified by clinical evaluation with neurophysiology. We do not typically test patients for multiple genetic causes of CMT simultaneously, although we did identify 11 patients with multiple genetic causes of CMT. It is our current policy to only consider performing genetic testing in clinically affected family members of a proband if their phenotype is atypical for the type of CMT in the family. In addition, we do not test asymptomatic minors with a family history of CMT, either by electrophysiology or genetic testing owing to the chance for increased psychological harm to the child.[29] We do routinely perform limited NCSs, though not needle electromyogram (EMG), on symptomatic children with CMT. Because nerve conduction changes, including slowing, are often uniform and detectable in early childhood in CMT,[17,18] testing of a single nerve is often adequate to guide genetic testing or determine whether a symptomatic child is affected in a family with CMT.

SPECIFIC FORMS OF CMT
CMT1

CMT1 includes five types of CMT that are caused by four genes when mutated. This group includes most people with CMT (over 70%). These genes are essential to Schwann cell function and the formation of myelin sheaths surrounding the axon, though they interact in different ways and thus are phenotypically heterogeneous.[30]

CMT1A

CMT1A is the most common type of CMT, affecting 55% of genetically defined patients.[24] It is caused by a 1.4 megabase (Mb) duplication at 17p11.2 including the PMP22 gene, created by unequal crossing over of homologous chromosomes.[31,32] People with CMT1A typically have the classic CMT phenotype, with normal age of onset for walking, development of symptoms in the first two decades, pes cavus, and slowly progressive motor and sensory neuropathy, which rarely progresses to wheelchair use later in life.[24,33] People with CMT1A have distinctive length dependent sensorimotor demyelinating neuropathies. One study found that more than 90% of patients with CMT1A had MNCV in the ulnar nerve between 16 and 35 m/s or less.[24]

CMT1A is an autosomal dominant condition, and most patients will have a family history. However, there is a de novo rate of about 10%.[34] Therefore, people without family history with ulnar MNCV under 35 m/s should first be screened for the *PMP22* duplication before proceeding with other genetic testing.[24] Once one person in a family has been genetically shown to have CMT1A, first and second-degree family members can be screened by MNCV. If other family members are shown to have the characteristically slowed conductions, it can be assumed that that person also has CMT1A without needing genetic testing.

HNPP

HNPP is caused by the reciprocal deletion of the 1.4 Mb stretch of chromosome 17p11.2 containing the *PMP22* gene.[35] A small percentage of people with HNPP have this phenotype due to a frameshift, splice site, or point mutation of the *PMP22* gene (www.molgen.ua.ac.be/cmtmutations). HNPP is the third most common type of CMT, affecting about 9.1% of genetically diagnosed patients,[24] with a de novo rate of about 20%.[36] The hallmark feature of HNPP is transient and recurrent motor and sensory mononeuropathies. These typically occur at entrapment sites, such as the carpal tunnel, ulnar groove, and fibular head.[37] These palsies may last hours, days, or weeks, or occasionally longer. For some people, HNPP can progress to long-term peripheral neuropathy phenotypically indistinguishable from CMT1, in which patients may require ankle-foot orthoses or wrist splints.[37] HNPP can be distinguished electrodiagnostically by marked slowing of the ulnar and sural sensory nerve conduction velocities, with or without reduced SNAP, and relatively preserved MNCV.[38] Distal motor latencies, particularly in the median and peroneal nerves, are typically prolonged, often out of proportion with the reduction of velocity.[39] Conduction block and focal slowing often occur at entrapment sites, particularly during a palsy episode.[37]

CMT1B

CMT1B is caused by mutations in the *MPZ* gene[40] located at chromosome 1q22, which encodes for *MPZ*, a major component of the myelin sheath. It affects about 8.5% of people with genetically defined CMT.[24] People with CMT1B usually present in a bimodal distribution. One group develops a severe, early onset, demyelinating neuropathy and the other group develops a late onset, milder, axonal neuropathy. Age of onset of symptoms is useful in determining the subtype of CMT. Most people with early onset CMT1B will have delayed walking and MNCV less than 15 m/s.[24] Those with late onset CMT1B will walk at a normal age and usually have MNCV greater than 35 m/s.[24]

CMT1C

CMT1C is caused by mutations in the *SIMPLE* gene at chromosome 16p13.3-p12.[41] The phenotype of CMT1C seems similar to that of CMT1A, with onset between the first and third decades and MNCV between 16 and 25 m/s,[42,43] as well as progressive sensorimotor nerve involvement. *SIMPLE* mutations are a rare cause for CMT, making up 0.6% to 1.2% of demyelinating CMT cohorts.[24,42]

CMT1D

CMT1D is caused by mutations in the *EGR2* gene at chromosome 10q21.1-q22.1.[44] Patients typically present in infancy with severe symptoms and may have congenital hypomyelination (hypotonia, delayed motor milestones, MNCV<10 m/s).[45] Cranial nerve involvement may also be present.[45,46] Recessive inheritance has also been described with this gene causing CMT4E, which seems to have a similar phenotype.

CMT1E

Point mutations in the *PMP22* gene cause CMT1E or HNPP, depending on the function of the mutation. Those with CMT1E tend to have earlier onset and more severe symptoms than those with CMT1A, but this is not invariable.[47,48] MNCV in severely affected patients are markedly reduced, usually less than 10 m/s.[47] Onset within the first 2 years of life presenting with delayed walking is not uncommon. CMT1E is a rare form of CMT, accounting for about 1% of people with genetically confirmed CMT.[24]

CMT2

CMT2A

CMT2A is caused by mutations in the *MFN2* gene.[49] This is the most common type of CMT2, accounting for approximately 21% of axonal CMT.[25] People with CMT2A usually, though not always, have a severe phenotype, with onset in infancy or early childhood and usually needing a wheelchair for ambulation by 20 years of age.[25,49] It may be difficult to perform NCSs and obtain responses for those with severe muscle atrophy and thus people who have severe symptoms without recordable potentials should be screened for CMT2A. The minority of patients may present with a mild or moderate axonal phenotype.[25] There are many polymorphisms in *MFN2* so that care must be taken to ensure that mutations are disease-causing. Most disease-causing mutations are in the GTPase domain, coiled-coil domains, or in other evolutionary conserved regions of the protein.[25]

CMT2B

CMT2B is caused by mutations in the *RAB7* gene.[50] This type of CMT is distinguished by distal sensory loss that often leads to foot ulcerations and subsequently infections and amputations[50–53] in addition to typical motor signs. Nerve conductions often have reduced amplitude with normal or near-normal velocities.[50–53] Sensory loss is often severe such that patients may be clinically indistinguishable from those with hereditary sensory and autonomic neuropathy (HSAN) type 1.

CMT2C

CMT2C is caused by mutations in the *TRPV4* gene.[54–56] CMT2C is characterized by a predominantly motor axonal neuropathy and vocal cord and diaphragmatic paresis, often presenting with hoarseness or stridor.[54–57] Sensorineural hearing loss and bladder urgency and incontinence have been reported.[54] CMT2C is allelic with spondylometaphyseal dysplasia, metatropic dysplasia, and brachyolmia, and thus may have some overlapping characteristics such as short statures and scoliosis.[55,58]

CMT2D

CMT2D is an axonal neuropathy caused by mutations in the *GARS* gene.[59] People with CMT2D typically have upper extremity weakness greater than and/or before lower extremity weakness and wasting, with a split-hand appearance of more atrophy in the FDI and thenar eminences and less so in the hypothenar eminence.[59,60] CMT2D is allelic with distal spinal muscular atrophy type V (dSMA-V), with the distinguishing feature being lack of sensory involvement in dSMA-V.[60]

CMT2E

CMT2E is caused by mutations in the neurofilaments light polypeptide (*NEFL*) gene.[61] NCSs may be axonal or in the demyelinating range.[62–64] Those with demyelinating conductions may have a severe early onset or a childhood presentation.[64] This is considered an axonal form of CMT because neurofilaments are components of the axon, not myelin.[65]

CMT2F

CMT2F is caused by mutations in the *HSPB1* gene, a member of the heat shock protein (HSP)-27 superfamily.[66] Most people with mutations in this gene have distal hereditary motor neuropathy (dHMN), a pure motor phenotype,[67,68] though some will have sensory findings on examination and electrophysiology.[69] Impairment typically begins in the distal legs and progresses slowly to the distal arms and then proximal legs.[68] There has been one report of presumed AR inheritance with mutations in this gene.[68]

CMT2L

CMT2L is caused by mutations in the *HSPB8* gene, also a member of the *HSP* superfamily, and is also known as *HSP22*.[70] Mutations in this gene have also been found to cause dHMN type II.[71] Scoliosis and proximal weakness have been reported.[72] Mutations in this gene are a rare cause of CMT.

CMT2K

CMT2K is caused by heterozygous mutations in the *GDAP1* gene, though recessive forms of CMT with mutations in this gene are called CMT4A and are likely more common.[73] Thus far, five mutations have been found to cause CMT2K: 358 C>T (p. R120W),[74,75] 469A>C (p.T157P) 75,[66] 678A>T (p.R226S),[76] 101C>G (p.S34C),[76] and 23delAG (p.G10fs).[76] Phenotypes range from mild adult onset and slowly progressive to severe childhood onset.[73–76] One study found that 3 out of 11 families with CMT2 had a dominantly inherited mutation in *GDAP1*,[76] indicating that this may be a significant cause of axonal CMT.

CMT4

CMT4A

CMT4A is caused by two recessive mutations in the *GDAP1* gene.[73] People with CMT4A typically have an early onset and severe sensorimotor neuropathy[73,77] that may be demyelinating or axonal in presentation.[78,79] Phenotype is typically severe, with first symptoms being noted in childhood and eventual progression to wheelchair not uncommon.[79,80] Vocal cord paralysis or hoarseness has also been reported.[79,80] Nerve conductions have been described as axonal or demyelinating, which has led to some confusion about the cell type of origin for the disease. *GDAP1* is a nuclear encoded gene that plays a role in mitochondrial fission or fragmentation, as opposed to *MFN2*, the causal gene for CMT2A, which plays an important role in mitochondrial fusion.

CMT4B1

CMT4B1 is caused by mutations in the myotubularin-related protein (*MTMR*)-2 gene.[81] Patients typically have demyelinating MNCV.[82] Onset is usually in childhood and causes distal weakness that progress proximally, often leading to wheelchair use by adulthood.[83] Diaphragmatic and facial weakness may occur.[84,85]

CMT4B2

CMT4B2 is caused by mutations in *SBF2*, also known as *MTMR13*.[86,87] Nerve conductions are usually demyelinating.[86,87] Onset is typically in childhood, though later than in CMT4B1.[87] Nerve biopsies showing focally folded myelin are characteristic of CMT4B1 (*MTMR2* mutations) and CMT4B2 (*MTMR13* mutations).

CMT4C

CMT4C is caused by mutations in the *SH3TC2* gene.[88] In addition to demyelinating sensorimotor neuropathy, scoliosis or kyphoscoliosis are hallmark features of this condition,[88–92] though not universally present. Patients often present in childhood with delayed walking, distal weakness, foot deformities, or scoliosis.[88–91,93] Cranial nerve involvements may also be present.[90,91,93] Although prevalence numbers are not known in all populations, there is evidence that CMT4C may be the most common of the AR-inherited neuropathies.[92]

CMT4F

CMT4F is caused by mutations in the *PERIAXIN* gene (*PRX*).[94,95] Patients have demyelinating conductions and severe early onset sensorimotor neuropathy.[94,96] Sensory ataxia may be present,[94,96,97] as might scoliosis.[96] Many sequence changes in the *PRX* gene have been found to be benign variants (www.molgen.ua.ac.be/cmtmutations), and variants of uncertain significance within the gene should be further investigated before determining if they are disease-causing mutations.

CMT4J

CMT4J is caused by mutations in the *FIG4* gene.[98] Patients may have demyelinating conductions and a severe motor phenotype, possibly asymmetric, with onset in early childhood. Rapid progression to a wheelchair in adulthood has been described for patients who were only mildly affected in their first two decades of life.[98,99] Early death has been reported (47 years of age).[99] Abnormalities on EMG may be similar to those seen in motor neuron disease, including fibrillations, positive waves, and reduced motor unit action potentials of long durations. However (see previous discussion), NCS may be in the demyelinating range despite these EMG changes.[99]

CMTX

CMT1X

CMT1X is caused by mutations in the *GJB1* gene, encoding the protein Cx32.[6] CMT1X is the second most common form of CMT, found in at least 10% of all patients.[24] Men typically have more severe symptoms than women with the condition,[100] and tend to have marked atrophy of the intrinsic hand muscles and all compartments of the calf muscles. Most men will have symptoms in childhood, though about 20% have a later age of onset.[24] Men with CMT1X have been reported to have transient stroke-like episodes with MRI changes following a stressor.[101] Whereas two out of three women with CMT1X will have slowly progressive mild symptoms, one out of three do have moderate neuropathy more similar to men with the condition.[100] Men with MNCV often present between 25 and 45 m/s, whereas women usually have MNCV greater than 35 m/s.[24]

HSAN

The HSANs are characterized by a predominant (although not always exclusive) sensory presentation. Patients may develop distinct clinical phenotypes according to the genetic abnormality, including distal lower limb sensory loss and neuropathic pain, congenital insensitivity to pain, or pure autonomic dysfunction. Most HSAN syndromes are AR and early-onset, although some can be autosomal dominant. HSAN subtypes are described in **Table 2**.

dHMNs

The dHMNs are inherited neuropathies that are exclusively motor in nature but are similar to CMT in any other way. Specifically, they are also length-dependent and

Table 2
Classification of the hereditary sensory and autonomic neuropathies

Type	Inheritance	Gene or Locus	Specific Phenotype
HSAN I	AD	SPTLC1	Mainly sensory, sensory complications, motor involvement variable, men may be more severely affected
CMT2B	AD	RAB7A	Sensorimotor, sensory complications, no pain
HSAN IB	AD	3p22–p24	Sensory, cough, gastroesophageal reflux
HSAN II	AR	WNK1	Severe sensory complications, mutilations, onset first 2 decades
HSAN III	AR	IKBKAP	Familial dysautonomia or Riley-Day syndrome, prominent autonomic, absence fungiform papillae of the tongue
HSAN IV	AR	NTRK1	Congenital insensitivity to pain with anhidrosis, severe sensory, anhidrosis, mental retardation, unmyelinated fibers mainly affected
HSAN V	AR	NTRK1	Congenital insensitivity to pain with mild anhidrosis, no mental retardation, small myelinated fibers mainly affected
HSAN V	AR	NGFB	Congenital insensitivity to pain, minimal autonomic, no mental retardation, mainly unmyelinated fibers affected
Channelopathy-associated insensitivity to pain	AR	SCN9A	Congenital insensitivity to pain

Abbreviations: AD, autosomal dominant; IKBKAP, inhibitor of kappa light polypeptide gene enhancer in B cells, kinase complex-associated protein; NGFB, nerve growth factor beta polypeptide; NTRK1, neurotrophic tyrosine kinase receptor type 1; RAB7, RAB7, member RAS oncogene family; SCN9A, sodium channel, voltage-gated, type IX, alpha subunit; SPTLC1, serine palmitoyltransferase, long-chain base subunit-1.

From Reilly MM, Shy ME. Diagnosis and new treatments in genetic neuropathies. J Neurol Neurosurg Psychiatry 2009;80(12):1304–14. Copyright 2009, from BMJ Publishing Group Ltd; with permission.

usually slowly progressive. Some of the dHMNs are actually caused by mutation in genes that are also related to CMT. **Table 3** is a description of dHMN subtypes and their main features.

Inherited Neuropathies in Multisystem Genetic Disorders

Inherited neuropathies can be part of a more generalized genetic disease that affects other neurologic and nonneurologic systems. Examples of genetic neurologic disorders that can present with peripheral neuropathies are the spinocerebellar ataxias and the hereditary spastic paraplegias. Metabolic disorders are another cause of multisystem diseases that also affect the peripheral nervous system. This group includes some leukodystrophies (metachromatic, Krabbe, adrenoleukodystrophy),

Table 3
Classification of the dHMNs

Type	Inheritance	Gene or Locus	Specific Phenotype
dHMN I	AD	Unknown	Juvenile-onset dHMN
dHMN II	AD	HSPB1 (HSP27)	Adult-onset typical dHMN, CMT2F
dHMN II	AD	HSPB8 (HSP22)	Adult-onset typical dHMN, CMT2L
dHMN III	AR	11q13	Early onset, slowly progressive
dHMN IV	AR	11q13	Juvenile onset, diaphragmatic involvement
dHMN V	AD	GARS	Upper limb onset, slowly progressive, CMT2D
dHMN V	AD	BSCL2	Upper limb onset, ± spasticity lower limbs, Silver-Russell syndrome
dHMN VI	AR	IGHMBP2	Spinal muscle atrophy with respiratory distress, infantile-onset respiratory distress
dHMN VIIA	AD	2q14	Adult onset, vocal cord paralysis
dHMN VIIB	AD	DCTN1	Adult onset, vocal cord paralysis, facial weakness
dHMN, ALS4	AD	SETX	Early onset, pyramidal signs
dHMN J	AR	9p21.1–p12	Juvenile onset, pyramidal features, Jerash
Congenital distal SMA	AD	12q23–12q24	Antenatal onset, arthrogryposis

Abbreviations: AD, autosomal dominant; BSCL2, Berardinelli-Seip congenital lipodystrophy 2 (seipin); DCTN1, dynactin1; IGHMBP2, immunoglobulin mu binding protein 2; SETX, sentaxin; SMA, spinal muscular atrophy.
From Reilly MM, Shy ME. Diagnosis and new treatments in genetic neuropathies. J Neurol Neurosurg Psychiatry 2009;80(12):1304–14. Copyright 2009, from BMJ Publishing Group Ltd; with permission.

peroxisomal diseases (Fabry, Refsum), lipoprotein deficiencies (Tangier, Cerebrotendinous xanthomatosis), porphyrias, mitochondrial diseases, and the familial amyloid neuropathies. A comprehensive review of these conditions is beyond the scope of this article; however, it is important to include this group of diseases in the differential diagnosis of patients with inherited neuropathies and signs of dysfunction beyond the peripheral nervous system.

THERAPEUTIC STRATEGIES AND FUTURE DIRECTIONS

Despite the great improvement in our biologic understanding of inherited neuropathies, derived mostly from developments in molecular biology and transgenic animal models in the last 25 years, there is still no treatment available for any type of CMT. Physical therapy, occupational therapy, and a few orthopedic procedures are still the cornerstone of CMT treatment.

A dedicated, multidisciplinary rehabilitation team can significantly contribute to the management of patients with CMT and improve functionality and quality of life. Physical therapy strategies to maintain muscle strength and tone, prevent muscle contractures, and improve balance are a common need for most patients with CMT. Orthotics are also an important component of treating these patients, providing support and improving balance for ambulation. Occupational therapy focused on developing tools and strategies to help patients with activities of daily living will benefit patients with CMT, especially those with hand weakness. Tendon lengthening and tendon transfers can benefit a subset of CMT patients with muscle contractures and tendon shortening and patients with significant weakness in functionally relevant muscles, respectively; however, the optimal timing of such procedures is still controversial.

Reducing the expression of *pmp22* in Schwann cells (hence treating the overexpression of *pmp22*) is a biologic strategy being tested to treat CMT1A. High-dose ascorbic acid (vitamin C) was shown to decrease *pmp22* levels and symptoms in mice with CMT1A, so that they were able to stay on a rotating rod longer, cross a beam more rapidly, and grip for longer than untreated mice.[102] Several studies have been performed in humans with CMT1A, testing different doses of vitamin C (1–4 g/d) for up to 2 years. Unfortunately, all studies failed to meet their primary outcome measures and did not show a significant effect on phenotype.[103–106] Progesterone antagonists have also been shown to decrease *pmp22* expression in a rat model of CMT1A, improving their phenotype (specifically, the axonal loss seen during disease progression).[107,108] Unfortunately, onapristone, the compound shown to have therapeutic effects in this study, is toxic to humans. Efforts to develop bioequivalent compounds with a better safety profile are ongoing.

Recent studies have demonstrated the role of ER accumulation of misfolded proteins and UPR activation in the pathogenesis of several animal models of CMT associated with point mutations in myelin-related genes, including *pmp22*[8] and *MPZ*.[9,10] Furthermore, treatment with an agent that relieves ER stress (curcumin) improved the phenotype of both models.[11,12] Therefore, compounds that either relieve ER stress or reduced UPR activation are promising therapeutic strategies to treat patients with mutations that cause misfolded proteins to accumulate in the ER of Schwann cells.

Treatment strategies for axonal forms of CMT have not been as easily identified as for demyelinating forms. Recently, histone deacetylase-6 inhibitors have been shown to correct axonal transport defects in a mouse model of CMT2F associated with point mutations in the *HSPB1* gene, rescuing the axonal loss and clinical phenotype of these mice.[109] It remains to be shown whether this same strategy could be useful in other forms of axonal CMT, but correcting axonal transport defects may be a common treatment option for most of these CMT types.

Two new technologies recently developed hold enormous potential in the search for compounds to treat CMT: cellular reprogramming and high-throughput drug screening. Cellular reprogramming is a technique that allows the generation of specific cell types (including stem cell–like cells, neurons, and glia) by genetically modifying readily available somatic cells such as fibroblasts or lymphocytes.[110,111] Using this technology, researchers are able to generate unlimited supplies of patient-specific cell lines for use in mechanistic studies and drug development.[112] These patient-specific cells lines will be particularly useful when combined with high-throughput screening of drug libraries containing thousands of compounds. In these highly automated platforms, the process of identifying compounds capable of correcting certain disease-related cell phenotypes is streamlined, allowing for a faster target selection of compounds to be tested in phase 1 animal studies. The use of patient-derived human cells offer the theoretical advantage of a more translational platform, which could facilitate the process of moving from phase 1 studies to human clinical trials. Whether this is actually true, remains to be proven. A recent study using cellular reprogramming successfully generated human neural crest progenitors derived from a patient with HSAN type III.[113] These cells are the precursors of sensory and autonomic neurons, the cell types most affected by this condition. Interestingly, patient-derived neural crest precursors expressed very low levels of normal inhibitor of kappa light polypeptide gene enhancer in B cells, kinase complex-associated protein (*IKBKAP*) transcript, while also displaying marked defects in neuronal differentiation and migration. The investigators were also able to find compounds that, at least partially, rescued this phenotype, validating this platform for drug discovery in inherited neuropathies.

SUMMARY

Although CMT is a genetically heterogeneous condition, it is often possible to deter-mine the type of CMT a person has by distinguishing characteristics. The prevalence of the various mutations, inheritance pattern, nerve conductions, and age of onset should be taken into account when deciding what genetic testing should be ordered. New genes causing CMT continue to be found, prevalence continues to be studied, and recommendations for testing will continue to evolve over time. Our increasing understanding of biologic processes involved in CMT has offered new therapeutic targets for drug development and new tools recently developed hold the promise of even faster drug discovery in CMT.

ACKNOWLEDGMENTS

MES is supported in part by research grants from the NINDS/ORD, Muscular Dystrophy Association, and the Charcot-Marie-Tooth Association. The authors would like to thank Luis Saporta for artwork prepared for this article.

Case study

A 25-year-old man with no family history of neuropathy had been weak since infancy. He was able to stand independently by 3 years of age but was never able to run normally and always had an abnormal gait. He is currently only able to walk if wearing ankle-foot orthoses. He also has pronounced weakness with fine movements of his fingers and is unable to button his clothes, cut his own food or perform activities such as turning a key in his front door. His neuro-logical function has been relatively stable since his teenage years. Nerve conduction studies showed markedly slowed NCVs (<10 m/s) in his upper extremities; NCV in his legs were unob-tainable at routine recording sites. Compound muscle amplitude potentials were significantly reduced in the arms and absent in the legs. Sensory nerve action potentials were absent in the arms and legs. Genetic testing revealed an Arg98Cys mutation in *MPZ* (myelin protein zero) leading to a diagnosis of severe CMT1B.

Comment: In North America, if one has a genetically diagnosable form of CMT it is likely that the causal mutation is in one of four genes (PMP22, MPZ, GJB1 or MFN2) unless the family history strongly suggests an autosomal recessive inheritance pattern (multiple affected siblings with no parents affected). CMT1A, the most common form of CMT typically has NCV around 20 m/sec in the arms and a classic CMT phenotype with normal early milestones and gradual weakness developing in the first two decades of life. Delayed early milestones and NCV<10 m/s are suggestive of an early onset form of CMT1B. GJB1 mutations causing CMT1X typically have intermediately slowed NCV (35-45 m/s) with an x-linked inheritance. MFN2 mutations cause the most frequent form of CMT2. Another group of patients with CMT1B often present symptoms in adulthood, with intermediate to normal NCV.

REFERENCES

1. Skre H. Genetic and clinical aspects of Charcot-Marie-Tooth's disease. Clin Genet 1974;6(2):98–118.
2. Dyck PJ, Oviatt KF, Lambert EH. Intensive evaluation of referred unclassified neuropathies yields improved diagnosis. Ann Neurol 1981;10:222–6.
3. Trapp BD, Pfeiffer SE, Anitei A, et al. Cell biology and myelin assembly. In: Lazzarini RA, editor. Myelin biology and disorders. San Diego (CA), London: Elsevier Academic Press; 2003. p. 29–56.
4. Niemann A, Berger P, Suter U. Pathomechanisms of mutant proteins in Charcot-Marie-Tooth disease. Neuromolecular Med 2006;8(1–2):217–42.

5. Li J. Hypothesis of double polarization. J Neurol Sci 2008;275(1–2):33–6.
6. Bergoffen J, Scherer SS, Wang S, et al. Connexin mutations in X-linked Charcot-Marie-Tooth disease. Science 1993;262(5142):2039–42.
7. Krajewski KM, Lewis RA, Fuerst DR, et al. Neurological dysfunction and axonal degeneration in Charcot-Marie-Tooth disease type 1A. Brain 2000;123(7):1516–27.
8. Colby J, Nicholson R, Dickson KM, et al. PMP22 carrying the trembler or trembler-J mutation is intracellularly retained in myelinating Schwann cells. Neurobiol Dis 2000;7:561–73.
9. Pennuto M, Tinelli E, Malaguti M, et al. Ablation of the UPR-mediator CHOP restores motor function and reduces demyelination in Charcot-Marie-Tooth 1BMice. Neuron 2008;57:393–405.
10. Saporta MA, Shy BR, Patzko A, et al. MpzR98C arrests Schwann cell development in a mouse model of early-onset Charcot-Marie-Tooth disease type 1B. Brain 2012;135(7):2032–47.
11. Khajavi M, Shiga K, Wiszniewski W, et al. Oral curcumin mitigates the clinical and neuropathologic phenotype of the Trembler-J mouse: a potential therapy for inherited neuropathy. Am J Hum Genet 2007;81:438–53.
12. Patzko A, Bai Y, Saporta M, et al. Curcumin derivatives promote Schwann cell differentiation and improve neuropathy in R98C CMT1B mice. Brain 2012;135(12):3551–66.
13. Harding AE, Thomas PK. Genetic aspects of hereditary motor and sensory neuropathy (types I and II). J Med Genet 1980;17(5):329–36.
14. Harding AE, Thomas PK. The clinical features of hereditary motor and sensory neuropathy types I and II. Brain 1980;103(2):259–80.
15. Thomas PK, Harding AE. Inherited neuropathies: the interface between molecular genetics and pathology. Brain Pathol 1993;3(2):129–33.
16. Michels VV, Dyck PJ. Mendelian inheritance and basis of classification of hereditary neuropathy with neuronal atrophy and degeneration. In: Dyck P, Thomas PK, Lambert EH, et al, editors. Peripheral neuropathy. 2nd edition. Philadelphia: W.B. Saunders Company; 1984. p. 1512–24.
17. Lewis RA, Sumner AJ. The electrodiagnostic distinctions between chronic familial and acquired demyelinative neuropathies. Neurology 1982;32(6):592–6.
18. Lewis RA, Sumner AJ, Shy ME. Electrophysiological features of inherited demyelinating neuropathies: a reappraisal in the era of molecular diagnosis. Muscle Nerve 2000;23(10):1472–87.
19. Ginsberg L, Malik O, Kenton AR, et al. Coexistent hereditary and inflammatory neuropathy. Brain 2004;127(1):193–202.
20. Dubourg O, Tardieu S, Birouk N, et al. The frequency of 17p11.2 duplication and Connexin 32 mutations in 282 Charcot-Marie-Tooth families in relation to the mode of inheritance and motor nerve conduction velocity. Neuromuscul Disord 2001;11(5):458–63.
21. England JD, Gronseth GS, Franklin G, et al. Practice parameter: the evaluation of distal symmetric polyneuropathy: the role of laboratory and genetic testing (an evidence-based review). Report of the American Academy of Neurology, the American Association of Neuromuscular and Electrodiagnostic Medicine, and the American Academy of Physical Medicine and Rehabilitation. PM R 2009;1(1):5–13.
22. England JD, Gronseth GS, Franklin G, et al. Practice parameter: evaluation of distal symmetric polyneuropathy: role of laboratory and genetic testing (an evidence-based review). Report of the American Academy of Neurology, American

Association of Neuromuscular and Electrodiagnostic Medicine, and American Academy of Physical Medicine and Rehabilitation. Neurology 2009;72(2):185–92.

23. Burgunder JM, Schols L, Baets J, et al. EFNS guidelines for the molecular diagnosis of neurogenetic disorders: motoneuron, peripheral nerve and muscle disorders. Eur J Neurol 2011;18(2):207–17.

24. Saporta AS, Sottile SL, Miller LJ, et al. Charcot-Marie-Tooth disease subtypes and genetic testing strategies. Ann Neurol 2011;69(1):22–33.

25. Feely SM, Laura M, Siskind CE, et al. MFN2 mutations cause severe phenotypes in most patients with CMT2A. Neurology 2011;76(20):1690–6.

26. Krajewski KM, Shy ME. Genetic testing in neuromuscular disease. Neurol Clin 2004;22(3):481–508, v.

27. Shy ME, Chen L, Swan ER, et al. Neuropathy progression in Charcot-Marie-Tooth disease type 1A. Neurology 2008;70(5):378–83.

28. Shy ME, Siskind C, Swan ER, et al. CMT1X phenotypes represent loss of GJB1 gene function. Neurology 2007;68(11):849–55.

29. Points to consider: ethical, legal, and psychosocial implications of genetic testing in children and adolescents. American Society of Human Genetics Board of Directors, American College of Medical Genetics Board of Directors. Am J Hum Genet 1995;57(5):1233–41.

30. Kamholz J, Menichella D, Jani A, et al. Charcot-Marie-Tooth disease type 1: molecular pathogenesis to gene therapy. Brain 2000;123(Pt 2):222–33.

31. Lupski JR, de Oca-Luna RM, Slaugenhaupt S, et al. DNA duplication associated with Charcot-Marie-Tooth disease type 1A. Cell 1991;66(2):219–32.

32. Raeymaekers P, Timmerman V, Nelis E, et al. Duplication in chromosome 17p11.2 in Charcot-Marie-Tooth neuropathy type 1a (CMT 1a). The HMSN Collaborative Research Group. Neuromuscul Disord 1991;1(2):93–7.

33. Sheth S, Francies K, Siskind CE, et al. Diabetes mellitus exacerbates motor and sensory impairment in CMT1A. J Peripher Nerv Syst 2008;13(4):299–304.

34. Blair IP, Nash J, Gordon MJ, et al. Prevalence and origin of de novo duplications in Charcot-Marie-Tooth disease type 1A: first report of a de novo duplication with a maternal origin. Am J Hum Genet 1996;58(3):472–6.

35. Chance PF, Alderson MK, Leppig KA, et al. DNA deletion associated with hereditary neuropathy with liability to pressure palsies. Cell 1993;72(1):143–51.

36. Infante J, Garcia A, Combarros O, et al. Diagnostic strategy for familial and sporadic cases of neuropathy associated with 17p11.2 deletion. Muscle Nerve 2001;24(9):1149–55.

37. Stogbauer F, Young P, Kuhlenbaumer G, et al. Hereditary recurrent focal neuropathies: clinical and molecular features. Neurology 2000;54(3):546–51.

38. Andersson PB, Yuen E, Parko K, et al. Electrodiagnostic features of hereditary neuropathy with liability to pressure palsies. Neurology 2000;54(1):40–4.

39. Li J, Krajewski K, Shy ME, et al. Hereditary neuropathy with liability to pressure palsy: the electrophysiology fits the name. Neurology 2002;58(12):1769–73.

40. Hayasaka K, Himoro M, Sato W, et al. Charcot-Marie-Tooth neuropathy type 1B is associated with mutations of the myelin P0 gene. Nat Genet 1993; 5(1):31–4.

41. Street VA, Bennett CL, Goldy JD, et al. Mutation of a putative protein degradation gene LITAF/SIMPLE in Charcot-Marie-Tooth disease 1C. Neurology 2003; 60(1):22–6.

42. Latour P, Gonnaud PM, Ollagnon E, et al. SIMPLE mutation analysis in dominant demyelinating Charcot-Marie-Tooth disease: three novel mutations. J Peripher Nerv Syst 2006;11(2):148–55.

43. Saifi GM, Szigeti K, Wiszniewski W, et al. SIMPLE mutations in Charcot-Marie-Tooth disease and the potential role of its protein product in protein degradation. Hum Mutat 2005;25(4):372–83.

44. Warner LE, Mancias P, Butler IJ, et al. Mutations in the early growth response 2 (EGR2) gene are associated with hereditary myelinopathies. Nat Genet 1998;18(4):382–4.

45. Vandenberghe N, Upadhyaya M, Gatignol A, et al. Frequency of mutations in the early growth response 2 gene associated with peripheral demyelinating neuropathies. J Med Genet 2002;39(12):e81.

46. Pareyson D, Taroni F, Botti S, et al. Cranial nerve involvement in CMT disease type 1 due to early growth response 2 gene mutation. Neurology 2000;54(8): 1696–8.

47. Boerkoel CF, Takashima H, Garcia CA, et al. Charcot-Marie-Tooth disease and related neuropathies: mutation distribution and genotype-phenotype correlation. Ann Neurol 2002;51(2):190–201.

48. Russo M, Laura M, Polke JM, et al. Variable phenotypes are associated with PMP22 missense mutations. Neuromuscul Disord 2011;21(2):106–14.

49. Zuchner S, Mersiyanova IV, Muglia M, et al. Mutations in the mitochondrial GTPase mitofusin 2 cause Charcot-Marie-Tooth neuropathy type 2A. Nat Genet 2004;36(5):449–51.

50. Verhoeven K, De Jonghe P, Coen K, et al. Mutations in the small GTP-ase late endosomal protein RAB7 cause Charcot-Marie-Tooth type 2B neuropathy. Am J Hum Genet 2003;72(3):722–7.

51. Auer-Grumbach M, De Jonghe P, Wagner K, et al. Phenotype-genotype correlations in a CMT2B family with refined 3q13-q22 locus. Neurology 2000;55(10): 1552–7.

52. De Jonghe P, Timmerman V, FitzPatrick D, et al. Mutilating neuropathic ulcerations in a chromosome 3q13-q22 linked Charcot-Marie-Tooth disease type 2B family. J Neurol Neurosurg Psychiatry 1997;62(6):570–3.

53. Kwon JM, Elliott JL, Yee WC, et al. Assignment of a second Charcot-Marie-Tooth type II locus to chromosome 3q. Am J Hum Genet 1995;57(4):853–8.

54. Landoure G, Zdebik AA, Martinez TL, et al. Mutations in TRPV4 cause Charcot-Marie-Tooth disease type 2C. Nat Genet 2010;42(2):170–4.

55. Chen DH, Sul Y, Weiss M, et al. CMT2C with vocal cord paresis associated with short stature and mutations in the TRPV4 gene. Neurology 2010;75(22): 1968–75.

56. Deng HX, Klein CJ, Yan J, et al. Scapuloperoneal spinal muscular atrophy and CMT2C are allelic disorders caused by alterations in TRPV4. Nat Genet 2010; 42(2):165–9.

57. Dyck PJ, Litchy WJ, Minnerath S, et al. Hereditary motor and sensory neuropathy with diaphragm and vocal cord paresis. Ann Neurol 1994;35(5):608–15.

58. Klein CJ, Cunningham JM, Atkinson EJ, et al. The gene for HMSN2C maps to 12q23-24: a region of neuromuscular disorders. Neurology 2003;60(7):1151–6.

59. Antonellis A, Ellsworth RE, Sambuughin N, et al. Glycyl tRNA synthetase mutations in Charcot-Marie-Tooth disease type 2D and distal spinal muscular atrophy type V. Am J Hum Genet 2003;72(5):1293–9.

60. Sivakumar K, Kyriakides T, Puls I, et al. Phenotypic spectrum of disorders associated with glycyl-tRNA synthetase mutations. Brain 2005;128(Pt 10):2304–14.

61. Mersiyanova IV, Perepelov AV, Polyakov AV, et al. A new variant of Charcot-Marie-Tooth disease type 2 is probably the result of a mutation in the neurofilament-light gene. Am J Hum Genet 2000;67(1):37–46.

62. Georgiou DM, Zidar J, Korosec M, et al. A novel NF-L mutation Pro22Ser is associated with CMT2 in a large Slovenian family. Neurogenetics 2002;4(2):93–6.
63. Yoshihara T, Yamamoto M, Hattori N, et al. Identification of novel sequence variants in the neurofilament-light gene in a Japanese population: analysis of Charcot-Marie-Tooth disease patients and normal individuals. J Peripher Nerv Syst 2002;7(4):221–4.
64. Jordanova A, De Jonghe P, Boerkoel CF, et al. Mutations in the neurofilament light chain gene (NEFL) cause early onset severe Charcot-Marie-Tooth disease. Brain 2003;126(Pt 3):590–7.
65. Perez-Olle R, Leung CL, Liem RK. Effects of Charcot-Marie-Tooth-linked mutations of the neurofilament light subunit on intermediate filament formation. J Cell Sci 2002;115(Pt 24):4937–46.
66. Evgrafov OV, Mersiyanova I, Irobi J, et al. Mutant small heat-shock protein 27 causes axonal Charcot-Marie-Tooth disease and distal hereditary motor neuropathy. Nat Genet 2004;36(6):602–6.
67. Chung KW, Kim SB, Cho SY, et al. Distal hereditary motor neuropathy in Korean patients with a small heat shock protein 27 mutation. Exp Mol Med 2008;40(3):304–12.
68. Houlden H, Laura M, Wavrant-De Vrieze F, et al. Mutations in the HSP27 (HSPB1) gene cause dominant, recessive, and sporadic distal HMN/CMT type 2. Neurology 2008;71(21):1660–8.
69. Solla P, Vannelli A, Bolino A, et al. Heat shock protein 27 R127W mutation: evidence of a continuum between axonal Charcot-Marie-Tooth and distal hereditary motor neuropathy. J Neurol Neurosurg Psychiatry 2010;81(9):958–62.
70. Tang BS, Zhao GH, Luo W, et al. Small heat-shock protein 22 mutated in autosomal dominant Charcot-Marie-Tooth disease type 2L. Hum Genet 2005;116(3):222–4.
71. Irobi J, Van Impe K, Seeman P, et al. Hot-spot residue in small heat-shock protein 22 causes distal motor neuropathy. Nat Genet 2004;36(6):597–601.
72. Tang BS, Luo W, Xia K, et al. A new locus for autosomal dominant Charcot-Marie-Tooth disease type 2 (CMT2L) maps to chromosome 12q24. Hum Genet 2004;114(6):527–33.
73. Baxter RV, Ben Othmane K, Rochelle JM, et al. Ganglioside-induced differentiation-associated protein-1 is mutant in Charcot-Marie-Tooth disease type 4A/8q21. Nat Genet 2002;30(1):21–2.
74. Sivera R, Espinos C, Vilchez JJ, et al. Phenotypical features of the p.R120W mutation in the GDAP1 gene causing autosomal dominant Charcot-Marie-Tooth disease. J Peripher Nerv Syst 2010;15(4):334–44.
75. Claramunt R, Pedrola L, Sevilla T, et al. Genetics of Charcot-Marie-Tooth disease type 4A: mutations, inheritance, phenotypic variability, and founder effect. J Med Genet 2005;42(4):358–65.
76. Crimella C, Tonelli A, Airoldi G, et al. The GST domain of GDAP1 is a frequent target of mutations in the dominant form of axonal Charcot Marie Tooth type 2K. J Med Genet 2010;47(10):712–6.
77. Senderek J, Bergmann C, Ramaekers VT, et al. Mutations in the ganglioside-induced differentiation-associated protein-1 (GDAP1) gene in intermediate type autosomal recessive Charcot-Marie-Tooth neuropathy. Brain 2003;126(Pt 3):642–9.
78. Nelis E, Erdem S, Van Den Bergh PY, et al. Mutations in GDAP1: autosomal recessive CMT with demyelination and axonopathy. Neurology 2002;59(12):1865–72.

79. Sevilla T, Cuesta A, Chumillas MJ, et al. Clinical, electrophysiological and morphological findings of Charcot-Marie-Tooth neuropathy with vocal cord palsy and mutations in the GDAP1 gene. Brain 2003;126(Pt 9):2023–33.

80. Boerkoel CF, Takashima H, Nakagawa M, et al. CMT4A: identification of a Hispanic GDAP1 founder mutation. Ann Neurol 2003;53(3):400–5.

81. Bolino A, Muglia M, Conforti FL, et al. Charcot-Marie-Tooth type 4B is caused by mutations in the gene encoding myotubularin-related protein-2. Nat Genet 2000; 25(1):17–9.

82. Houlden H, King RH, Wood NW, et al. Mutations in the 5' region of the myotubularin-related protein 2 (MTMR2) gene in autosomal recessive hereditary neuropathy with focally folded myelin. Brain 2001;124(Pt 5):907–15.

83. Parman Y, Battaloglu E, Baris I, et al. Clinicopathological and genetic study of early-onset demyelinating neuropathy. Brain 2004;127(Pt 11):2540–50.

84. Tyson J, Ellis D, Fairbrother U, et al. Hereditary demyelinating neuropathy of infancy. A genetically complex syndrome. Brain 1997;120(Pt 1):47–63.

85. Verny C, Ravise N, Leutenegger AL, et al. Coincidence of two genetic forms of Charcot-Marie-Tooth disease in a single family. Neurology 2004;63(8):1527–9.

86. Senderek J, Bergmann C, Weber S, et al. Mutation of the SBF2 gene, encoding a novel member of the myotubularin family, in Charcot-Marie-Tooth neuropathy type 4B2/11p15. Hum Mol Genet 2003;12(3):349–56.

87. Azzedine H, Bolino A, Taieb T, et al. Mutations in MTMR13, a new pseudophosphatase homologue of MTMR2 and Sbf1, in two families with an autosomal recessive demyelinating form of Charcot-Marie-Tooth disease associated with early-onset glaucoma. Am J Hum Genet 2003;72(5):1141–53.

88. Senderek J, Bergmann C, Stendel C, et al. Mutations in a gene encoding a novel SH3/TPR domain protein cause autosomal recessive Charcot-Marie-Tooth type 4C neuropathy. Am J Hum Genet 2003;73(5):1106–19.

89. Gooding R, Colomer J, King R, et al. A novel Gypsy founder mutation, p.Arg1109X in the CMT4C gene, causes variable peripheral neuropathy phenotypes. J Med Genet 2005;42(12):e69.

90. Colomer J, Gooding R, Angelicheva D, et al. Clinical spectrum of CMT4C disease in patients homozygous for the p.Arg1109X mutation in SH3TC2. Neuromuscul Disord 2006;16(7):449–53.

91. Azzedine H, Ravise N, Verny C, et al. Spine deformities in Charcot-Marie-Tooth 4C caused by SH3TC2 gene mutations. Neurology 2006;67(4):602–6.

92. Lassuthova P, Mazanec R, Vondracek P, et al. High frequency of SH3TC2 mutations in Czech HMSN I patients. Clin Genet 2011;80(4):334–45.

93. Houlden H, Laura M, Ginsberg L, et al. The phenotype of Charcot-Marie-Tooth disease type 4C due to SH3TC2 mutations and possible predisposition to an inflammatory neuropathy. Neuromuscul Disord 2009;19(4):264–9.

94. Boerkoel CF, Takashima H, Stankiewicz P, et al. Periaxin mutations cause recessive Dejerine-Sottas neuropathy. Am J Hum Genet 2001;68(2):325–33.

95. Guilbot A, Williams A, Ravise N, et al. A mutation in periaxin is responsible for CMT4F, an autosomal recessive form of Charcot-Marie-Tooth disease. Hum Mol Genet 2001;10(4):415–21.

96. Marchesi C, Milani M, Morbin M, et al. Four novel cases of periaxin-related neuropathy and review of the literature. Neurology 2010;75(20):1830–8.

97. Kabzinska D, Drac H, Sherman DL, et al. Charcot-Marie-Tooth type 4F disease caused by S399fsx410 mutation in the PRX gene. Neurology 2006;66(5): 745–7.

98. Chow CY, Zhang Y, Dowling JJ, et al. Mutation of FIG4 causes neurodegeneration in the pale tremor mouse and patients with CMT4J. Nature 2007;448(7149): 68–72.
99. Zhang X, Chow CY, Sahenk Z, et al. Mutation of FIG4 causes a rapidly progressive, asymmetric neuronal degeneration. Brain 2008;131(Pt 8):1990–2001.
100. Siskind C, Murphy SM, Ovens R, et al. Phenotype expression in women with CMT1X. J Peripher Nerv Syst 2011;16:102–7.
101. Siskind C, Feely SM, Bernes S, et al. Persistent CNS dysfunction in a boy with CMT1X. J Neurol Sci 2009;279(1–2):109–13.
102. Passage E, Norreel JC, Noack-Fraissignes P, et al. Ascorbic acid treatment corrects the phenotype of a mouse model of Charcot-Marie-Tooth disease. Nat Med 2004;10(4):396–401.
103. Verhamme C, de Haan RJ, Vermeulen M, et al. Oral high dose ascorbic acid treatment for one year in young CMT1A patients: a randomised, double-blind, placebo-controlled phase II trial. BMC Med 2009;7:70.
104. Burns J, Ouvrier RA, Yiu EM, et al. Ascorbic acid for Charcot-Marie-Tooth disease type 1A in children: a randomised, double-blind, placebo-controlled, safety and efficacy trial. Lancet Neurol 2009;8(6):537–44.
105. Micallef J, Attarian S, Dubourg O, et al. Effect of ascorbic acid in patients with Charcot-Marie-Tooth disease type 1A: a multicentre, randomised, double-blind, placebo-controlled trial. Lancet Neurol 2009;8(12):1103–10.
106. Pareyson D, Reilly MM, Schenone A, et al. Ascorbic acid in Charcot-Marie-Tooth disease type 1A (CMT-TRIAAL and CMT-TRAUK): a double-blind randomised trial. Lancet Neurol 2011;10(4):320–8.
107. Sereda MW, Meyer zu Hörste G, Suter U, et al. Therapeutic administration of progesterone antagonist in a model of Charcot-Marie-Tooth disease (CMT-1A). Nat Med 2003;9(12):1533–7.
108. Meyer zu Hörste G, Prukop T, Liebetanz D, et al. Antiprogesterone therapy uncouples axonal loss from demyelination in a transgenic rat model of CMT1A neuropathy. Ann Neurol 2007;61(1):61–72.
109. d'Ydewalle C, Krishnan J, Chiheb DM, et al. HDAC6 inhibitors reverse axonal loss in a mouse model of mutant HSPB1-induced Charcot-Marie-Tooth disease. Nat Med 2011;17(8):968–74.
110. Takahashi K, Yamanaka S. Induction of pluripotent stem cells from mouse embryonic and adult fibroblast cultures by defined factors. Cell 2006;126(4): 663–76.
111. Dimos JT, Rodolfa KT, Niakan KK, et al. Induced pluripotent stem cells generated from patients with ALS can be differentiated into motor neurons. Science 2008;321(5893):1218–21.
112. Saporta MA, Grskovic M, Dimos JT. Induced pluripotent stem cells in the study of neurological diseases. Stem Cell Res Ther 2011;2(5):37.
113. Lee G, Papapetrou EP, Kim H, et al. Modelling pathogenesis and treatment of familial dysautonomia using patient-specific iPSCs. Nature 2009;461(7262): 402–6.

Index

Note: Page numbers of article titles are in **boldface** type.

W

Moving?

Make sure your subscription moves with you!

To notify us of your new address, find your **Clinics Account Number** (located on your mailing label above your name), and contact customer service at:

Email: journalscustomerservice-usa@elsevier.com

800-654-2452 (subscribers in the U.S. & Canada)
314-447-8871 (subscribers outside of the U.S. & Canada)

Fax number: 314-447-8029

Elsevier Health Sciences Division
Subscription Customer Service
3251 Riverport Lane
Maryland Heights, MO 63043

*To ensure uninterrupted delivery of your subscription, please notify us at least 4 weeks in advance of move.

Printed and bound by CPI Group (UK) Ltd, Croydon, CR0 4YY

13/10/2024

01773497-0001